Oncology for Nurses and Health Care Professionals

Volume 1

Pathology, Diagnosis and Treatment

Oncology for Nurses and Health Care Professionals

Volume 1

Pathology, Diagnosis and Treatment

edited by

ROBERT TIFFANY

Director of Nursing, The Royal Marsden Hospital, London

London
GEORGE ALLEN & UNWIN
Boston Sydney

First published in 1978

GEORGE ALLEN & UNWIN LTD
40 Museum Street, London WC1A 1LU

British Library Cataloguing in Publication Data

Oncology for nurses and health care professionals.
Vol. 1: Pathology, diagnosis,
1. Cancer
I. Tiffany, Robert
616.9′94 RC261 78-40350

ISBN 0-04-610009-1
ISBN 0-04-610010-5 Pbk.

Typeset in 11 on 13 point Baskerville
and printed in Great Britain
by William Clowes & Sons Limited
London, Beccles and Colchester

Preface

Cancer is one of the major health problems of our times. A cancer patient is not merely an individual with a diseased body; he is also a person with a thinking mind and a stirring soul. He has attitudes and aptitudes, interests and instincts, hopes and dreams, which are all affected by his condition. There is a need for a close partnership of all who are engaged in different aspects of caring for the cancer patient if we are to achieve a health care system that will meet the demands of this philosophical framework.

The purpose of this book is to provide a concise and comprehensive introduction to oncology for nurses and other health care professionals. The presentation of the various subjects was entrusted to a team of authors chosen for their expertise in their own profession and oncology. Although each chapter reflects the unique point of view of its author or authors, they share the same commitment to total patient care based upon a multidisciplinary approach to meet this objective. A certain amount of overlap and repetition may at times be apparent to the reader. The content of each volume has been arranged so that each chapter may stand in its entirety, enabling the book to be used for reference purposes. A detailed reading list is given at the end of each chapter to assist the reader in further study of the theme taken by the author.

The book as a whole should be of particular value to trained health care professionals wishing to continue and develop their work in oncology, and to those taking courses of study in oncology such as are approved by the Joint Board of Clinical Nursing Studies.

As editor, I owe thanks to a large number of people for the completion of this project. It is my pleasure to thank the contributors for their willing co-operation and my colleagues in the Department of Nursing Studies at the Royal Marsden Hospital for their continued help and support. I am indebted to my secretary, Miss June Bailey, for all her help and assistance, and without whom this book would not have been possible.

Robert Tiffany

Contents

List of Tables

Chapter 1

The Cancer Cell

L. M. COBB
M.R.C.Path., M.R.C.V.S., Ph.D.
Head of Department of Environmental Physiology
Huntingdon Research Centre

Normal Cells

Before we can understand how cancer cells differ from normal cells we must first look at the structure and function of the normal cell. There is no such thing in the body as a typical cell; instead there are many different cell types which vary according to their functions. A cell is not visible to the naked eye, but twenty average-size cells (e.g. leucocytes), placed side by side would just be visible.

All cells have the same basic structure of a nucleus enclosed by a nuclear membrane and surrounded by cytoplasm, which is in turn surrounded by a thin cell membrane. Although the nucleus is more or less spherical, the shape of the surrounding cytoplasm varies greatly giving rise to cuboidal, pyramidal, columnar or squamous cells. The nucleus carries a vast amount of coded information. In fact, each nucleus carries sufficient information to carry out the functions of any cell in the body. The vast amount of information stored in the nucleus is coded on the deoxyribonucleic acid (DNA). Long strands of DNA are coiled up to form the chromosomes. This genetic information is conveyed from the nucleus to the cytoplasm by the intervention of a particular type of ribonucleic acid (RNA) called messenger RNA. In the cytoplasm the information is translated with the co-operation of other RNA molecules, when protein synthesis occurs. When it is necessary for more cells to be produced, the cytoplasm and nucleus will divide to produce two identical cells. In order for the daughter cells to be exactly like the parent cell from which they arise, the chromosones within the nucleus must duplicate before cell division or mitosis. The cell goes through a complex sequence of events prior to and in preparation for this division, but it is not within the scope of this chapter to go into further detail (see Chapter 10).

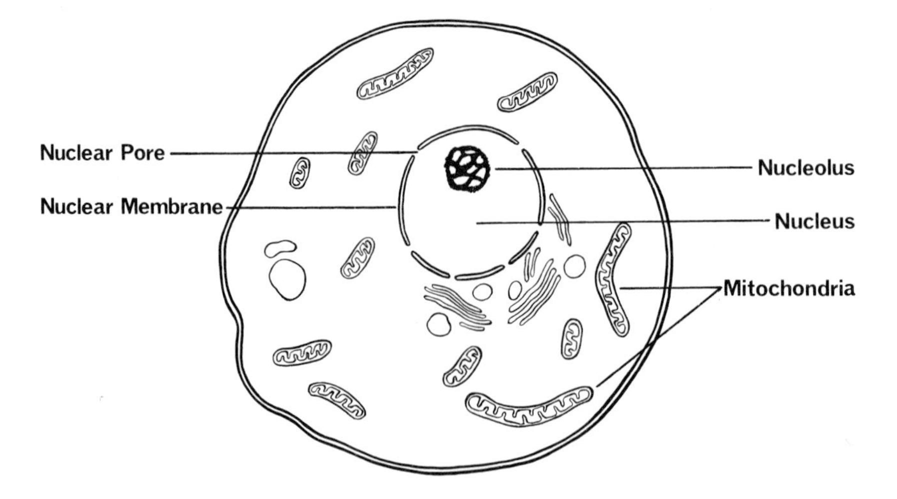

Figure 1.1 Diagram to show the structures in all living cells.

GROWTH

The basic unit of an organism, including man, is the individual cell. Growth of the organism begins with the fertilized ovum and increase in size is achieved by cell division. At each division a parent cell gives rise to two daughter cells. This is true for initial growth and for replacement and repair. It has been suggested that the term growth is not very precise because it could mean only the enlargement of a cell and therefore many biologists prefer the term proliferation. Cellular proliferation is a normal, indeed essential property of any organism. Proliferation rates vary widely between different tissues and are influenced by the rate and extent of cell loss. There is a very rapid rate of proliferation during early embryonic life which slows down with the maturity and development of the organism. By adult life there will be some tissues with no proliferative activity, such as certain types of nerve and muscle cells. Others will maintain a high level of proliferation throughout life, such as bone marrow and the epithelial lining of the gastrointestinal tract. Others, such as the skin, will proliferate at a moderate rate according to the demand for new cells. This proliferation rate can also be increased considerably when necessary, as in wound healing.

The processes which cause a cell to duplicate the chromosomes and subsequently divide, remain to be established. It has been proposed that in some tissues, if not all, the cells principally concerned with the growth of the organ (germinal cells) are constantly in a state in which they are prepared to divide. They are, however, prevented from doing so by chemical inhibitors (chalones). When the level of these inhibitors in the surrounding fluids falls, then the cells divide. For example, the outer layer of skin cells which are continuously shed, are normally replaced from the basal layer of dividing cells. These basal cells are to some extent inhibited by a chemical produced by the upper, more mature, cells. If the upper cells of an area of skin are destroyed, the inhibitor they produce will no longer be available to inhibit the basal cells, which therefore divide to produce new cells to repair the damage.

Any tissue in which a large number of cells show duplication of chromosomes and subsequent cell division, is said to have a high mitotic activity. This can be seen on microscopic examination of a section of the basal layer of the skin, following damage to the superficial layers. The mitotic index, a measurement of mitotic activity, is the percentage of cells in an area which are undergoing mitosis. The amount of mitotic activity in normal tissue varies greatly. At one end of the scale are the neurones which divide only in the foetus and are, therefore, never seen in mitosis in the adult. At the other end of the scale there are tissues such as hair, intestinal mucosa and bone marrow which have a high mitotic index. A mitotic index of one indicates that one nucleus in one hundred is observed to be in the process of duplication.

DIFFERENTIATION

To develop into the various organs with widely different structure and function, cells must specialize. At the beginning of this chapter, the point was made that there was no single typical cell. The process by which cell differences arise during development so that cells of the various tissues take on definite characteristics, is known as differentiation. Starting from one cell, the fertilized ovum, a whole series of different cell populations arise during embryonic development. This is a result of a combination of proliferation and differentiation. Differentiation may be defined as progression along the pathway of specialization in activity of a cell. Such specialized activity is thought to be regulated by the DNA; various parts of the DNA code being repressed or de-repressed may disallow or allow the expression of the messenger in that part of the code. As stated earlier, each nucleus carries sufficient information to carry out the functions of any cell in the body. Almost all the information available in any one cell is repressed. It is thought, therefore, that by the process of de-repression of limited areas in the code, cells differentiate into their particular tissue types. The exact mechanism of differentiation by de-repression is not known. In the adult organism, a very large number of different cell populations exist. These can be classified on anatomical and/or biochemical

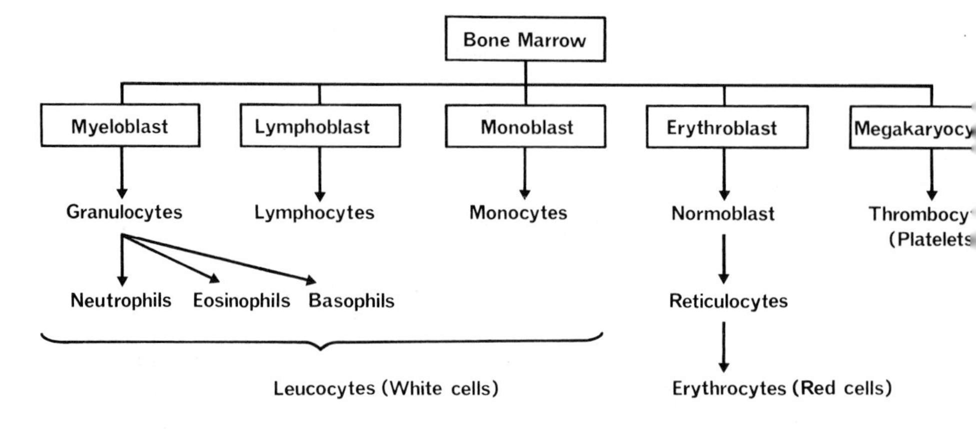

Figure 1.2 Process of differentiation for the production of circulating blood cells.

grounds, i.e. liver cells, skin cells, connective tissue cells etc. The process of differentiation is not confined to developmental growth. In adult life it is the same process of differentiation that enables a variety of mature blood cells to be produced from a single bone marrow stem cell.

CONTACT INHIBITION

The nature and mechanism of contact inhibition is not fully understood. It probably depends on some property of the cell's surface, the cell membrane. It is also thought to be involved in the normal recognition of self since if two different types of normal cells are brought into contact they may show inhibition on meeting each other. For example, following a fracture of the femur, growth will occur if a space is allowed between the two ends of broken bone (traction). On meeting, the cells recognize 'self', growth ceases and union takes place. If, however, a different tissue is placed between the two ends of bone, growth will cease and there is a recognition of 'non-self' and union will not take place. If normal cells are explanted into a suitable nutrient medium in a glass container, they will show active movement and proliferate. When, however, the surface area is covered, then both active movement and proliferation will cease. The hallmark of cellular activity is order and control maintaining a constant balance. The factors which initiate and terminate the whole process are as yet not fully understood. It is when one or more cells escape from this control that the process of malignancy begins. Growth becomes uncontrolled, disorderly and invasive and the normal equilibrium is disturbed to a greater or lesser extent.

Malignant Cells

A malignant cell can arise as a result of a change in any one of the cell types of the body. A cancer is a new growth which is not controlled by the normal growth-regulating mechanisms. The most obvious fact about tumours is that they form a mass of tissue extending beyond the confines of the organ from which they arise. High mitotic activity can be seen in most tumours. It would be wrong, however, to imply that the relationship between growth rate (as indicated by the mitotic index) and the malignancy of a tumour is in any sense a direct one. It is the popular belief that cancer cells grow faster than normal cells; this is not always true. In the adult normal tissues do not grow, they maintain a steady number of cells. In many tissues this is achieved without much proliferation because there is not much cell loss (e.g. liver). In other tissues this is achieved by maintaining a fast rate of cell division which balances a fast rate of cell loss (e.g. bone marrow). Neither tissue *grows*, they are both maintained in a steady state. There is no need for cancer cells to proliferate rapidly to produce a tumour. It is enough that new cells are produced when cells they might be replacing are not differentiating, ageing and dying and therefore tumour cells will accumulate. It requires only a slow proliferation in numbers to gradually outgrow controlled normal cell populations. Cancer cells may also take a longer period of time during mitosis and this may account in part for the appearance of more mitotic figures. One of the essential features of cancer cells is that they lose their normal differentiated state. This loss of differentiation manifests itself in two ways: loss of function; inappropriate function. In the former the process may go through various stages, beginning as a well-differentiated tumour, the cells of which function in a very similar style to those of the tissue in which they arise. Later, the tumour cells may progress to moderately differentiated and eventually undifferentiated (anaplastic) cells, that is they have lost the appearance and function of the cells of the tissue in which they arose. Some tumours, however, are anaplastic from their conception. This loss of the appearance and function of the normal cell by the cancer cell is clearly illustrated with malignant melanoma. The cancer cell in this case arises from the normal pigment-producing cell in the skin (melanocyte). The initial cancer cells still retain the ability to produce pigment and therefore colonies of them in the skin are observed as small black nodules. However, with the progression of the tumour there is gradual loss of normal function and the cells may no longer produce pigment and appear as pink or white nodules. Inappropriate function occasionally arises in some tumours. In the nucleus of malignant cells inhibitors may fail to be effective, so that a malignant cell derived from one tissue carries out functions normally allotted to cells of other tissues. For example, parathormone, which is normally produced by the parathyroid gland, can sometimes be produced by the cells of kidney tumours. Malignant cells in the bronchus can sometimes produce hormones associated with the pituitary gland.

Loss of contact inhibition and loss of the characteristic to recognize 'self' from 'non-self' enables malignant cells to infiltrate surrounding tissue and eventually spread to distant organs of the body (metastasize). These secondary growths are termed metastases.

Table 1.1 *Differences between normal and malignant cell systems*

	Normal	*Malignant*
Growth	1. Controlled and co-ordinated 2. Control mechanisms regulate development and maintenance of cell populations	Loss of control and co-ordination allowing tumour formation
Differentiation	Cells well differentiated with specialist functions	Loss of differentiation with loss of function and adoption of inappropriate function
Contact Inhibition	Cells display contact inhibition and recognize other cells as 'self' or 'non-self'. They do not infiltrate adjacent tissues	Loss of contact inhibition and loss of ability to recognize 'self' from 'non-self' resulting in infiltration and dissemination

THE SPREAD OF CANCER

Direct Invasion

The tumour not only expands in size but infiltrates between the surrounding tissue cells. Normal tissue will eventually be disorganized and destroyed. Resistance to this infiltration varies, being less in loose connective tissue but greater in bone and cartilage. Structural and functional change may follow. The surface of the skin and other organs may become breached and the resulting ulcer secondarily infected. Erosion of a large blood vessel may cause serious, even fatal, haemorrhage. A tumour in the bowel or oesophagus may cause obstruction and direct spread from the cervix to the ureters may result in renal failure. Pain will occur when nerve endings are involved.

Lymphatic Spread

The walls of the lymphatics are so delicate they offer little resistance to the invading cancer cells which easily grow into them. Once inside the lymphatic vessel malignant cells may grow as a column or be broken off and carried as an embolus to the draining lymph node. The embolus may then grow steadily inside the node, slowly destroying it and converting it into a new mass of cancerous tissue. Eventually another embolus of tumour breaks off and passes to another node repeating the process. The node may become hard and palpable and eventually attached to the surrounding tissue. The flow of lymph may be stopped or reversed producing lymphoedema. Cells which reach the thoracic duct will enter the general circulation and can be deposited in any part of the body.

Blood Spread

In addition to entering the blood-stream from the lymphatics, tumour cells can invade vessels directly. Capillaries have weak, thin walls and do not offer great resistance. As the tumour extends along the lumen of the blood vessel, single cells, or groups of cells may separate off from the main mass of cells. Not all cancer cells breaking away will be able to form metastases. Only a small percentage will survive to establish a proliferating cell system in their new environment.

Cavity Spread

Occasionally a tumour may spread from one structure to another across cavities, such as carcinoma of the stomach to the ovary. Also cells may be carried along natural channels; as for example when cells from a tumour of the renal pelvis are carried down the ureter to form deposits in the bladder.

It is the metastases that are usually the cause of death in patients where treatment has proved unsuccessful. Cancer cells from the bronchus that have metastasized to the liver may cause sufficient liver damage that the patient goes into liver failure. Cancer cells from bones

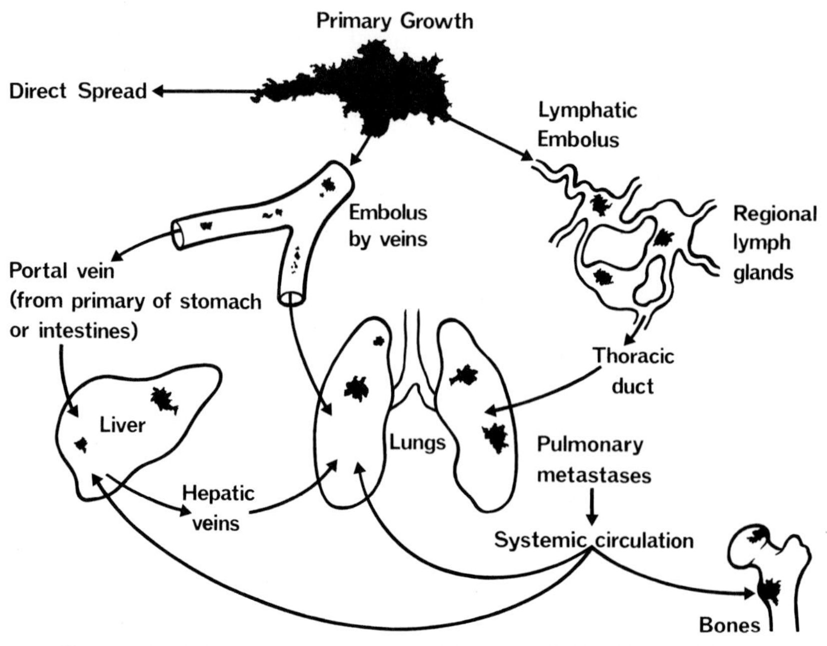

Figure 1.3 Schematic representation of the spread of malignant disease.

that have metastasized to the lungs may by local growth so interfere with the interchange of gases that the patient goes into respiratory failure.

SUMMARY

Cancer cells have certain well-known characteristics. In the early stages of tumour growth the cancer cells often resemble the original cell from which the cancer was derived. With the growth of the tumour mass, the cells start to differ markedly from the original cell. The cancer cell has the ability to infiltrate into the tissues and spread throughout the body. The cancer becomes a 'parasite' in the host organism and if not eradicated will usually lead to the death of the host organism.

Bibliography

Capra, L. G. (1972) *The Care of the Cancer Patient*. William Heinemann Medical Books Ltd.

Harris, R. J. C. (ed.) (1970) *What we know about Cancer*. George Allen & Unwin.

Sutton, P. M. (1965) *The Nature of Cancer*. English Universities Press.

Walter, J. (1971) *Cancer and Radiotherapy: A Short Guide for Nurses and Medical Students*. London: J. & A. Churchill.

Chapter 2

The General Pathology of Tumours

N. F. C. GOWING
M.D., B.S., F.R.C.Path.
Department of Histopathology
Royal Marsden Hospital
London

Definition and Nature of Tumours

Etymologically, the word *tumour* means a swelling. Thus, the *Oxford English Dictionary* gives one definition as 'an abnormal or morbid swelling or enlargement in any part of the body of an animal or plant'. However, by common usage, most clinicians and pathologists use tumour synonymously with *neoplasm*. Of course, there are many pathological swellings which are not truly neoplastic: for example, inflammatory lesions, cysts and certain congenital malformations. Abnormal swellings occur very frequently in the female breast; some of these are malignant tumours and some are benign tumours, but many are not neoplasms at all but simple tissue proliferations probably resulting from hormonal stimulation. Thus, it becomes necessary to frame a definition of a tumour (neoplasm) in the limited sense that the word is now used. Many definitions have been proposed, but the one quoted here is that suggested by Professor R. A. Willis: 'A tumour is an abnormal mass of tissue, the growth of which exceeds and is uncoordinated with that of the normal tissues, and persists in the same excessive manner after cessation of the stimuli which evoked the change.'

From this definition it will be seen that true neoplasms differ in certain very important respects from other tumefactions such as inflammatory swellings. In its early stages the swelling of an inflammatory lesion (such as that following invasion of the body by bacteria) results from dilation of blood vessels and the passage of fluid and cells from the blood into the tissue spaces. However, cellular proliferation in excess of normal does occur later, fibroblasts and vascular endothelial cells being those mainly involved. If the bacteria (the 'stimuli which evoked the change') are eliminated, the excessive cellular proliferation rapidly subsides. If there has been much tissue destruction, complete return to normal is not possible and a permanent swelling composed of fibrous scar tissue remains. However, such a residual lesion displays no power of continued growth.

The sequence of events in the genesis of neoplasia is different. First, contact of the tissues with a tumour-evoking agent, such as a carcinogenic chemical, often produces no apparent effect for a considerable time; in man this latent period between exposure to the agent and the development of the tumour may be measured in years or even decades. Second, the tumour does not regress if exposure to the carcinogen ceases. Indeed, in patients with chemically induced neoplasms, particularly those occurring as occupational hazards, often years have passed since the patient was in contact with the carcinogen. In other words, the carcinogen has produced in the cells a persisting capacity for sustained excessive proliferation – the growth 'persists in the same excessive manner after cessation of the stimuli which evoked the change'. It must be added that the precise nature of this change in the cells is still not known.

Neoplasms may be divided into two broad groups, benign or malignant. Malignant tumours are characterized by their ability to infiltrate and destroy the normal tissues in their neighbourhood; furthermore they are usually capable of dissemination to distant sites where they establish secondary deposits, a process known as metastasis. Malignant tumours are those which are grouped together as 'cancer'; however 'cancer' should not be regarded as a single disease, but rather as a collection of disparate, although allied, disorders.

These statements have to be qualified slightly in view of the fact that malignant neoplasms occasionally undergo spontaneous regression. However, this is such a rare event that it does not impinge significantly on the tumour problem, nor does it obviate the general validity of the propositions outlined. It is sometimes stated that neoplasms are autonomous growths. Clearly, no tumour can be strictly autonomous since it relies on its host (the body of the patient) for its blood supply and nutrients. But apart from this obvious point, there is evidence that certain neoplasms remain partly responsive to controlling factors, especially hormones. Thus, some breast cancers regress if the hormonal milieu is altered by ablative procedures, such as adrenalectomy or oophorectomy, or by the administration of androgens or oestrogens. However, with the passage of time, tumours may become less and less responsive to such hormonal control: that is to say there is a tendency, a progression, towards autonomy.

Classification of Tumours

The modern classification of tumours is based on their histogenesis, which means that they are given specific names according to the tissues or cells from which they arise. They are further subdivided into benign and malignant categories. Before discussing the detailed nomenclature of neoplasms, it is desirable to point out certain difficulties which preclude our fitting all growths into neat histogenetic and behavioural groups.

First, there are a number of tumours whose histogenesis is unknown or uncertain, but which nevertheless merit specific names because they form clearly defined entities, each having its own particular microscopic pattern, age and sex incidence, preferential sites of origin, natural history and response to therapy. Some of these tumours have been named after the workers who first clearly described them: for example, *Ewing's sarcoma of bone, Hodgkin's disease, Kaposi's sarcoma, Paget's disease of the skin* and *Burkitt's lymphoma.* Others are given descriptive titles, based on their microscopic structure and sometimes also on their anatomical site of origin: *epithelioid sarcoma, alveolar soft-part sarcoma* and *clear-cell sarcoma of tendons and aponeuroses.*

Second, highly malignant tumours may lose all resemblance to the normal tissues from which they arise, so that they show no characteristic microscopic pattern to indicate their origin. The extent to which a neoplasm resembles the normal tissue from which it is derived is called its degree of differentiation. A neoplasm is said to be *well differentiated* if the resemblance to normal tissue is close; *poorly differentiated* if the resemblance is only vague. Intermediate degrees of differentiation are also recognized. Tumours which have lost all similarity to the corresponding normal tissue are said to be *dedifferentiated, undifferentiated,* or *anaplastic.* All anaplastic tumours, whatever their origin, are composed of undifferentiated and often rapidly dividing cells so that they all tend to acquire similar microscopic appearances; this phenomenon is called *convergence.*

Third, it must be stressed that the terms benign and malignant are relative rather than absolute. Between perfectly benign tumours which grow very slowly and display no tendency to recur after simple excision, and highly malignant growths which disseminate and kill within a few months, there is an infinite gradation of behaviour patterns. Some tumours have a tendency to recur locally although they rarely if ever metastasize: others metastasize widely while the primary growth is still small and clinically undetected. Furthermore, tumours which are benign in a pathological sense may nevertheless kill the patient if they develop in an area where they can press on some vital structure such as the brain.

THE CONCEPT OF PREMALIGNANCY AND CARCINOMA *IN SITU*

There are a number of tissue changes which are said to be premalignant or precancerous. A *precancerous lesion* may be defined as one which, although not itself malignant, is statistically more liable to undergo malignant change than is the corresponding normal tissue. Examples of precancerous lesions are ulcerative colitis, skin damaged by ultraviolet rays or ionizing radiation, chronic arsenical skin lesions, and certain benign tumours such as adenomatous polyps of the large intestine.

A tissue may display the cytological changes of malignancy, but without invasion of adjacent structures. This phenomenon is known as *carcinoma in situ*. It can be recognized only in epithelium, and is also called *intraepithelial carcinoma* or *intramucosal carcinoma*. It represents an early, curative stage in the development of a cancer, and its recognition is clearly of great importance. In certain situations, such as the urinary tract and cervix uteri, cytological screening is a valuable method for its detection. Sometimes epithelium displays cytological changes which suggest neoplastic development but fall short of definite malignancy; this phenomenon is called *dysplasia* and the epithelium involved is said to be *dysplastic*. It is probable that dysplasia can progress to intra-epithelial carcinoma which in turn can evolve to invasive carcinoma.

TUMOUR NOMENCLATURE BASED ON HISTOGENESIS

The tissues of the body comprise four main groups: (1) epithelium; (2) connective tissues, including lymphoid and haemopoietic (blood-cell forming) tissues; (3) muscle; and (4) nervous tissue. Tumours arising from these various tissues will be considered in turn.

1. *Epithelial Tumours*

In epithelium the constituent cells are closely applied and adherent to one another, there being very little intercellular material. Epithelium forms sheets which cover the skin surface and line the respiratory, alimentary and genitourinary tracts. Epithelial cells are also disposed as solid masses, or hollow vesicles or tubules, as in the liver, kidney, endocrine glands, exocrine glands and gland ducts.

A benign tumour arising from surface epithelium is called a *papilloma*. Growths of this type may develop from the skin surface (epidermis), the epithelium lining the urinary tract (especially the bladder), the epithelial lining of the alimentary canal, the epithelium of the respiratory tract and the ducts of glands. The term *papilloma* may be qualified by an appropriate adjective depending upon the precise origin and microscopic pattern of the particular tumour. For example, those showing keratin formation and resembling the epidermis in structure are called *squamous cell papillomas*; and those arising from the transitional epithelium of the urinary tract are called *transitional cell papillomas*. A benign tumour of glandular epithelium is called an *adenoma*. Adenomas may arise from either endocrine or exocrine glands; they occur in such sites as the pituitary, thyroid, salivary glands, adrenals, pancreatic islets, sweat glands and the intestinal mucosa.

All malignant neoplasms of epithelium, either surface or glandular, are designated *carcinomas*. Carcinomas are very common and form a clinically important group of tumours. Those arising in the skin, lung, breast, stomach, large intestine, bladder and cervix uteri are among the most frequently encountered malignant growths in man. Carcinomas are subdivided into special types according to their microscopic appearances and the particular sort of epithelium from which they originate. For example, the epithelium covering the skin, and lining the mouth, pharynx, oesophagus and larynx is stratified squamous in type, and carcinomas arising from it usually show the formation of prickle cells and keratin; they are called *squamous cell carcinomas*. Most carcinomas of the cervix uteri are also of this type. Malignant tumours arising from the (transitional) epithelium of the urinary tract (renal pelves, ureters, bladder and urethra) are called *transitional cell carcinomas*; this term is also applied to neoplasms of similar histological appearances, arising from the mucosa of the nasal cavity and paranasal sinuses. Many transitional cell carcinomas of the urinary tract grow from the epithelial surface in the form of delicate frond-like projections. Such a growth pattern is described as *papillary*. It should be noted that whereas a *papilloma* is by definition a benign tumour, the adjective papillary is simply descriptive of the configuration of a lesion, which may be either benign or malignant. The term *adenocarcinoma* is used when a tumour shows a glandular pattern microscopically.

There are many other terms which are applied to various special types of epithelial neoplasms, and the most important of these will be listed and defined:

Cystadenoma – a benign tumour of glandular origin forming fluid-filled cavities (cysts) large enough to be seen with the naked eye.

Papillary cystadenoma – similar to a cystadenoma, but also featuring papillary processes growing from the epithelium lining the cysts. The adjective *serous* or *mucous* (mucinous) may be used as further descriptive refinements depending upon whether the fluid in the cysts is slightly viscid (like serum) or markedly viscid and jelly-like (mucinous).

Cystadenocarcinoma and papillary cystadenocarcinoma – the malignant counterparts of cystadenomas. Again the tumours may be further qualified as either *serous* or *mucinous*. Both benign and malignant tumours of this group commonly arise in the ovary.

Mucoid carcinoma – an adenocarcinoma which produces so much mucin that it appears soft, translucent and jelly-like to the naked eye. Such tumours occur especially in the breast and large intestine.

'Oat-cell' carcinoma – a tumour composed of small spheroidal and ovoid cells which have darkly staining nuclei and scanty cytoplasm. So-called because the shape of the cells is reminiscent of oat grains. These tumours occur mainly in the lung, although similar growths occasionally develop in other organs.

Medullary (or encephaloid) carcinoma – a tumour which is soft because it is highly cellular and contains very little fibrous supporting stroma. An important variant is *medullary carcinoma with lymphoid stroma*, a neoplasm which occurs in the breast and has a relatively good prognosis. Microscopically, there is an intense infiltration of the tumour with lymphoid cells which may indicate a defence reaction on the part of the host. *Medullary carcinoma with amyloid stroma* is a special type of tumour arising in the thyroid gland. In this instance the dense stroma may render the neoplasm firm rather than soft – an example of the vagaries of terminology!

Scirrhous carcinoma – this simply means a hard carcinoma, the firm consistency being due to the presence of a dense fibrous stroma with a relative sparsity of cells within the growth. The term is applied mainly to a common type of breast carcinoma, but it is now used less often than it was in the past.

Giant-cell carcinoma – a tumour characterized microscopically by large cells with multiple nuclei. Such growths occur in the lungs, thyroid and occasionally elsewhere.

Intraduct carcinoma – this is a form of *in situ* carcinoma of the breast in which cancer cells distend the ducts from which they arise but without penetrating their walls. Very often, both intraduct and invasive growth patterns are seen together in the same neoplasm. Although it is possible for intraduct carcinoma to arise in other glands, the term is used almost exclusively in relation to the breast.

Intralobular carcinoma – like intraduct carcinoma, this is a form of *in situ* breast carcinoma, but instead of developing within the ducts, the neoplasm originates in the small secretory units (acini) which are grouped together to form the mammary lobules. Intralobular and infiltrating growth may be present in the same tumour.

2. *Tumours of Connective Tissue and Muscle*

Neoplasms arising from connective tissue and muscle are grouped together because they have a number of features in common. However, tumours of the haemopoietic and lymphoid systems have certain very special characteristics, and they merit separate consideration.

(*a*) *Tumours of muscle and of connective tissues other than haemopoietic and lymphoid.* Microscopically, muscle is of two main types, smooth and striated. Striated muscle fibres are characterized by bands which cross the cells at right angles to their long axes. Such cross-striations are lacking in smooth muscle. Striated muscle is also known as voluntary or skeletal muscle because the large muscles which are attached to the bones, and which are under voluntary control, are of this type. Smooth muscle is sometimes called involuntary because it forms contractile tissue not under conscious control, such as the musculature of the stomach and intestines. However, it should be noted that heart muscle is cross-striated. Connective tissues are subdivided into a number of special types: (i) fibrous tissue, in which bundles of tough collagen fibres run between the cells; (ii) adipose tissue which stores fat; (iii) bone, in which the fibrous component is hardened by the deposition of calcium; (iv) cartilage; and (v) synovial tissue which lines joint cavities. It is also convenient to group the endothelial cells, which line blood vessels and lymphatics, with the connective tissues for the purpose of tumour classification.

There is no generic term for benign tumours of muscle and connective tissues: each tumour receives a different name depending upon the type of tissue from which it is derived. All malignant tumours of connective tissue and muscle are known as *sarcomas*; these are subdivided and receive special names according to their tissue of origin.

Nomenclature of connective tissue and muscle tumours

Tissue of origin	*Benign tumours*	*Malignant tumours*
Fibrous tissue	Fibroma	Fibrosarcoma
Adipose (fatty) tissue	Lipoma	Liposarcoma
Bone	Osteoma	Osteosarcoma
Cartilage	Chondroma	Chondrosarcoma
Synovium	Benign synovioma	Synovial sarcoma
Blood vessel endothelium	Haemangioma	Haemangiosarcoma
Lymph vessel endothelium	Lymphangioma	Lymphangiosarcoma
Smooth muscle	Leiomyoma	Leiomyosarcoma
Striated muscle	Rhabdomyoma	Rhabdomyosarcoma

As indicated earlier, this list has to be enlarged by the addition of certain special types of neoplasm which have characteristic microscopic features but whose precise tissue or cell of origin is not at present known. These special types include: *alveolar soft-part sarcoma, epithelioid sarcoma, clear-cell sarcoma of tendons and aponeuroses* and *Ewing's sarcoma* of bone. Furthermore, the classification is oversimplified in other ways. For example, a considerable number of benign tumours of bone and cartilage are recognized, other than simple osteomas and chondromas. Depending on their microscopic appearances, a variety of special benign growths have been delineated and named: *osteoid osteoma, benign chondroblastoma, chondromyxoid fibroma* and *benign osteoblastoma.* Another neoplasm of bone, not listed in the above table, is the *giant-cell tumour* which can be either benign or malignant; this tumour features multinucleated cells similar to those normally involved in bone resorption (osteoclasts), and for this reason the alternative name of *osteoclastoma* is sometimes used. A further useful refinement of classification is to divide malignant tumours into subtypes according to their degree of aggressiveness. Thus, liposarcomas may be subdivided into well-differentiated, myxoid, pleomorphic, and round cell types, the degree of aggressiveness increasing in the order given. Subtypes of rhabdomycosarcoma are also recognized.

(*b*) *Tumours of haemopoietic and lymphoid tissue.* Haemopoietic tissue produces cells which circulate in the blood-stream: the erythrocytes (red cells), the granular leukocytes (white cells) comprising the neutrophils, eosinophils and basophils, and the monocytes (large white cells). Also present in the blood-stream are the non-nucleated platelets (produced by the megakaryocytes of the bone marrow) and another form of white cell, the lymphocytes (derived from lymphoid tissue). In the normal adult, haemopoietic tissue is confined to the marrow of certain bones, especially those of the skull, the vertebral column, the thoracic cage, the pectoral girdle and the pelvic girdle. In the foetus, haemopoiesis occurs also in the marrow of the long bones and in the liver and spleen. In certain disease states, these other sites may again become active in postnatal life. The lymphoid tissue is widely scattered through the body, occurring in the following anatomical locations: (i) as encapsulated, rounded or ovoid masses, the lymph nodes, which are situated mainly in the neck, axillae, groin, thorax and abdomen; (ii) as non-encapsulated masses or nodules, in the oropharynx (the tonsils), the back of the tongue (lingual tonsil), the nasopharynx and the walls of the small and large intestines; (iii) the white pulp (Malpighian bodies) of the spleen; and (iv) the thymus. The lymphoid tissue produces cells (lymphocytes) which play a vital role in the resistance of the body to infection. Some lymphocytes differentiate into plasma cells (plasmacytes) which secrete soluble substances (antibodies or immunoglobulins) concerned with neutralizing the effects of microbial invasion: others destroy micro-organisms by coming into more direct contact with them (cell-mediated immunity).

The classification and nomenclature of tumours of the haemopoietic and lymphoid systems is still the subject of much discussion and controversy, and no universally agreed terminology has yet been devised. However, this confusion involves tumours of lymphoid tissue rather than those of the haemopoietic cells. Before outlining a classification, it is desirable to emphasize certain facts: (1) no benign tumours of the haemopoietic and lymphoid tissues are currently recognized; (2) many neoplasms of these tissues do not present as localized tumour masses, but develop as generalized cellular proliferations in the bone marrow (or lymphoid tissue) with diffuse infiltration of other organs (such as the spleen, liver and kidneys) and the appearance of large numbers of neoplastic cells in the blood-stream: such a process is called *leukaemia* when the white blood cells are involved and *erythraemia (polycythaemia rubra)* when the red cells are implicated; (3) sometimes a neoplasm features both a localized mass (or masses) and a leukaemic blood picture: the tumour mass may appear before the leukaemic manifestation, or the leukaemia may develop first and the tumefaction develop later.

Leukaemias are classified according to the cell type which proliferates and appears in the peripheral blood, and they are also divided into acute and chronic varieties depending upon the clinical tempo of the disease:

Cell type	*Acute*	*Chronic*
Granular leukocytes	Myeloblastic leukaemia	Myelocytic leukaemia
Monocytes	Acute monocytic leukaemia	Chronic monocytic leukaemia
Lymphocytes	Lymphoblastic leukaemia	Lymphocytic leukaemia

Occasionally there is a neoplastic proliferation of both the red cell and white cell precursors with the appearance in the peripheral blood of atypical erythroblasts (primitive red cells) and myeloblasts (primitive white cells). This condition may run an acute or chronic course and is known as *erythroleukaemia, erythraemic myelosis* or *di Guglielmo's disease*. Rarely, megakaryocytes are the main proliferating cell type; the bone marrow becomes infiltrated with large numbers of these cells which are also found in extramedullary tissues and organs (especially the spleen and liver). This is called *megakaryocytic myelosis.* As mentioned, tumour masses sometimes develop in patients with leukaemia. In lymphoblastic and lymphocytic leukaemias such tumours are appropriately called *malignant lymphomas (vide infra).* With regard to the granulocytic leukaemias, tumours appear most often in the acute (myeloblastic) type and are composed mainly of primitive myeloblasts, so that *myeloblastoma* is a suitable designation. However, the term *chloroma* is often used because these tumours frequently have a characteristic green colour.

Malignant lymphomas usually present as lymph node enlargements, but extranodal tissue, such as the tonsils, the intestinal lymphoid nodules, the thymus and the spleen, may be the primary site. Other rarer sites of presentation are bone, brain, skin, thyroid, testis and ovary. Wherever the initial manifestation may be, lymphomas tend to involve the lymphoid tissues of the body more and more widely as the disease progresses. The classification and nomenclature of lymphoid tumours is still confused and a number of different schemes have been suggested. However, there is basic agreement that terminology should be based on: (i) the cell type of which the tumour is composed; (ii) the degree of cellular differentiation; and (iii) the cellular arrangement, which may be either follicular (nodular) like that of some cells in normal lymphoid tissue, or diffuse. There are also certain special types which have been given eponyms. A simple scheme of classification is as follows:

1. Well-differentiated lymphocytic lymphoma.
2. Poorly-differentiated lymphocytic lymphoma.
3. Lymphoplasmacytoid, where there is differentiation towards plasma cells. Since plasma cells normally produce antibodies (immunoglobulins) tumours showing such differentiation may be associated with increased amounts of immunoglobulin in the blood.
4. Histiocytic lymphoma. Histiocytes are related to the monocytes (large mononuclear cells) of the blood, but are found in lymphoid tissue and in the connective tissues throughout the body. They are capable of ingesting particulate matter both living and non-living and are also known as macrophages.
5. Undifferentiated lymphoma, where the cells show no feature characteristic of a particular type.
6. Follicular (or nodular) lymphomas. Here the tumour cells are arranged as spheroidal aggregates, similar to the follicles of normal lymphoid tissue.

7. Hodgkin's disease. This is a special type of malignant lymphoma, the precise cell of origin being at present unknown. Microscopically, it features a mixture of different cells (lymphocytes, histiocytes, eosinophils, plasmacytes, fibroblasts) among which are varying numbers of characteristic multinucleated giant cells known as Reed–Sternberg cells. Hodgkin's disease is subdivided into four histological types: (a) lymphocytic predominant; (b) nodular sclerosing; (c) mixed cellularity; and (d) lymphocytic depletion. Type (a) is characterized by large numbers of lymphocytes and few Reed–Sternberg cells. Type (b) has broad bands of fibrous connective tissue splitting the tissue into cellular nodules. In type (c) there is a moderate number of Reed–Sternberg cells, with a mixture of histiocytes, plasma cells, lymphocytes and eosinophils. Type (d) has large numbers of Reed–Sternberg cells but very few lymphocytes or other cells. Type (a) has the best prognosis and type (d) the worst.
8. Burkitt's lymphoma is another special tumour type. It affects especially children between 2 and 14 years of age and often presents as a swelling of the jaw, either upper or lower. It has a remarkable geographical distribution, being particularly prevalent in equatorial Africa, although some cases have been recognized in other parts of the world. The epidemiology of the disease was thought to indicate a viral aetiology, probably with the participation of an insect vector. However, further studies have shown the problem to be more complex and multiple causative factors are likely to be involved.

Although the term malignant lymphoma has been widely adopted, it should be noted that tumours of the lymphocytic type are also called *lymphosarcoma*, and those of the histiocytic and undifferentiated types, *reticulum cell sarcoma*.

3. *Tumours of Neural Tissue*

Within the nervous system there are two main types of cells: the nerve cells proper (*neurocytes*) which are responsible for the transmission of nerve impulses, and the supporting cells. In the central nervous system the supporting elements are known collectively as neuroglia. There are three sorts of glial cells: astrocytes, oligodendrocytes and ependymal cells. The astrocytes and oligodendrocytes are found among the neurocytes and the bundles of nerve fibres derived from them. Ependymal cells line the cavities (ventricles) which contain cerebrospinal fluid. A fourth type of cell known as *microglia* belongs to the monocyte/macrophage series and is not of nervous tissue origin. When tumours arise from microglia, they are really malignant lymphomas although they are often called *microgliomas*. Another structure in the brain from which tumours sometimes arise is the choroid plexus which secretes cerebrospinal fluid and is arranged as vascular fringes projecting into the ventricles; the tumours are either papillomas or carcinomas. The peripheral nerves have a special type of supporting cell, the neurilemmal (or Schwann) cell, and there is also a connective tissue component with fibrocytes.

Tumours of neurocytes are extremely rare in the central nervous system; indeed some authorities deny their existence in this site. Most arise from nerve cells situated outside the brain and spinal cord. The adrenal medulla and the sympathetic ganglia of the abdomen and upper thoracic region are the usual sites of origin. Benign tumours of neurocytes are composed of fully differentiated nerve cells and are called *ganglioneuromas*; this term is derived from the name given to the large neurocytes of the sympathetic ganglia, *ganglion cells* or *gangliocytes*. Malignant tumours of nerve cells are called *neuroblastomas*, indicating that the growths are composed of embryonic nerve cells or neuroblasts. Neuroblastoma is one of the important common tumours of childhood. Sometimes a tumour is composed of a mixture of neuroblasts and mature ganglion cells; the term *ganglioneuroblastoma* may then be used.

Tumours of glial origin receive the generic name of *glioma*, but they are subdivided, according to the cell type, into *astrocytoma*, *oligodendroglioma* and *ependymoma*. It is not practical to divide glomas sharply into benign and malignant forms, since even the best differentiated of these growths are unencapsulated and tend to invade adjacent normal tissue. The usual practice is to grade them according to the degree of malignancy as judged by histological criteria. A system of four numerical grades is commonly employed. Grade 1 refers to a high degree of differentiation and low malignancy, grade 4 tumours are poorly differentiated and highly malignant, and grades 2 and 3 are intermediate. The most malignant types of astrocytoma often exhibit marked irregularity in the size and shape of the cells, with large multinucleated forms and many mitotic figures; *glioblastoma multiforme* is the name sometimes given to such a tumour. Even the highly differentiated, relatively benign, slowly growing gliomas are difficult to cure because of their infiltrative tendency and impracticality of complete surgical excision. However, there is a group of well-differentiated, often cystic, cerebellar astrocytomas of childhood, in which the prognosis is quite favourable. Many patients with this special type of tumour have been cured by surgery. Also classified with the gliomas is an embryonal tumour of childhood, the cerebellar *medulloblastoma*; this is a highly malignant, but radiosensitive tumour. Yet another special type of neural tumour is the *retinoblastoma*; this arises in the eye from embryonic retinal tissue and, like other embryonal tumours, affects mainly young children. Retinoblastomas may show a familial and hereditary incidence, and bilateral growths sometimes occur.

Tumours of the pineal body are of several types. The pineal body is a small structure attached by a stalk to the roof of the third ventricle. Microscopically it is composed of special cells, pinealocytes, and glial cells. Tumours of the pinealocytes are called *pinealomas*, while the glial cells may give rise to gliomas. The pineal is also one of the sites where teratomas and other germ cell tumours occur *(vide infra)*.

Tumours of peripheral nerves arise either from the special sheath cells (Schwann cells or neurilemmal cells) or from fibroblasts. The former give rise to *neurilemmomas* (also called *Schwannomas* or *neurinomas*) and the latter to *neurofibromas*. The malignant counterparts are *malignant neurilemmoma* and *neurofibrosarcoma*. The lesion known as *traumatic*, or *amputation neuroma* is not a true tumour but consists of a tangle of nerve fibres which sprout from the severed end of a nerve; sheath cells also proliferate. Traumatic neuromas may form painful nodules in operation scars or amputation stumps.

Although not of nervous tissue origin, it is convenient to consider in this section those tumours which arise from the membranes covering the brain and spinal cord, the meninges. Such tumours have characteristic microscopic appearances and are called *meningiomas*. Most are benign, but malignant variants do occur.

The different tumour types discussed in this section may be tabulated as follows:

Tumours of neurocytes
Benign – ganglioneuroma
Malignant – neuroblastoma

Tumours of glial cells
From astrocytes – astrocytoma
From oligodendrocytes – oligodendroglioma
From ependymal cells – ependymoma
From embryonal cells – medulloblastoma

Tumours of the choroid plexus
Benign – papilloma
Malignant – carcinoma

Tumours of embryonal retinal tissue
Retinoblastoma

Tumours of the pineal body
Pinealoma
Glioma

Tumours of the meninges
Benign – meningioma
Malignant – malignant meningioma; meningeal sarcoma

Tumours of peripheral nerves
From neurilemmal (Schwann) cells
Benign – neurilemmoma (Schwannoma, neurinoma)
Malignant – malignant neurilemmoma
From sheath fibroblasts
Benign – neurofibroma
Malignant – neurofibrosarcoma
From regenerating neurofibrils
Traumatic (amputation) neuroma; not a true neoplasm.

4. *Miscellaneous Special Tumours*

To be considered here are a number of neoplasms which do not fit readily into the preceding sections and which require some further discussion.

(*a*) *Carcinoid tumours*. These are neoplasms of epithelial type and of low grade malignancy. The term 'carcinoid' was introduced (1907) in the belief that they were not malignant, although histologically they appeared to be infiltrating epithelial tumours, i.e. they were 'carcinoma-like'. It is now appreciated that they are capable of disseminating widely, despite their slow rate of growth. Common sites of origin are the vermiform appendix and the small intestine, where they arise from special cells known as Kultchitsky or argentaffin cells. The term *argentaffin* refers to the presence of cytoplasmic granules which are blackened by silver salts. The alternative name *argentaffin carcinoma* has been used for carcinoid tumours. However, similar neoplasms arise in the stomach, large intestine and bronchi, and the argentaffin reaction is often negative in tumours in these situations. Carcinoids can produce soluble products which are absorbed into the blood-stream and may result in a characteristic collection of signs and symptoms, the *carcinoid syndrome*. The syndrome includes diarrhoea, paroxysmal flushing, attacks of breathlessness due to broncho-constriction, and structural changes in the cardiac valves.

(*b*) *Germ cell tumours*. A number of important types of tumour are thought to be derived from germ cells, both in men and women. Such neoplasms arise most frequently in the gonads (testis and ovary), but they can also develop primarily in other parts of the body, particularly the retroperitoneum, the anterior mediastinum and the pineal region. One type of germ cell tumour is called a *seminoma* when it affects the testis and *dysgerminoma* when it arises in the ovary. Seminoma and dysgerminoma are microscopically identical. Tumours of this type arising in the anterior mediastinum or pineal region, have received a variety of names: seminoma, seminomatous tumour, germinoma, atypical teratoma.

Teratomas are tumours in which the germ cells manifest their potentiality to produce multiple tissues of different types. Thus, microscopic examination of such a tumour may reveal a mixture of epithelium, cartilage, bone, smooth muscle, striated muscle, nervous tissue etc. Highly organized structures can also develop; for example, skin with sweat glands and hairs, and teeth. Teratomas may be either benign or malignant. Ovarian teratomas are usually benign, and are often cystic, the cyst being lined by skin with abundant hair, and the lumen containing sebaceous material; such benign teratomas are commonly referred to as 'dermoid cysts'. On the other hand, most testicular teratomas are malignant. A special variety of germ cell tumour which has been studied extensively in the last decade, is the *endodermal sinus tumour or yolk sac tumour*. Growths of this sort have a microscopic pattern reminiscent of certain structures in the normal yolk sac. They occur especially in the testes of infants and young children, but also in the ovary and occasionally elsewhere.

(*c*) *Choriocarcinoma* (Chorion-epithelioma). This is a malignant tumour arising from trophoblast, the foetal component of the placenta. Thus, it may occur in pregnant women, originating from the foetus but metastasizing in the mother. However, choriocarcinomas can also arise in teratomas, both gonadal and extragonadal. Gestational choriocarcinoma is a tumour which has yielded very satisfactorily to modern chemotherapy, but testicular choriocarcinoma responds poorly and is an extremely aggressive neoplasm with a very poor prognosis. Non-gestational choriocarcinomas are a type of germ cell tumour.

(*d*) *Malignant melanomas*. These tumours arise from melanocytes, the pigment-producing cells of the skin and eye. Benign lesions composed of melanocytes comprise the common naevi or moles of the skin. Malignant melanomas arise mainly in the skin and eye, less commonly in the nasal cavity, the mouth and the anal canal. They are often heavily pigmented, but pigment production is variable and may be absent.

(*e*) *Embryonic tumours of the viscera*. These growths arise from immature embryonic tissue which is 'committed' to develop into visceral structures such as those of the kidney or liver. Embryonic tumours of the kidney are called *nephroblastoma (or Wilms's tumour)*; those of the liver, *hepatoblastoma*. Such neoplasms occur especially in children. Microscopically, they may display different types of tissues, both epithelial and non-epithelial, but the variety is more limited than it is in teratomas. *Mesodermal mixed tumours* of the uterus (and ovary) histologically show a similar mixture of tissues, but they occur in middle-aged and elderly women rather than children.

(*f*) *Tumours of chromaffin tissue and paraganglia*. Chromaffin tissue is so named because fixation in chrome salts produces a brown pigment in the cytoplasm of the tissue cells. Embryologically the tissue is derived from neuroectoderm and is closely associated with the sympathetic nervous system. It produces the hormones epinephrine and norepinephrine. The largest discrete masses of chromaffin tissue are the medullae of the adrenal glands; smaller collections are scattered along the sympathetic nervous system chain, especially in the abdomen. These extramedullary masses of tissue are called paraganglia. Tumours of adrenal chromaffin tissue have been called *chromaffinomas*, but the term *phaeochromocytoma* is now generally employed. Tumours of similar structure outside the adrenal, arising from the chromaffin paraganglia, are called *chromaffin paragangliomas*. There is evidence that some paraganglia, especially those in the head and neck and upper thorax, act as chemoreceptors, that is to say they respond to certain changes in the chemistry of the blood and mediate appropriate physiological adjustments. For this reason the term *chemodectoma* was suggested, and has been widely used for tumours of these structures. However, there is now a consensus of opinion against the term chemodectoma, with the suggestion that all tumours of paraganglia should be called paragangliomas, the adjectives chromaffin or non-chromaffin being added as appropriate. Phaeochromocytomas and paragangliomas are usually benign, but malignant variants do occur.

The Naked-Eye Appearances of Neoplasms

TUMOUR SIZE

It might be thought that the size of a tumour would be simply a function of time, and that all neoplasms would tend to grow larger as their age increased. While this is true in general, the situation is often more complex. For example, a tumour may kill the patient by widespread metastasis, although the primary growth remains tiny, microscopic or indeed undetectable; or a malignant tumour may kill by involvement of some vital structure while it is still quite small. Very occasionally a neoplasm may regress spontaneously. The largest tumours one sees are those which are benign or of low grade malignancy, slowly growing and in such a situation that they can expand freely without causing any symptoms severe enough to make the patient seek early medical advice. For example, some benign cystic tumours of ovary, which can expand freely in the abdominal cavity, reach an enormous size.

SHAPE AND OUTLINE

Tumours which are able to expand or infiltrate freely in all directions tend to be spheroidal, but there are many situations in which this shape cannot be retained. A tumour growing within an elongated muscle belly often takes the form of an ellipsoid. If growing against a bone, one surface may become flattened or concave. A tumour involving the wall of a hollow tubular viscus, such as the oesophagus or intestine, often extends circumferentially, causing narrowing of the lumen and eventually complete obstruction. Tumours frequently involve epithelial surfaces, such as the skin or the mucous membranes of internal organs, and a variety of different growth patterns may then be seen. For example, ulceration of the tumour may produce a crater with raised edges (Fig. 2.1); the tumour may form a protruding nodule attached to the surface by a stalk, a form of growth known as *polypoid* and the nodule being called a polyp; the neoplasm may grow outward as finger-like protrusions, a pattern described as *villous* or *papillary* (Fig. 2.2).

The periphery of a tumour may be sharply demarcated from the surrounding normal tissue and some are enclosed in fibrous tissue capsules which may be thin and delicate or measure up to a few millimetres in thickness. Even malignant tumours sometimes show partial encapsulation, although careful examination will reveal penetration of the capsule at one or more points. On the other hand, the limits of a

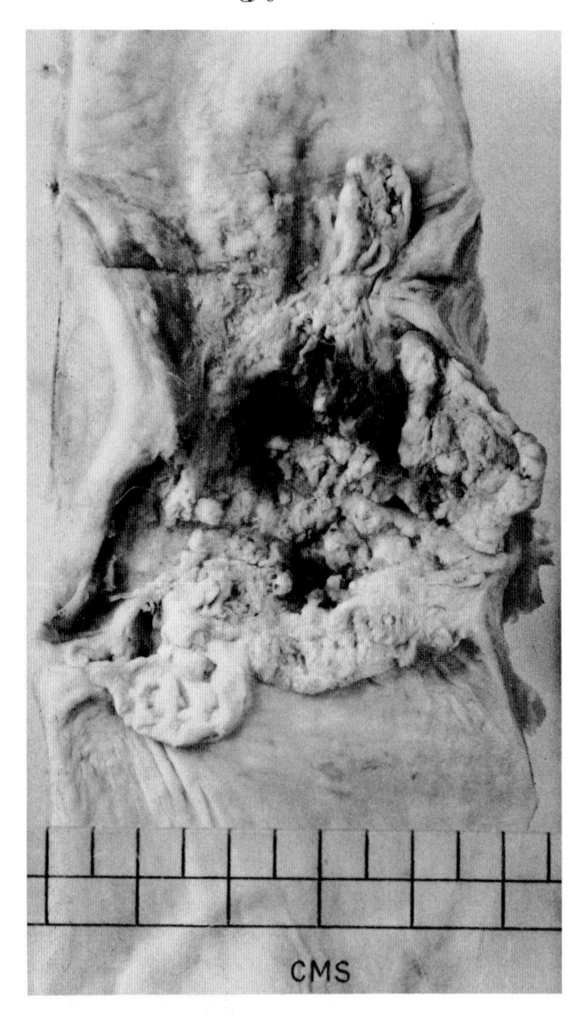

Figure 2.1 Ulcerated carcinoma of the oesophagus. The gullet has been opened longitudinally to display the large ulcerated neoplasm with raised everted edges.

growth may be very poorly defined, the tumour tissue merging imperceptibly with the normal; this feature is especially marked in certain well-differentiated astrocytomas of the brain. Some carcinomas of the stomach infiltrate diffusely, producing generalized thickening of the gastric wall but no localized tumour mass. Other carcinomas, for example the common types occurring in the breast, display very irregular outlines with grey strands of tissue extending into the adjacent mammary tissue; it was the presence of such claw-like extensions around tumours that led to the introduction of the word *cancer* (Latin, a crab).

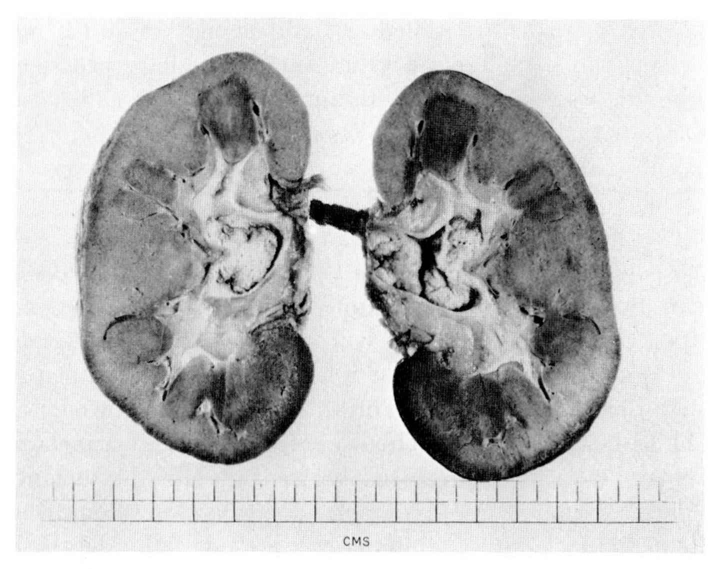

Figure 2.2 Papillary carcinoma of the renal pelvis. The kidney has been hemisected and, in both halves, a papillary tumour can be seen, almost filling the pelvis.

CONSISTENCY

This is extremely variable. Tumours which are very cellular and have little stroma are quite soft and are sometimes described as *encephaloid* or *medullary*. Fibrous tissue stroma imparts a degree of firmness to a tumour and when such stroma is abundant and dense the growth will be hard; such tumours are said to be *scirrhous*, a term which is used most frequently in respect of certain breast cancers. An even greater degree of hardness is imparted by calcification or bone formation. Tumours arising from bone-producing cells may be extremely hard, sometimes even denser than normal bone, but neoplasms of other types may calcify or bone may form in their stroma.

Some tumours produce large amounts of mucin, a glairy, jelly-like substance. When abundant, mucin imparts a glistening translucent appearance to a neoplasm. Carcinomas producing much mucin are called *mucoid* or *colloid cancers*; the term mucoid is preferred. Another phenomenon which can greatly affect the consistency of a tumour is necrosis, the death of cells still situated within the living body. When extensive, necrosis can lead to marked softening, or indeed liquefaction, of a tumour. Cyst formation is another factor contributing to the variability of the gross appearance. Some neoplasms, especially those arising in the ovary, are predominantly cystic and display thin-walled loculi filled with liquid which may be glairy and mucoid, or more watery. Such growths are called *cystadenomas* if they are benign, or *cystadenocarcinomas* if malignant. Quite often, papillary processes protrude into the cyst cavities, the tumours then being called *papillary cystadenomas* or *papillary cystadenocarcinomas*.

COLOUR

The basic colour of a cellular tumour is grey, but there are many factors which can modify it. The blood supply to a tumour may be sparse or abundant. Moderate vascularity will impart a pinkish tinge. Highly vascular tumours are dark red, and if haemorrhage occurs the pigment in the shed blood breaks down to produce patches of brown coloration (Fig. 2.3). Other pigments which may colour tumours are melanin and lipochromes. Melanin is produced by special cells, the melanocytes. Benign and malignant tumours of melanocytes vary in colour from light brown to deep black, although sometimes the cells fail to synthesize the pigment and the tumours remain uncoloured; an unpigmented tumour of melanocytes is called an *amelanotic* (or *achromic*) *melanoma*. Tumours of other sorts are sometimes secondarily pigmented with melanin; two common examples are *basal cell papilloma* and *basal cell carcinoma* of the skin. Lipochromes (carotenoids) are not synthesized in the body, but are ingested with certain food substances which contain them. These pigments are readily fat soluble and they become concentrated in cells and tissues rich in fat. Tumours coloured yellow by lipochromes include those derived from adipose tissue cells – lipoma and liposarcoma. However, there are also a number of other tumours whose cells often contain abundant fat and which therefore accumulate lipochrome pigment. These include certain adenomas and carcinomas of the kidney, adenomas and carcinomas of the adrenal cortex, and some ovarian tumours.

The Microscopic Structure of Tumours

Microscopically we can distinguish two components within a tumour: the actual proliferating neoplastic cells and their products; and a supporting connective-tissue stroma. The proportion of these two elements is very variable. In some tumours the stroma is extremely scanty, in others it is very abundant.

The appearance of the neoplastic cells will depend on the histogenesis of the growth and the degree of differentiation. Benign tumours and slowly growing malignant tumours may be well differentiated, and

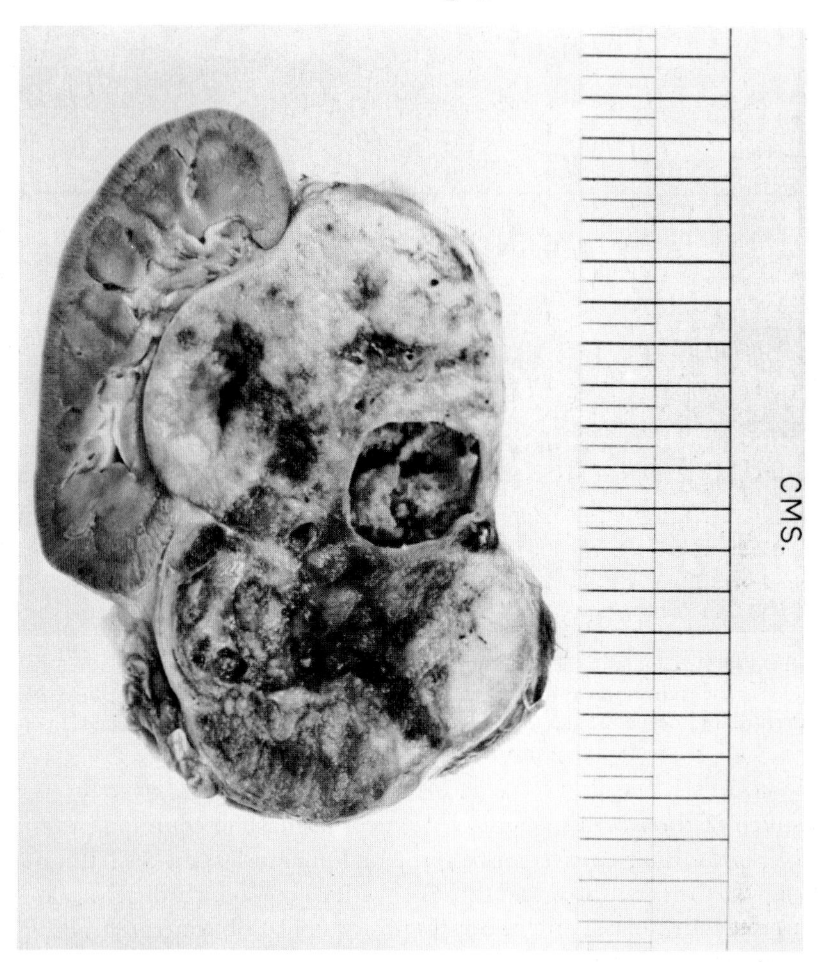

Figure 2.3 Renal cortical carcinoma ('hypernephroma'). The cut surface of a hemisected kidney showing a large tumour mass. The paler areas were yellowish (lipochrome pigment) and the dark patches were red or brown (blood pigment).

resemble fairly closely the normal tissue from which they arise. Thus, differentiated neoplasms of glandular origin, will show well-formed epithelial tubules, acini or cell cords (Fig. 2.4). Malignant neoplasms display various degrees of divergence from the normal. The cells and their nuclei may vary considerably in size and shape (*pleomorphism*), and the nuclear–cytoplasmic ratio is often increased. Sometimes the tumour cells are much larger than their normal counterparts and they may contain multiple nuclei (tumour giant cells). Mitotic figures may be numerous and are often abnormal. The degree of differentiation shown by a tumour is the basis of *grading*, whereby some estimate can

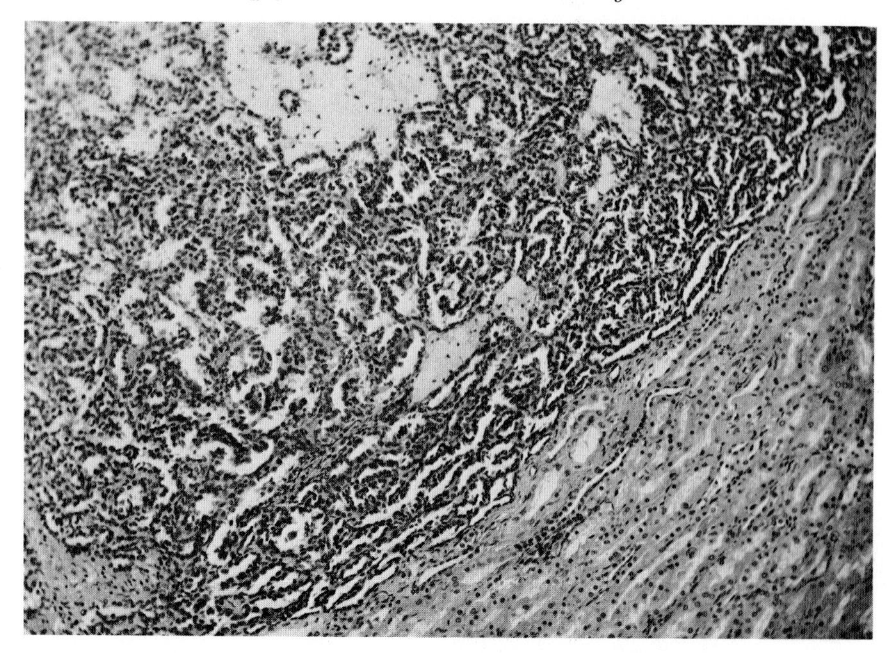

Figure 2.4 Adenoma of the renal cortex. A photomicrograph showing normal renal tubules in the right lower third and the adenoma occupying the rest of the field. Note the irregularity of the tubules forming the tumour compared with the normal tubules. (Section stained with haematoxylin and eosin × 160.)

be given of the aggressiveness of the neoplasm. The common practice is to use a numerical system of three or four grades, grade 1 tumours being well differentiated and those of grades 3 or 4 poorly differentiated. A more accurate assessment of prognosis may be obtained if grading is combined with *staging*. By staging is meant an estimate of the extent to which the neoplasm has spread. A number of different staging systems have been suggested. One which is widely used is known as TNM. This is based on the extent or size of the local tumour mass (T), the degree of involvement of the regional lymph nodes (N) and the presence or absence of distant metastases (M).

The stroma of most tumours consists of fibrous connective tissue and blood vessels, but the relative amount of connective tissue and the degree of vascularity are very variable. Highly malignant tumours may have very scanty stroma and the blood vessels supplying them are often thin-walled and delicate, so that haemorrhage into such growths is not uncommon. Sometimes the stroma is infiltrated with inflammatory cells of various types: lymphocytes, plasma cells, macrophages, neutrophil polymorphs, eosinophils and mast cells, in varying proportions. In certain tumours, for example carcinoma of the breast, the

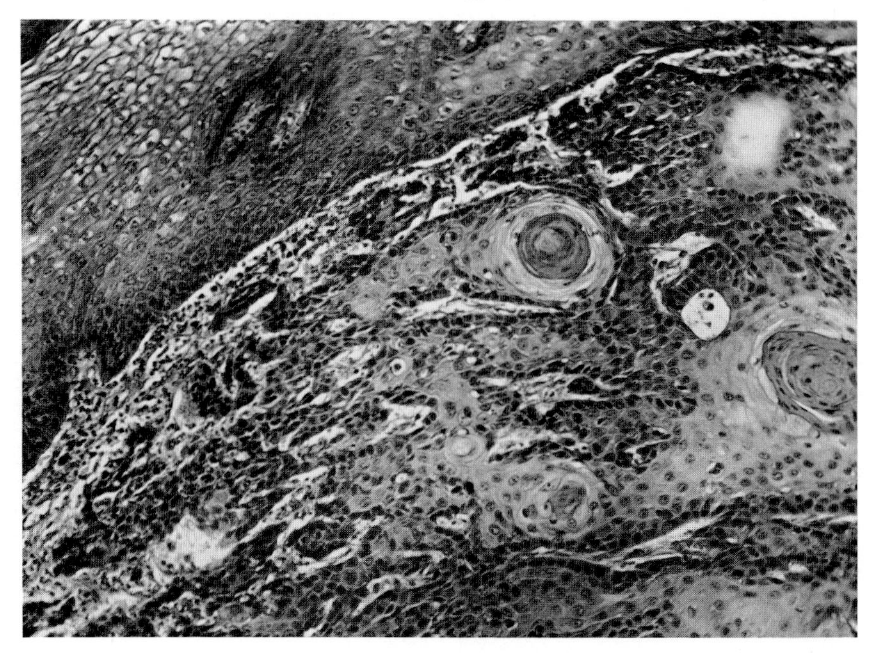

Figure 2.5 Squamous cell carcinoma of the pharynx. A photomicrograph showing the tumour infiltrating beneath the normal surface epithelium, which is situated in the left upper third of the field. Note that the neoplasm is forming concentric whorls of keratin. (Section stained with haematoxylin and eosin × 160.)

presence of many inflammatory cells may represent a defence reaction by the body, and there is evidence that a very dense inflammatory-cell infiltrate is associated with an improved prognosis. Calcification in tumours has already been mentioned; it may occur either in the stroma or in dead tumour cells. Another change which is occasionally seen in the stroma is bone or cartilage formation. Bone and cartilage are seen more often in tumours of osteoblasts or chondroblasts, but they are then the product of the tumour cells and not of the stroma.

The Spread of Malignant Tumours

It has already been emphasized that benign tumours grow by expansion, compressing the surrounding normal tissue from which they are sharply demarcated and often separated by capsules. Malignant tumours, on the other hand, infiltrate and destroy surrounding tissues and usually have the propensity to spread to distant sites and establish secondary deposits in other organs and tissues (Fig. 2.5). The process whereby a malignant tumour disseminates and establishes such secondary growths is known as *metastasis*. Dissemination can take place along a number of different routes: the lymphatics, blood vessels, serous cavities and cerebrospinal fluid pathways.

LYMPHATIC SPREAD

This is extremely important, especially with carcinomas. Columns of tumour cells invade the walls of small lymphatic vessels, and cell clusters break free and are carried in the lymph stream towards the regional lymph nodes. In the lymph nodes, the carcinoma cells are arrested and grow, producing a secondary tumour mass. Spread may occur progressively from node to node, until a whole group or chain of lymph nodes is involved. By such progressive spread along lymphatic pathways, the neoplastic cells may eventually enter the thoracic duct or the right lymphatic duct from which the lymph is finally discharged into the subclavian veins at the root of the neck; further spread of the tumour can then take place by the blood-stream.

BLOOD-STREAM SPREAD

Tumours invade veins much more readily than arteries. The direction of spread will therefore be determined by the venous drainage from the tissue or organ in which the neoplasm has arisen. Blood from the stomach, small intestine, most of the large intestine, the gall-bladder, spleen and pancreas is drained by the portal system to the liver. Tumours arising in these organs will therefore tend to spread to the liver, and indeed secondary deposits in the liver very commonly develop from such neoplasms as carcinoma of the stomach, large intestine or pancreas.

From most other organs and tissues, and from the liver itself, the venous blood flows towards the right side of the heart and then through the pulmonary arteries to the lungs. Thus, sarcomas arising in bone or in the soft tissues of the trunk or limbs usually develop their initial blood-borne secondaries in the lungs. The pulmonary veins carry blood from the lungs to the left side of the heart which pumps it into the arterial system and distributes it throughout the body. Consequently, malignant growths arising in the lungs are often disseminated through the systemic blood-stream to many organs. Once secondary growths are established they can involve the veins of the organ in which they have developed, so that the further pattern of spread may be complex and dissemination may eventually be very widespread.

SPREAD THROUGH SEROUS CAVITIES

The serous membranes (pleural, pericardial and peritoneal) are often invaded by tumours. The irritation produced by the neoplasm leads to an outpouring of excess serous fluid in which groups of cancer cells can be transported. This very often leads to extensive 'seeding' of the serous membranes by innumerable secondary deposits. Such a phenomenon may be seen in the pleural membranes in carcinomas of the lung, and in the peritoneal membranes in carcinoma of the stomach or ovary.

SPREAD THROUGH CEREBROSPINAL FLUID PATHWAYS

The cerebrospinal fluid is secreted into the ventricles of the brain and passes into the subarachnoid space covering the brain and spinal cord: the fluid is absorbed into the large venous sinuses. One type of tumour which may spread through the cerebrospinal fluid is the medulloblastoma arising in the cerebellum of children or young adults; it sometimes disseminates to produce numerous small deposits on the surface of the spinal cord.

Chapter 3

The Aetiology of Human Cancers

R. L. CARTER
M.A., D.M., D.Sc., M.R.C.Path.
Institute of Cancer Research, and
Royal Marsden Hospital, Surrey
and
A. MUNRO NEVILLE
M.D., Ph.D., M.R.C.Path.
Unit of Human Cancer Biology,
Ludwig Institute for Cancer Research, in
conjunction with Royal Marsden Hospital, London

Cancer is a diverse group of diseases, and it is as futile to look for a single cause as a single cure. Instead, it is more realistic to try and identify the separate links in a whole chain of interacting 'causes' – differing for various kinds of cancer, varying in their origin, potency and mode of action, and operating over a broad time-scale such that twenty, thirty, forty or more years may elapse before a particular cancer declares itself clinically.

Whatever the tissue from which a cancer develops, the ultimate target for carcinogenic action is the genetic material – deoxyribonucleic acid or DNA – which makes up part of the chromosomes in the nuclei of human and mammalian cells. Details of the complex interactions between carcinogens and DNA, and their immediate consequences, are beyond the scope of this account, and we shall confine ourselves to a discussion of some of the carcinogens and the tumours with which they are associated.

Most human cancers are thought to arise as a consequence of the interplay of several factors which can be considered in two broad categories: intrinsic and extrinsic.

Intrinsic factors
- Genetic susceptibility
- Hormonal status

Extrinsic factors
- Chemicals
- Physical agents (ionizing and ultraviolet radiations)
- Viruses

Intrinsic Factors

GENETIC ASPECTS

Congenital cancers, apparent at or shortly after birth, are excessively rare. Examples include nephroblastoma, neuroblastoma and acute leukaemia. More commonly encountered are situations where there is an *inherited predisposition* to develop one or more forms of cancer, usually inherited as a Mendelian recessive characteristic. Various clinical patterns have been described.

1. Diseases in which tumour susceptibility is inherited as part of a syndrome with chromosomal abnormalities:
   Down's syndrome (acute leukaemia);
   Klinefelter's syndrome (carcinoma of male breast).
2. Diseases in which tumour susceptibility is inherited as part of a syndrome with immunological abnormalities:
   Ataxia telangiectasia; Wiskott–Aldrich syndrome } (mainly leukaemias and lymphomas, but also some epithelial and mesenchymal tumours).
3. Diseases in which tumour susceptibility is inherited as part of a syndrome without chromosomal or immunological abnormalities:
   Xeroderma pigmentosum (cancers of skin and subcutaneous tissues);
   Polyposis coli (carcinoma of colon);
   Neurofibromatosis (glioma, meningioma, etc.).
4. Tumour susceptibility unaccompanied by a syndrome:
   Retinoblastoma;
   Some cases of phaeochromocytoma;
   Multiple endocrine adenomatosis types I and II.

Only a small proportion of human cancer shows any predictable mode of inheritance. Some of the common cancers, particularly of the breast and stomach, are sometimes encountered in several members of one family; but such occurrences appear to be random and follow no clear genetic pattern. In certain circumstances it may be difficult to distinguish between genetic susceptibility and a shared (postnatal) exposure to some exogenous cancer-inducing agents. This problem can sometimes be clarified by investigating cancer incidence in special groups such as homozygous twins and immigrants. Changing death rates for certain cancers have, for example, been observed in Japanese migrating to California. Among the fatal cancers affecting the Japanese in Japan, gastric cancer is common, colorectal cancer much less common and breast cancer is rare. This pattern changes in Japanese who move to California where, within the span of one generation, their incidence of gastric cancer has slowly fallen, the incidence of colorectal cancer has risen and the incidence of breast cancer has also risen (albeit very slowly). Genetic factors in these individuals thus appear to be outweighed by exogenous factors in the development of three forms of cancer – though no light is thrown on the possible nature of the exogenous factors concerned.

A number of genetically-determined 'markers' have been described in human populations which have been linked with a predisposition to develop various diseases. A few such associations have been described in cancer – blood group A and gastric cancer, certain leucocyte antigens (HLA) and nasopharyngeal cancer – and it is likely that this field will grow in the future.

HORMONAL ASPECTS

There is extensive evidence in laboratory animals that hormones are implicated in the development of tumours of the breast and certain endocrine glands. The situation is more complex in man, but three general statements can be made.

1. There is no evidence that endogenous hormones, alone, are carcinogenic in man. Given the often vital physiological functions of such hormones, this is hardly surprising. On the other hand, it is argued that the *balance* of certain hormones, and their metabolites, may reflect a *predisposition* to develop certain cancers particularly of the breast. Deranged biosynthesis of hormones has been demonstrated in several endocrine tumours, particularly of the adrenals and gonads; but such abnormalities are the consequence of the tumour rather than its cause.
2. Some established tumours are sensitive to hormones. The best documented examples are carcinomas of the breast and prostate, and hormonal manipulation – by ablation of endocrine glands and by giving exogenous hormones – forms a basic mode of clinical management. The proportion of hormone-sensitive tumours varies and, in most patients, initially sensitive tumours become hormone-resistant and thus escape from control.
3. There is some evidence that exogenous hormones or hormone-like substances may, under very specific circumstances, be carcinogenic. Examples include oestrogens and stilboestrol and these are discussed later.

Extrinsic Factors

These consist of chemical agents, physical agents and viruses.

CHEMICALS AS HUMAN CARCINOGENS

Chemical agents are widely thought to be the most important extrinsic factors in the aetiology of many human cancers. They may be considered in two groups – occupational and non-occupational.

Table 3.1 *Extrinsic factors claimed to be predisposing causes of cancer*

Target tissue	*Suspected agent*
Skin	1. Chronic exposure to solar rays 2. X-rays 3. Chemicals: arsenic; saltpetre; processed oils and paraffins; tar and pitch 4. Soot
Nasal sinuses	1. Wood 2. Chemicals: arsenic
Lower lip	1. Chronic exposure to solar rays 2. Tobacco and prolonged heat
Tongue	1. Tobacco 2. Snuff 3. Poor oral hygiene 4. Syphilis
Pharynx	1. Excessive use of tobacco and alcohol
Lung	1. Tobacco 2. Chemicals: arsenic; asbestos; chromium; nickel 3. Radioactive substances 4. Coal tar fumes
Oesophagus	1. Heavy consumption of strong alcohol 2. Tobacco
Stomach	1. Diet
Bladder	1. Chemicals: aniline dyes; benzidene 2. Tobacco 3. Infestation (Bilharziasis)
Cervix	1. Coitus (hygiene)

Occupational carcinogens

Several chemicals encountered in occupational contexts induce tumours in man (see Table 3.1). A few examples will be described with particular reference to four target organs – skin, bladder, lungs and paranasal sinuses.

Skin. The first example of an occupational cancer was published in 1775 when the English surgeon, Percivall Pott, described cancers of the skin and scrotum in chimney sweeps. Pott seems to have suspected that *soot*, despite its lack of physical irritancy, was responsible for the development of these cancers; he also recognized that prolonged exposure for many years was necessary before the cancers developed.

A later example of occupational cancers of the skin and scrotum was provided by exposure to *mineral oils*, first in the 1870s among shale oil workers in Lanarkshire and then, at the turn of the century, in the Lancashire cotton spinners who used mineral oils to lubricate their spindles. As a result of legislation, altered industrial practice and a declining cotton industry, these cancers are now rarely seen, but mineral oil cancers have recently reappeared in a fresh occupational context. Cancers of the skin and scrotum are increasingly being described among toolsetters who use mineral oils to lubricate and cool automatic lathes. These workers may also have an increased incidence of cancers of the respiratory and upper alimentary tracts, suggesting that the carcinogenic hazards of mineral oils include inhaled and swallowed droplets as well as direct skin contact. But more work is required to confirm and clarify these possible additional risks.

Bladder. An increased incidence of bladder cancer among workers in the chemical industry was first described in Germany in 1895. Similar observations were subsequently made in workers in other countries and in other industries, notably rubber and cable making, and suspicion focused on a group of chemicals known as the *aromatic amines*. The epidemiology of these cancers was extensively studied in the chemical industry in England in the 1950s, and much is now known of their natural history. It was found, for example, that the proportion of men who developed bladder cancer increased with the degree of occupational exposure to β-naphthylamine, a potent carcinogenic aromatic amine. The mean latent period between exposure and diagnosis of bladder cancer (the induction period) was fifteen to twenty years with extreme ranges of five to forty-five years. Despite this long latent period, the average age at onset of bladder cancer in chemical workers was characteristically earlier (by an average of about twenty years) than in a matched control group of bladder cancer patients with no known exposure to occupational carcinogens.

Although most of the carcinogenic aromatic amines encountered occupationally are absorbed through the skin, tumours do not develop locally at the point of initial contact. Absorbed aromatic amines are metabolized in the body and it is certain metabolites, excreted in the urine (and therefore in prolonged contact with the bladder), which are the active carcinogens.

Lungs and respiratory tract. An increased incidence of lung cancer, and sometimes of more proximal parts of the respiratory tract and in other sites, has been observed in several occupational contexts:

Metals and organometallic compounds
- Asbestos
- Arsenic
- Nickel
- Chromates

Alkylating agents
- Mustard gas
- Chloro-ethers

Radioactive ores
- Radium
- ?Haematite

The carcinogenic hazards of asbestos illustrate some of the difficulties posed by occupational carcinogens. Asbestos is a complex mixture of natural fibrous silicates which vary greatly in biological activity. Crocidolite (blue asbestos) is a potent carcinogen, while amosite is less so. Occupational exposure to asbestos is generally incurred during mining, milling and manufacture of asbestos-containing materials, or during contact with asbestos in special contexts such as in dockyards. It commonly involves inhalation or ingestion of a mixture of asbestos fibres, inconstant in composition, thus reinforcing the difficulty of defining particular carcinogenic hazards in terms of particular forms of asbestos.

Occupational exposure to asbestos is associated with an increased incidence of bronchial cancers and of mesotheliomas, which develop from the mesothelial cells lining the pleural and peritoneal cavities. Mesotheliomas are rare and many of them are linked with occupational exposure to asbestos. Such tumours thus serve as valuable 'marker' lesions in epidemiological studies.

Recent investigations have shown that the carcinogenic effects of asbestos on the bronchi are greatly enhanced by cigarette smoking, indicating that these two carcinogenic stimuli powerfully reinforce each other. (A similar potentiating effect of cigarette smoke is suspected in the lung cancers associated with exposure to arsenic.) Gastrointestinal cancers may also be more common in asbestos workers, presumably as a consequence of swallowing fibres, but more substantiating evidence is required.

The mode of action of carcinogenic asbestos fibres is unknown though current work stresses the probable importance of the physical characteristics of the fibres – their shape, length and diameter.

Paranasal sinuses. A proportion of cancers of the paranasal sinuses, particularly those arising in the ethmoids, are occupational in origin. Though less rare than mesotheliomas, some of these tumours are still sufficiently uncommon to serve as 'marker' lesions, suggesting exposure to a suspected occupational carcinogen. Two examples are cited. A high incidence of sinus carcinoma (and also bronchial carcinoma) was observed in the 1920s among refiners of nickel-containing ores in South Wales. The refining process was phased out, and both these nickel-associated cancers have virtually disappeared from the area. More recently, the normally rare adenocarcinomas of the ethmoid sinuses have been described in furniture makers and in workers exposed to leather dusts. Inhaled hardwood dusts are suspected in the furniture industry but other materials may be implicated: no carcinogen has yet been identified.

Non-occupational Carcinogens

Some of the chemicals considered as occupational carcinogens may also be encountered outside a strictly occupational context:

Polycyclic aromatic hydrocarbons, asbestos, arsenic
Tobacco smoke
Drugs
Naturally occurring carcinogens – ?aflatoxin

Polycyclic aromatic hydrocarbons, notably benzo(a)pyrene, are invariably formed during the combustion of organic material and can be widely demonstrated in urban air, cigarette smoke and foodstuffs. The amounts present are minute and the hazards which they present are uncertain. *Arsenic* is naturally present in drinking water in certain parts of the world and such areas are characterized by a high incidence of skin cancers. The hazards of non-occupational exposure to *asbestos* are controversial. Populations living near the South African crocidolite mines were found in the 1960s to have an increased incidence of mesothelioma, but it must be stressed that improved dust control was introduced in these mines over the forty or more years that such tumours take to develop. In more representative environments, most urban adults have asbestos bodies and fibres in their lungs but there is no current evidence that this finding can be linked with any excessive morbidity or mortality.

Tobacco smoke. Most observers consider that the carcinogenic effects of tobacco smoke for man are established beyond any reasonable doubt, even though the identity of the carcinogenic components and their mode of action are unclear.

Increasing mortality from lung cancer in smokers first became apparent in continental Europe in the 1920s, and in England and Wales in the 1930s. Full documentation emerged from extensive retrospective and prospective studies made in the United Kingdom and the United States in the fifties and early sixties. The salient features are well known. The increased incidence of lung cancer among smokers varies in different parts of the world but is consistently greater in men than women. It is associated more strongly with cigarettes than pipes or cigars. A dose–response relationship exists linking the incidence of lung cancer to the number of cigarettes smoked and the duration of the smoking habit. Lung cancer is commoner among people who habitually inhale cigarette smoke. It is commoner in urban than in rural communities. Lastly, the incidence of lung cancer falls in ex-smokers; about fifteen years after smoking the last cigarette the former smoker appears to be at no greater risk of developing lung cancer than an individual who has never smoked.

The significance of the sex difference and the 'urban factor' is disputed but both probably reflect the greater consumption of tobacco by men and by urban (as opposed to rural) populations; evidence incriminating a carcinogenic pollutant in urban air, such as benzo(a)-pyrene, is unconvincing. Cigarette smoking appears to potentiate the effects of other lung carcinogens. This effect is seen most clearly in the asbestos-associated lung cancers and it may also occur in relation to arsenic.

The incidence of cancers at other sites, notably oesophagus and bladder, is also increased by cigarette smoking; the mechanisms involved are still obscure.

Drugs. A number of drugs are now known to have induced cancer in man. Some examples are shown below:

Drug	*Target tissue*
'Thorotrast' Anabolic steroids ?Oral contraceptives	Liver
Chlornaphthazin	Bladder
Sodium arsenite (Fowler's solution)	Skin
Stilboestrol	Vagina of *foetus*

Much attention has been paid to stilboestrol which, given to pregnant women to prevent habitual abortion, has very occasionally acted transplacentally on the *foetus* and induced the rare adenocarcinomas of the vagina. These lesions are appearing after a latent period of about fifteen to twenty years.

Naturally-occurring carcinogens. Most of the chemical carcinogens so far discussed are associated with man living in a developed and predominantly industrial and urban society. Completely different problems in chemical carcinogenesis are encountered in more remote parts of the world where a simple rural existence may have continued, virtually unchanged, for many generations. Primary carcinoma of the liver (hepatocarcinoma) provides a good example.

This tumour shows a marked (a hundredfold) variation in its worldwide incidence. It is rare in Europe and North America but common among the indigenous inhabitants of parts of Africa (Mozambique, Kenya) and in the Far East (China, Thailand, Singapore, Papua – New Guinea). The incidence falls in Africans who change to an urban mode of life, whether in Africa itself or in the West. The common features of the high-incidence areas are poverty and a tropical or subtropical rural environment. Poverty is related not only to malnutrition but also to poor living conditions where infections such as viral hepatitis are common and where contamination of poorly stored food is likely to occur. Much attention has been paid to contamination of staple foodstuffs – rice, wheat, barley, soya beans, nuts – by the mould *Aspergillus flavus*. This mould synthesizes toxins (aflatoxins) which are potent liver carcinogens in experimental animals. Epidemiological studies have demonstrated aflatoxin contamination in food consumed in high-incidence areas of Mozambique, Kenya and Thailand, and established an overall correlation between levels of dietary aflatoxin and the incidence of liver cancer. Though still circumstantial, the evidence that the naturally occurring aflatoxin may be a carcinogen for the human liver in certain parts of the world is growing considerably.

PHYSICAL AGENTS AS HUMAN CARCINOGENS

The physical agents which act as human carcinogens are ionizing and ultraviolet radiations.

Ionizing Radiation

The first recorded examples of radiation-induced tumours in man were skin cancers in radiologists and makers of X-ray tubes who were unaware of the dangers to which they were exposed. A high incidence of lung cancer was subsequently described among men who mined radioactive ores in Saxony and Czechoslovakia. Another example of radium as a human carcinogen is provided by the bone sarcomas which developed in a group of girls in North America who applied luminous radium-containing paint to watch dials and instrument boards. They used fine brushes and, in the course of 'pointing' them between their lips, they swallowed considerable amounts of radium which were deposited and retained in the skeleton. More recently, increasing attention has been paid to radiation-associated cancers of the thyroid and bone marrow (leukaemias).

The thyroid cancers have been described in two principal contexts: among young adults who received therapeutic irradiation of the neck in infancy for what would not be regarded as totally unacceptable reasons (such as an enlarged thymus), and among the victims of the thermonuclear explosions in Hiroshima and Nagasaki, and in the Marshall Islands. The effective carcinogenic dose for the various kinds of irradiation for the human thyroid gland can be calculated with some accuracy; the latent period (20–25 years) is also known with reasonable precision. Both depend on the age of the patient and there is evidence that the thyroid in young children is more sensitive to ionizing radiation than the adult gland. Recent pathological studies have shown an unusually high incidence of clinically occult thyroid cancers among Japanese from Hiroshima and Nagasaki dying from conditions unconnected with the thermonuclear explosions of 1945. Despite extensive investigation, there is no evidence that internal irradiation of the thyroid with iodine-131 for the treatment of hyperthyroidism carries an enhanced risk of thyroid cancer.

Most of the radiation-induced leukaemias in man have developed among the survivors of the two Japanese thermonuclear explosions and in patients who received therapeutic irradiation for ankylosing spondylitis. A third, more controversial, group consists of children with acute leukaemia whose mothers had received diagnostic irradiation during the antenatal period. This association suggests that foetal bone marrow is, at certain stages, extremely sensitive to small doses of external irradiation. Continuing argument centres round two points – the true incidence of the association between antenatal irradiation and subsequent leukaemia, and the possible operation of additional factors which, acting on foetal tissues, also predispose to the subsequent development of leukaemia in childhood.

Ultraviolet (u.v.) Light

Prolonged exposure to intense sunlight over many years carries an increased risk of cancers of the exposed skin, particularly among fair-skinned Caucasians. A similar but less pronounced relationship exists in Caucasians between u.v. light and cutaneous melanoma. The carcinogenic effects of u.v. light are, however, best illustrated by the extremely rare condition of xeroderma pigmentosum. Inherited as a Mendelian autosomal recessive characteristic, the typical form of this disease is characterized by an inborn inability to repair the mild degree of damage which u.v. light inflicts on DNA. In normal individuals, such damage is easily and regularly repaired; in patients with xeroderma pigmentosum the damaged DNA accumulates and, after a latent period of about ten to fifteen years, multiple cancers of the exposed skin and subcutaneous tissues develop.

VIRUSES AS HUMAN CARCINOGENS

Although viruses are implicated in the aetiology of several tumours in experimental animals, there is no human cancer which has been shown unequivocally to be caused by a virus. A virus is, however, closely involved in Burkitt lymphoma and probably in carcinoma of the postnasal space, and viruses may play a part in the development of some leukaemias and lymphomas, carcinomas of the breast and cervix uteri, and (conceivably) in certain sarcomas. Here we shall confine ourselves to a single condition – Burkitt lymphoma.

This is an aggressive tumour which occurs in young children in parts of sub-Saharal Africa and in Papua – New Guinea. The distribution in Africa was mapped by Dennis Burkitt who drew attention to the climatic characteristics of the high-incidence areas (high temperature, high rainfall); later, space–time 'clustering' and 'drift' of cases were observed. In 1964, Epstein and Barr isolated a virus – the Epstein–Barr (EB) virus – from cells of a Burkitt lymphoma growing as a fresh culture in the laboratory. Methods were developed to detect anti-EB virus antibodies in serum, and several seroepidemiological surveys were carried out. Patients with Burkitt lymphoma were shown to have consistently high levels of anti-EB virus antibodies. But two anomalous findings emerged. Patients with one other, unrelated malignancy – cancer of the postnasal space – were also shown to have high levels of anti-EB virus antibodies in their serum; and the same antibodies were also present, at lower titres, in most apparently healthy adults living in temperate climates where Burkitt lymphoma or postnasal space cancer were virtually unknown. This paradox was partly resolved by the chance discovery that EB virus was the long-sought aetiological agent of infectious mononucleosis. More seroepidemiological surveys indicated that EB virus infection was sometimes associated with non-specific febrile illnesses (particularly in children) and that about one-third of EB virus infections were asymptomatic. The paradox therefore returns in a different form: How to associate the single EB virus with two forms of malignant disease (Burkitt lymphoma and cancer of the postnasal space), with the self-limiting and benign condition of infectious mononucleosis, and with trivial non-specific infections trailing off into completely 'silent' subclinical infections?

The current view is that the clinical pattern of EB virus-induced diseases is determined jointly by the virus *and by the host or patient.* The geographical studies of Mr Burkitt showed a close similarity between the distribution of Burkitt lymphoma and of holoendemic malaria; and it has been proposed that chronic severe malaria modifies host responses in some ill-defined way such that a subsequent infection with EB virus fails to elicit an effective antiviral response and Burkitt lymphoma develops as a progressive malignancy. In the absence of pre-existing malaria (and perhaps other severe debilitating conditions), almost all EB virus infections are self-limiting and Burkitt lymphoma hardly ever develops. EB virus-associated antigens and nucleic acids have been described in Burkitt lymphoma cells, and EB virus vaccines have been shown to protect against EB virus-associated lymphomas induced experimentally in Primates. The circumstantial links between the virus and the human tumour are quite strong though much still remains to be clarified.

One general concluding point may be made. Most human cancers arise from the operation of many factors. It is convenient to group these factors into the various categories that we have used in this chapter – extrinsic and intrinsic, chemicals and viruses and physical agents – but it is wrong to regard them as rigidly exclusive. The distinction between exogenous and endogenous chemicals is blurred by the fact that some chemical carcinogens are generated from innocuous non-carcinogenic precursors in the body, sometimes as a result of the host's own metabolism or by his normal bacterial flora in the gut. Chemicals and ionizing radiations may, in part, be carcinogenic because they activate latent oncogenic viruses. If we take one common form of cancer – breast cancer – it is probable that we are talking about a patient in whom a virus, hormones and chemicals are operating *together* in a genetically susceptible host. Despite the daunting complexity that is implied, it has to be accepted that the development of most human cancers is likely to be a multifactorial process.

References

Carter, R. L. and Symington, T. (1975) New trends in cancer 4 – chemical carcinogens in man, *Health Trends*, **7**, 47.

Symington, T. and Carter, R. L. (1976) *Scientific Foundations of Oncology*. London: William Heinemann Medical Books Ltd.

For detailed information see *I.A.R.C. Monographs on the Evaluation of Carcinogenic Risks of Chemicals to Man*. **1**–**9**. Lyons: International Agency for Research on Cancer.

Chapter 4

Systemic Manifestations of Malignant Tumours

PHILIP K. BONDY
M.D., F.R.C.P.
Cancer Research Campaign Professor of Medicine
Institute of Cancer Research
Consultant in Medicine
Ludwig Institute for Cancer Research
Honorary Consultant in Medicine
Royal Marsden Hospital
Surrey

Introduction

Cancer commonly produces disability and kills because the tumour mass is so large or so situated that it interferes with some vital function. Often, however, the major influence interfering with normal function is some factor produced by the tumour which has its effect at a distance.

Inappropriate Hormone Secretion

Neoplasms of the endocrine glands are often capable of producing hormonal products appropriate to the tissue of origin. Unlike normal tissues, however, such tumours are rarely under control of the feedback mechanisms which should keep endocrine secretion in balance. Thus tumours of the adrenal cortex may cause hyperadrenocorticism, hyperaldosteronism, masculinization or feminization; tumours of the ovary may cause precocious feminization or postmenopausal metrorrhagia; tumours of the parathyroid gland cause hypercalcaemia, etc. These effects may induce illness or death, but they are, in a sense, appropriate in view of the type of tissue in which the neoplasm arose. In some cases, such hormones are useful in diagnosing and following treatment of the tumour. For example the therapist finds it valuable to follow the production of chorionic gonadotrophin by tumours derived from placenta or placental rests such as choriocarcinoma or teratoma of the testis.

Most, perhaps all, cancers produce proteins or polypeptides which are not found in the normal tissue from which the cancer arose, or, if normally present, occur only in trace amounts. Such cancer-associated polypeptides are sometimes identical or so similar to physiological hormones, that they cause endocrine effects. In addition, some of the abnormal polypeptides are capable of producing immune reactions. These effects are considered later.

ADRENOCORTICOTROPHIC HORMONE (ACTH)

This is the commonest and one of the most dangerous inappropriate hormones produced by tumours. It is most commonly associated with small cell undifferentiated ('oat cell') carcinoma of the bronchus, carcinoid tumours and islet cell tumours of the pancreas but, more rarely, tumours of almost any other tissue may secrete this hormone. It produces uncontrolled stimulation of the adrenal cortex and consequent elevation of the plasma and urine cortisol levels. Acutely, this causes loss of body potassium through the kidneys, and metabolic alkalosis. This, combined with the low serum potassium level may cause cardiac arrhythmias. The well-known ability of excess corticosteroids to suppress the inflammatory reaction permits infections to progress unchecked and often unperceived. Cushings's syndrome occurs when the effect has persisted over a period of weeks or months. This is rare, however, in patients with bronchial carcinoma.

Treatment is urgent, since life expectancy is greatly shortened by this complication. Removal of the tumours will restore the metabolism to normal; but if this is impossible, drugs (e.g. aminoglutethimide) which block adrenal cortical function may be useful. Occasionally, bilateral adrenalectomy is justified.

ACTH itself is capable of increasing skin pigmentation and fragments of the ACTH molecule are even more potent in this respect. Thus patients with tumour-associated excess ACTH secretion almost always have excessive pigmentation. Sometimes pigmentation occurs without ACTH secretion. In addition, tumour-associated skin diseases (discussed later) may produce special types of skin pigmentation.

SYNDROME OF INAPPROPRIATE ANTIDIURETIC HORMONE

About one-third of 'oat cell' carcinomas of the bronchus produce vasopressin or some similar substance which inhibits excretion of water through the kidneys. As a result, the patient becomes overhydrated, the constituents of plasma and intracellular water are abnormally diluted and the osmotic pressure of the plasma falls. It is recognized in its mild form by inability to excrete ingested water. In advanced cases depressed plasma sodium concentration and low plasma osmolarity are associated with simultaneous excretion of concentrated urine. The resulting hypo-osmolarity of the brain can cause mental confusion, and, in advanced cases convulsions, coma and death.

In mild cases, there is no need for treatment, if fluid intake is moderately restricted. When disturbances of brain function occur, total water intake should be restricted to less than 1 litre per day. In extreme cases, intravenous administration of hypertonic saline, combined with restriction of fluid intake may be life-saving. Drugs which produce the syndrome of diabetes insipidus, such as lithium carbonate or some of the tetracycline antibiotics may be helpful. The best treatment is to eliminate the tumour.

GYNAECOMASTIA

Enlargement and engorgement of the male breast may occur in association with certain tumours, especially squamous cell carcinomas of the bronchus, carcinoma of the adrenal cortex or teratomas of the testis. In the case of the adrenal tumour, the cause is usually secretion of oestrogens by the neoplastic cells. With other types of cancer, the explanation is not so clear. In some instances, inappropriate secretion of prolactin has been postulated. Sometimes the abnormality is associated with secretion of the placental hormones, somatomammotrophin or chorionic gonadotrophin. The situation in patients with bronchial carcinoma is complicated by the well-known fact that any form of disease of the pleura can cause gynaecomastia, by mechanisms which are still obscure. The situation may become clearer in the near future because modern methods of measuring the various gonadotrophic hormones and prolactin will permit evaluation of the significant factors in enough patients to draw conclusions.

HYPERTHYROIDISM

The pituitary gland makes a thyrotrophic hormone, and so does the placenta. In view of the fact that many other pituitary and placental hormones are produced by tumours, it would be surprising if excess production of thyroid stimulating factor(s) did not also occur. Appreciable concentrations of placental thyrotrophin are often found in the plasma of patients with tumours of placental origin. In spite of this, actual hyperthyroidism appears to be extraordinarily rare. Indeed, only a handful of patients have been reported with this complication which has, in every reported instance, undergone remission when the tumour mass could be reduced. In all such cases it is critical to be sure that the patient did not have incidental simultaneous Graves's disease – a common disorder which might be expected to occur quite often in patients with another common disease – cancer.

POLYCYTHAEMIA

Most patients with cancer tend to be anaemic. Therefore, when a patient proves to have an elevated erythrocyte count and haemoglobin, one suspects that the tumour may be producing the hormone, erythropoietin, which stimulates the bone marrow to produce red blood cells. The normal source of this hormone is the kidneys, and most patients in which the polycythaemia has been recognized have had renal cell carcinomas.

Systemic Metabolic Derangements

HYPERCALCAEMIA

In mild form, elevated serum calcium causes constipation and lethargy; but when severe, it causes vomiting, dehydration, renal tubular damage and uraemia, mental confusion and cardiac arrhythmias. The commonest cause of elevated serum calcium concentrations is cancer, and the commonest cancer to cause this effect is mammary carcinoma. In almost every affected case of breast cancer, the high calcium level is due to microscopic or gross skeletal metastases. Serum calcium levels usually are only slightly elevated, but they can occasionally rise extremely rapidly especially after endocrine manipulation. A common cause of acute deterioration and sudden death in such patients is hypercalcaemia. The serum calcium may also be raised by a similar mechanism in patients with myeloma and, rarely, by other tumours.

In a few patients – especially those with squamous cell carcinoma of the bronchus or renal cell carcinoma (hypernephroma) – hypercalcaemia results from release by the tumour of parathyroid hormone, or a very similar polypeptide. In such patients the serum phosphate is depressed, whereas it is usually normal in patients with hypercalcaemia due to carcinoma of the breast or myeloma.

Hypercalcaemia can be treated acutely by forced hydration, corticosteroids, oral sodium phosphate and, in recalcitrant cases, mithramycin. These manoeuvres may provide temporary relief, but unless the tumour is brought under control, hypercalcaemia is likely to recur. In a few patients no manoeuvre seems to control the elevated calcium level, and the patient dies.

CACHEXIA AND ANOREXIA

Some patients lose weight rapidly and fade away in a few weeks or months in spite of energetic attempts to improve their nutrition. This situation is most common in cancer of the gastrointestinal tract and lung and it is rare with mammary cancer, although it may occur with any type of tumour. The neoplasm may be small and may not interfere with free passage of food through the gastrointestinal system. In experimental animals this situation may occur in spite of adequate calorie intake but all human patients with this syndrome in my experience have severe anorexia. Their weight loss is caused by self-imposed starvation. It seems likely that this profound and intractable loss of appetite is caused by a product of the tumour, but the nature of the product is not known.

HYPOGLYCAEMIA

Tumours can cause the blood glucose concentration to fall low enough to cause anxiety, sweating, mental confusion, convulsions or coma. The beta cells of the Islets of Langerhans normally produce insulin, and adenomas or carcinomas arising from these cells may produce inappropriate amounts of the hormone, thus reducing the blood glucose. Insulin has also been identified in other neoplasma, such as 'oat-cell' carcinomas of the lung, but in these cases it does not appear that the hormone was released into the circulation, since the patients did not have hypoglycaemia.

The blood glucose may be depressed in patients with bulky sarcomas, especially those arising in the retroperitoneal area. It is clear that these tumours do not contain or secrete insulin, though they may produce other types of substances with insulin-like activity. They may also interfere with the conversion of protein into glucose by the liver, or their metabolic rate may be so high that they use up glucose faster than it can be absorbed or produced by the liver. In all of these situations, the earliest abnormality of the metabolism is hypoglycaemia occurring after fasting – especially before breakfast in the morning. With advancing activity of the tumour, the hypoglycaemia may become constant. Intravenous administration of glucose may help temporarily, as may frequent feedings; but the only really satisfactory way to handle the situation is to destroy or remove the tumour. When this is possible, the metabolic derangement returns to normal; but when the tumour recurs, hypoglycaemia may be the earliest sign. Since it may be difficult to distinguish the symptoms of hypoglycaemia from those of cerebral metastases or oversedation, much care must be given to evaluating patients with confusion or mental deterioration.

CLUBBING AND HYPERTROPHIC PULMONARY OSTEOARTHROPATHY

It is common for tumours of the bronchus to be associated with swelling of the tips of the fingers and toes and excess production of tissue under the nail – a condition known as 'clubbing'. In some cases, in addition, subperiosteal bone may be laid down, especially along the tibia and fibula near the ankle, and the radius and ulna near the wrist. The involved areas are usually tender so the complaints may be confused superficially with arthritis. The periosteal change is most common with squamous cell carcinoma of the bronchus, but it may be seen with many other types of tumour. The changes are not, however, specific for carcinoma. Clubbing may occur congenitally (and without any implications of altered susceptibility to neoplasia), and it is common in patients with chronic pulmonary infections (e.g. bronchiectasis, tuberculosis), liver disease and, on occasion, in thyroid disease. It is not clear why clubbing occurs. Attempts have been made to explain this type of change as a result of excessive inappropriate secretion of growth hormone by the tumour, but the evidence of this connection is not convincing.

Immunological Manifestations

There is a common belief that patients with advanced cancer have impaired function of their immune mechanisms. The evidence for this belief rests on the reduced ability of standard antigens to produce skin reactions of the delayed hypersensitivity type (e.g. the tuberculin reaction), and on diminished ability of the patients' lymphocytes to be activated by specific and non-specific antigens. It is not clear that these observations have much to do with the total functioning immunity of the patient. Certainly, one should be highly sceptical of the popular dogma that the spread of cancer is prevented by surveillance by the body's immune system, and that spread is a result of breakdown of this surveillance. In spite of this, certain information justifies the suspicion that immunity may be modified in patients with cancer.

INFECTION

Infection is the commonest cause of death in patients with terminal cancer. Frequently this takes the form of pneumonia or septicaemia. Often the infection can be related to mechanical effects of the tumour – for example, infection of an obstructed segment of lung. In many instances, however, no explanation is available except the general debilitated state of the patient. I doubt whether a specific immune mechanism must be invoked. The combination of malnutrition, bone marrow suppression from chemotherapy or radiotherapy, and the mechanical effects of surgery probably are adequate to explain most infections. Yet it must be mentioned that certain diseases are associated particularly with specific infections. Thus herpes zoster is very common in patients with Hodgkin's disease, and cytomegalic virus often causes severe infections in leukaemias. These are tumours of the tissues which are directly involved in the immune reaction, however, and so their abnormalities of immune responses may not be representative of the abnormality in other types of tumour.

FEVER

Fever is also common in patients with tumours. Careful investigation has shown that in most instances, fever can be explained by infection. Sometimes necrosis of the tumour provides a suitable focus for bacterial growth. The fever may not respond to antibiotics because the blood supply to the necrotic area is too meagre to deliver adequate concentrations of the medicine. However, not all fevers in cancer patients can be explained by infection. Tumours of the kidney (Wilms's, and hypernephroma) are prone to produce fever without evidence of infection. Fever may be the presenting symptom in an appreciable portion of patients with lymphoma or leukaemia, and such patients may not have demonstrable infection.

AUTOIMMUNE DISEASE

A high proportion of patients with cancer have antibodies against smooth muscle, nucleoproteins or other components of the normal cells of the body. It is questionable whether these antibodies cause disease, in most cases, but a few circumstances are known where they are important. In patients with lymphoma, autoimmune haemolytic anaemia is a well-established complication. Increased red cell destruction is also frequently demonstrable in patients with leukaemia, and sometimes in association with solid tumours. The haemolytic process is sometimes associated with the presence of cold agglutinins. Membranous glomerulonephritis, though a rare complication, is a well-recognized problem in many solid tumours and leukaemia, but not in lymphomas. The disease arises from deposition of antigen/antibody complex in the glomeruli, where it may increase permeability and produce the nephrotic syndrome of severe proteinuria and oedema.

Skin Manifestations of Tumours

In addition to the lumps produced by metastases to the skin, and the specific tumours of the skin, such as squamous cell carcinoma, basal cell carcinoma, melanoma and mycosis fungoides, a number of changes may occur in the skin as a distant result of tumours or their products. It is possible that some or all of these changes are a reflection of autoimmune skin disease, but this is not proven at present.

POLYMYOSITIS AND DERMATOMYOSITIS

This is a rare disease, usually seen in late middle age. In its full-blown form it causes weakness and tenderness of the muscles, especially those of the shoulder girdle. A characteristic complaint is inability to raise the hands to the head to comb the hair. The hip girdle may also be affected, to such a degree that the patient may not be able to walk. In extreme cases, the patient may not be able to lift his head from the pillow, or swallow. Although smooth muscles are not affected, the myocardium may be damaged so congestive heart failure may occur. The muscle manifestations are sometimes seen alone, but are usually accompanied by a skin rash. This may be merely a faint violet flush of the cheeks and eyelids, or it may progress to a deep-red flush with local oedema involving the face, upper chest, back of the shoulders and arms and legs. It may be associated, as well, with a scaly maculopapular eruption of the wrists and knuckles. Small penetrating ulcers may form over knuckles or on fingertips leading to an appearance similar to that seen in advanced sclerodema. When the disease involves only the muscles, it is called 'polymyositis' but when the skin is involved as well, it is called 'dermatomyositis'. The disease can occur in the absence of demonstrable cancer, but often the disease is established. When either form of the disease is seen for the first time in a patient over the age of forty, there is an even chance that a tumour will be demonstrable. For this reason, patients who present with this disease should be investigated aggressively for the presence of carcinoma especially of the gastro-intestinal tract, lung or bladder. Other types of neoplasm may also be associated with the disease, but this is rare. The tumour may be small, so development of the skin manifestation may permit early diagnosis and cure. If this occurs, the muscle and skin manifestations disappear. If cure of the cancer is impossible, patients may still get a great deal of relief from corticosteroids or from drugs often used in cancer chemotherapy such as methotrexate.

ACANTHOSIS NIGRICANS

This consists of increased pigmentation and thickening especially of the skin of the axilla, and back of the neck, though other areas may also be involved. In its mildest form it may look superficially like a patch of dirt, but when further advanced, thickening of the skin may be quite striking. It does not appear to be associated in any way with the pituitary pigment-producing hormones mentioned earlier, although the congenital form may be associated with abnormalities of hypothalamic function. It occurs in three forms: a congenital form, seen in children and particularly florid in patients with systemic lipoatrophy (lipoatrophic diabetes); an 'acquired' form associated with obesity or medication with corticosteroids; and 'malignant' acanthosis nigricans. There is no difference between the three forms on examination of the skin, but the first two are not associated with cancer. When acanthosis nigricans appears for the first time in a non-obese middle-aged patient, there is a very high probability of an adenocarcinoma, especially of the stomach or other intraabdominal organ. In about a fifth of the cases, the skin lesions appear before the cancer can be recognized.

OTHER SKIN LESIONS

Other skin lesions which are often associated with cancer include ichthyosis, especially of the palms, increased skin thickness with hyperkeratosis (tylosis), pemphigoid, erythema gyratum repens and many others. Some of these are common in elderly people, and their association with cancer may be a coincidence rather than a causal relationship.

Neurological Manifestations

Usually, when a patient with cancer develops neurological symptoms it is because the tumour has spread to the brain or meninges. Metastases may be numerous and small, so brain scans and even the new computerized scanning X-ray methods may not be able to see them. Sometimes a diagnosis can be made by finding tumour cells in the spinal fluid. If the lesions are located in the proper region of the brain, it may be possible to identify a localized disorder, which helps to confirm the diagnosis of secondary deposits. If metastases involve the frontal lobes, however, bizarre behavioural changes may occur which must be distinguished from those associated with hypercalcaemia or plasma dilution caused by the syndrome of inappropriate secretion of antidiuretic hormone which have been discussed previously. The secondaries may cause serious organic functional deterioration which is difficult to distinguish from that caused by cerebral arteriosclerosis.

In some instances, however, degeneration of the nervous system may be a distant manifestation of the tumour. In these patients, even meticulous examination of the nervous system at autopsy fails to reveal metastatic deposits.

PERIPHERAL NEUROPATHY

Peripheral neuropathy is the commonest such manifestation, which may occur in as many as 1 per cent of patients with unselected solid tumours. It is much more commonly associated with carcinoma of the lung and ovary than with other types of tumour, but it can be seen with most types of cancer. It usually involves the distal portions of the limbs, and mainly causes paraesthesias, such as tingling, and anaesthesia. Sometimes there is motor involvement as well, which must be distinguished from the myositis previously described because the function of the muscles themselves, and their appearance on biopsy, are normal. Patients may complain of difficulty with walking or performing fine movements because of loss of sensory control. Pain may also occur and deep tendon reflexes may be lost. Many of these symptoms are like those produced by the chemotherapeutic agent, vincristine. Sorting out the exact cause may be very difficult in patients with cancer who have been treated with this drug.

PROGRESSIVE MULTIFOCAL LEUCOENCEPHALOPATHY

This may cause any kind of cerebral damage. Patients may show evidence of depressed intelligence, loss of memory, emotional lability or episodic fluctuations of consciousness. The cerebellum may be involved, in which case ataxia and tremor may be prominent. If the lower centres of the brain are affected, there may be difficulty in swallowing, changes in speech, nystagmus and ocular paralyses. It is not clear at present whether the disease is a result of autoimmunity, a virus infection of the central nervous system or the production of some form of neurotoxin by the tumour. It may be greatly improved or disappear when the primary tumour is brought under control, but this is unusual. It has been claimed that cytosine arabinoside is effective in treating this disease.

References

Klastersky, J., Weerts, D., Hensgens, C. and Debusscher, L. (1973) Fever of unexplained origin in patients with cancer, *European J. Cancer* **9**, 649.

Bondy, P. K. (1976) Systemic effects of neoplasia, in *Scientific Foundations of Oncology*, p. 557. T. Symington and R. L. Carter (eds.). London: William Heinemann Medical Books Ltd.

Rees, L. H. and Ratcliffe, J. G. (1974) Ectopic hormone production by non-endocrine tumours, *Clin. Endocrinol.*, **3**, 263.

Chapter 5

Radiological Investigations

C. A. PARSONS
F.R.C.S., F.R.C.R.
Consultant Radiologist
The Royal Marsden Hospital
London and Surrey

Diagnostic radiology has an important place in the management of malignant disease. It may be helpful in:

1. The diagnosis of the primary tumour.
2. Determining the extent of that tumour.
3. The demonstration of distant metastases.
4. Monitoring the response of the disease to treatment.
5. Serial follow-up to show early evidence of recurrence.

Usually a diagnosis of cancer has been reached before the patient is referred to an oncology centre. All radiological investigations undertaken at other hospitals prior to referral must be reviewed. The purpose of this is to confirm that the X-ray findings are compatible with the diagnosis and staging that has been made and to assess the development of the disease over a period of time, confirming its progressive nature and indicating the rate of advance.

All the investigations commonly seen in a department of general radiology are used from time to time in the specialized oncology diagnostic X-ray department; however, there is a great emphasis on some procedures. Lymphography and mammography, of which we carry out 1,200 and 6,000 per annum, respectively, at the Royal Marsden Hospital, are the prime examples. The availability of grey scale ultrasound and high quality isotope imaging techniques have made some radiological techniques partly redundant. In particular, angiography is required much less frequently than before. The introduction of com-

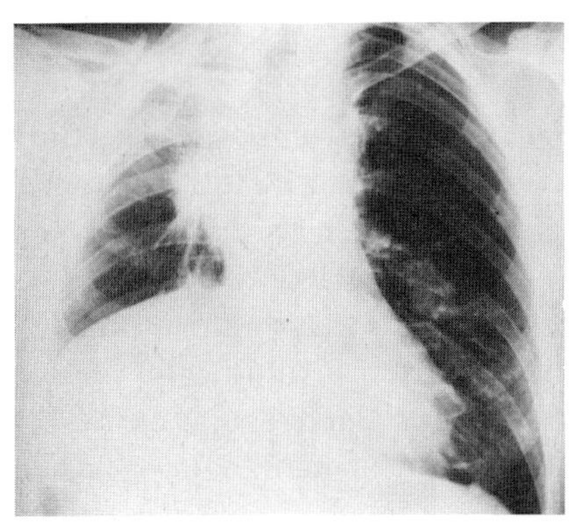

Figure 5.1 Unresectable carcinoma of right main bronchus after radiotherapy. Secondary deposit in left mid-zone. Note raised right diaphragm and trachea displaced to right.

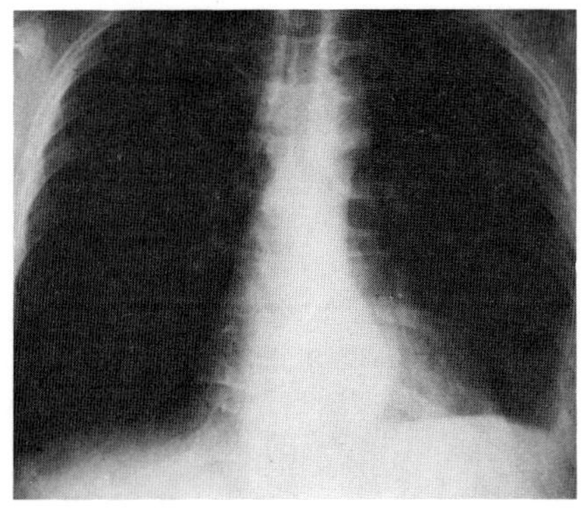

Figure 5.2 High Kv film shows 'mass' through heart to be an encysted effusion.

puterized axial tomography, EMI scanning, has provided a dramatic advance in the demonstration of brain tumours, and we anticipate a similar advance with the application of this technique to other organs.

Clinical radiology then is not a static unchanging subject but a field of endeavour in which change and progress are occurring at a remarkable rate.

The Chest

The most common single X-ray investigation of cancer patients is the chest film. This reflects the frequency of spread of secondary deposits to the lung and bony thoracic cage and the frequency of primary bronchial carcinomas and mediastinal tumours.

At the first visit three films are taken:

(*a*) a conventional exposure, Fig. 5.1, which will demonstrate the lungs and the ribs.
(*b*) a 'high kv' film, Fig. 5.2, which penetrates the rib and heart opacities allowing lung lesions to be seen through them more clearly. The air filled trachea and main bronchi will be clearly shown.
(*c*) a lateral film, to aid in localization of abnormalities already shown on the other two films, and to display areas such as the retrosternal region not clearly seen on the straight views.

CARCINOMA OF THE BRONCHUS

Carcinoma of the bronchus can be divided into two groups according to the site at which it occurs, central or peripheral. Small peripheral lung cancers may cause no symptoms, their discovery depending on a chest X-ray taken for some other purpose. A variety of appearances are commonly seen. The tumour may be shown as a rounded opacity, in which case it may be indistinguishable from a number of benign conditions. A notch in the outline of the lesion or an irregular or frankly spiculated appearance gives rise to suspicion of malignancy. As the peripheral bronchial carcinoma enlarges it may outgrow its blood supply so that the centre of the mass cavitates. A cavitating mass with craggy irregular walls is very likely to be a lung cancer, but similar appearances are found in other conditions such as lung abscess.

As the tumour grows it invades the structures around. Although the pleura forms a temporary barrier to local spread, eventually it will be breached and the underlying bone or another adjacent pulmonary lobe infiltrated. Rib destruction is commonly seen with tumours at the lung apex; these are known as Pancoast tumours. Tumours lying against the heart may invade the pericardium causing an effusion with rapid increase in the size of the heart outline, as seen on the chest film. Tumour cells metastasizing through the pulmonary lymphatics will cause enlargement of the hilar and paratracheal lymph nodes, and this may be more obvious on the X-ray than the peripheral tumour.

Tumours arising in the more centrally placed bronchi may be recognized as a mass, or may only be apparent because of changes which occur in the peripheral lung due to partial or complete blockage of the main bronchus by the tumour. The normal secretions from the peripheral bronchi cannot escape past the obstruction and this increases the likelihood of infection and pulmonary consolidation (Fig. 5.3). When complete obstruction occurs air is absorbed from the lung beyond the block causing its collapse. The effect this has on the appearance of the chest X-ray depends on the size of the bronchus which is obstructed. If this is a main bronchus, the whole of a lung or lobe will collapse and the surrounding mobile structures, the mediastinum and diaphragm, will move in to fill the space left by the collapsed lung. Radiotherapy will often produce a rapid improvement in this situation by shrinking the central tumour and allowing reaeration of the lung. Massive collapse is commonly accompanied by a pleural effusion (Fig. 5.4).

Tomography is often helpful in demonstrating the exact site of block in a central bronchus or in clearly defining the outline of a peripheral tumour (Fig. 5.5). A full description of tomography will be found in

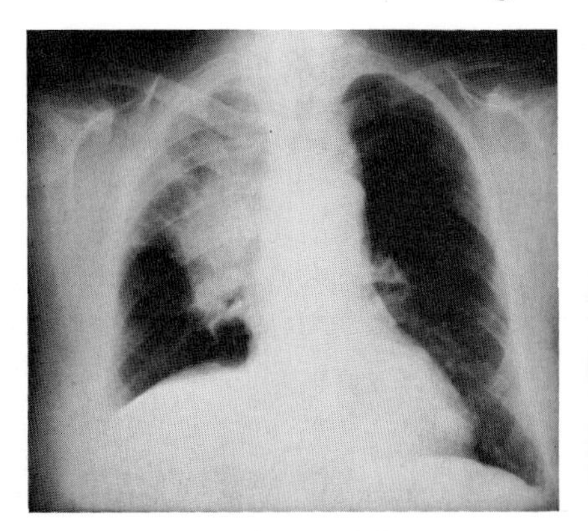

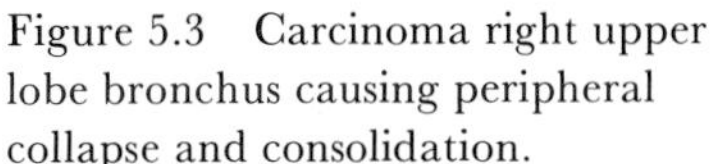

Figure 5.3 Carcinoma right upper lobe bronchus causing peripheral collapse and consolidation.

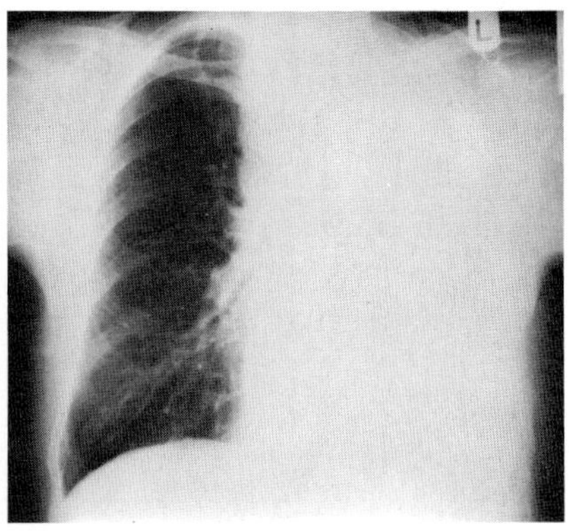

Figure 5.4 Collapse of the whole left lung and effusion. The mediastinum is displaced towards the opaque hemithorax.

Wright's book listed at the end of this chapter. In essence the technique requires that the tube producing the X-rays, and positioned above the horizontal patient, is connected by a rigid bar to the film in a sliding carriage below the table. The bar is pivoted at the vertical level of the lesion being investigated. During the exposure the tube and film move in opposite directions, the centre of the X-ray beam being directed through the lesion. The structures at the level at which the bar is pivoted will appear in focus on the developed film, but structures within the patient at levels above or below the pivot will be so blurred that they will not be visible on the film.

METASTASES TO THE LUNG

Metastases to the lung occur from a great variety of tumours; indeed, it is unwise to think of any tumour as never metastasizing to the lung. Typically, pulmonary secondary deposits are round opacities scattered

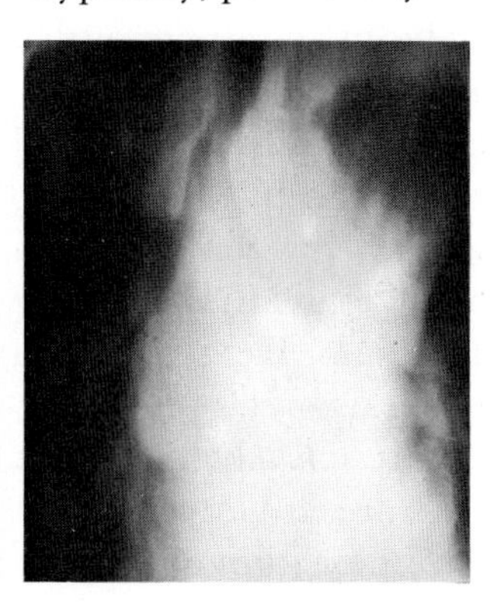

Figure 5.5 Tomography shows narrowing of left main bronchus by surrounding tumour.

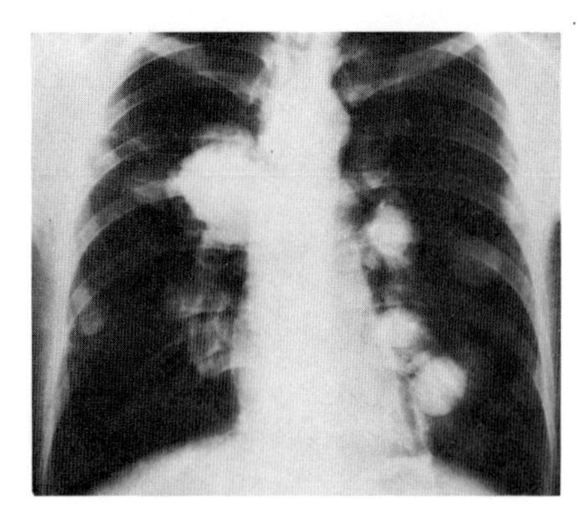

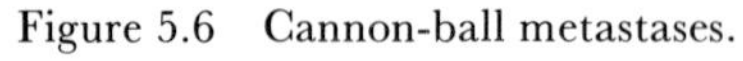

Figure 5.6 Cannon-ball metastases.

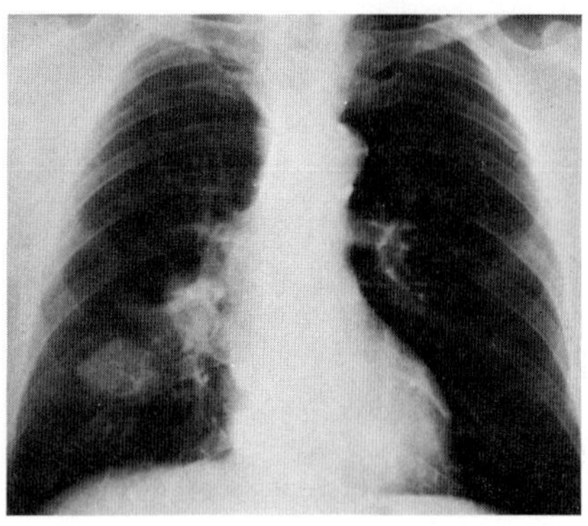

Figure 5.7 Enlargement of right hilar lymph nodes and adjacent pulmonary lymphomatous deposit.

throughout the lung fields (Fig. 5.6), but they may be ill-defined and irregular in outline. Without effective treatment deposits can be shown to enlarge by comparing chest films taken at intervals. Similarly, reduction in size or complete disappearance will accompany appropriate treatment. Pulmonary deposits may be single and huge, occupying the whole of a hemithorax, or multiple and minute. Occasionally one or several metastases will cavitate, usually following chemotherapy. Pleural deposits often coexist and may cause a pleural effusion. If the fluid of an effusion prevents the underlying lung being seen on a conventional chest X-ray, a further film should be taken with the patient lying on his side, when the fluid will run to the most dependent part of the chest, leaving the previously hidden lung on view. This is a decubitus film.

TUMOURS OF THE MEDIASTINUM

Tumours of the mediastinum are common. The mediastinum is the central area between the medial surfaces of the parietal pleura of the two lungs, and extends from the sternum anteriorly to the dorsal spine. The space is divided arbitrarily into regions, in each of which particular histological types of tumours occur. The anterior mediastinum lies in front of the pericardium. The tumours commonly found in this region include thyroid carcinomas, thymomas, lymphomas and teratomas. The middle mediastinum contains the heart, great vessels and main airways. Lymphomas involving the hilar and paratracheal lymph nodes and central bronchial carcinomas lie in this area. The posterior mediastinum is behind the pericardium and contains tumours of the

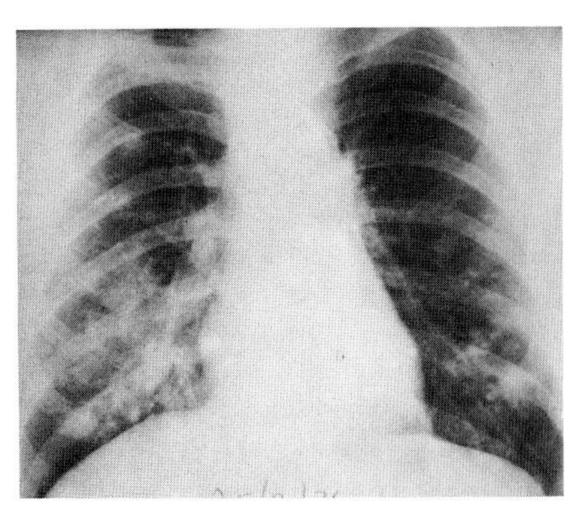

Figure 5.8 Pulmonary Hodgkin's disease.

oesophagus, neural tissue and masses associated with destructive deposits in the vertebrae.

Often the radiologist is unable to distinguish one mediastinal tumour from another. There are a number of features which may be helpful. Thyroid masses may be continued into the neck and contain nodules of calcium. Teratomas may contain calcium, bone or teeth. Neural tumours often erode the vertebral body or rib on which they lie.

The lymphomas deserve special mention since radiology plays a major role in staging the extent of the disease and it is upon this that treatment selection depends. The most common abnormality seen is mediastinal and hilar lymph node enlargement which often returns to normal appearance following chemotherapy or radiotherapy (Fig. 5.7). Lymphomatous pulmonary lesions are not often seen when the patient first presents but frequently develop during the course of the illness. They are often multiple small fluffy opacities which respond well to treatment but recur in crops over the course of several years (Fig. 5.8). Rarely the pulmonary lesions of lymphoma are large, occupying the whole of a segment or lobe of lung. Destructive bony deposits may be present in the ribs.

Tumours of the mediastinum and bronchus may compress and invade the great veins. The patient may be dyspnoeic due to obstruction of the venous return to the heart and have distended veins in the head, neck and arms. The obstructing lesion can be localized by superior vena cavography. The patient starves overnight prior to coming to the X-ray department. 40 ml of contrast medium (Conray 280) is injected over two to three seconds into the veins of each arm. Seven films are exposed at one-second intervals starting half-way through the injection. The contrast medium will opacify the veins from the arms,

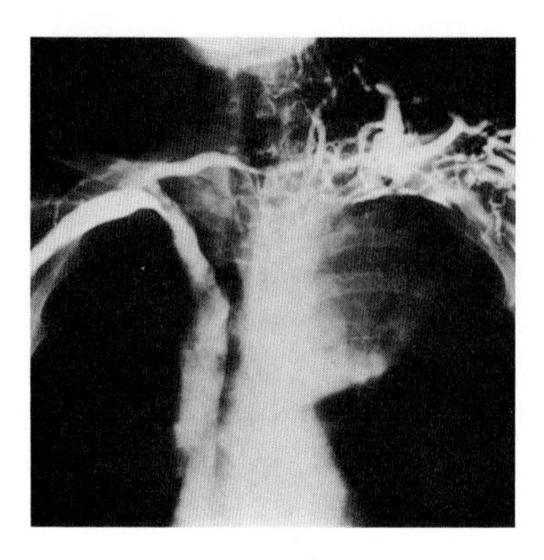

Figure 5.9 Superior vena cavagram showing complete obstruction to the left innominate vein with collateral vessels to left side of neck and chest wall.

the innominate veins, superior vena cava, pulmonary vessels and aorta in turn. Compression of the great veins will be shown and the alternative, collateral, pathways which the blood takes to return to the heart (Fig. 5.9). Tumour or thrombus may be present within the lumen of the opacified veins. In addition, by following the flow of contrast medium for seven seconds the effect of the mediastinal tumour on the blood supply to the lungs will be shown. Decreased perfusion may be caused by the tumour itself or by postradiation fibrosis. The investigation also helps in distinguishing that part of the hilar opacity which is due to vascular structures from tumour or lymph node masses.

Lymphography

There is little opportunity for the nurse in a general hospital to see this procedure, and yet it is extremely common in the specialist oncology unit. The investigation will be described in some detail because of its importance in evaluating patients with malignant diseases. Lymphography is undertaken in cancer patients for these reasons:

1. The diagnosis and staging of lymphomas.
2. The diagnosis and staging of some metastatic diseases.
3. To demonstrate the response of involved lymph nodes to treatment.
4. Serial follow-up films of the opacified nodes will show if tumour tissue within the nodes enlarges, indicating recurrence.
5. The thoroughness of lymph node excision at operation can be checked.
6. Investigation of non-specific symptoms which may be due to malignancy, such as unexplained pyrexia or pruritus.

THE PROCEDURE

The procedure can be undertaken on out-patients. In adults no patient preparation is required, but children under age ten need a general anaesthetic. The bladder should be emptied immediately prior to the procedure as the patient will be required to lie still for one to two hours. With the patient on an X-ray table the feet are cleaned with Chlorhexidine in spirit. 0·5 ml of a blue dye, Patent Blue Violet 2·5 per cent, is injected subcutaneously on the dorsum of each foot close to the base of the toes. Local analgesic is injected further up the foot to allow a small incision to be made. The lymphatic ducts are identified by the blue dye, which they take up. One lymphatic duct is dissected free of the surrounding tissues and isolated by passing a ligature around it. A fine needle SWG 30 is introduced into the lymphatic duct and tied firmly in place. The needle is connected by polythene tubing to a syringe containing 10 ml of an oily contrast medium, Ultrafluid Lipiodol. The oil is injected by pressure on the syringe piston by a pump. A variety of pumps exists from home-made arrangements to highly sophisticated rate-adjustable electric injectors. Whatever system is available, a flow rate of about 7 ml per hour is desirable so that the procedure is not unnecessarily prolonged for the patient.

As soon as the injection of contrast medium is started, X-ray films of the calves are exposed to confirm that the contrast medium is actually entering a lymphatic duct. Should a vein have been selected in error, the column of contrast medium is shown to fragment, with droplets collecting in groups or around the vein valves. When this occurs the injection must be stopped immediately since the oil would otherwise eventually all be distributed to the pulmonary capillaries. With appropriate experience this error is rare.

If there has been a previous operation on the leg or groin contrast medium may be discharged into the tissues from divided channels causing discomfort for several days. Lymphaticovenous communications may develop at the site of previous surgery so that oil may be diverted into the blood-stream. To avoid these complications control films should be taken when it is judged that the column of oil has reached the site of any previous operations.

When 5 ml of Lipiodol has been injected on each side, a film of the pelvis is taken to show the level the column of oil has reached. The further amount needed to attain the level of L4 vertebral body on that particular patient is estimated. When this has been given, the injection is stopped and the wounds sutured. Waterproof dressings are applied and the patient advised that no restrictions need be placed on their activities on account of the lymphogram. The sutures are removed by the patient's general practitioner or district nurse when the wounds have healed.

On completion of the injection the patient walks 250 metres to pump the oil up to the abdominal lymph channels and a film of the abdomen is taken. This shows the course followed by the pelvic and para-aortic lymphatics which may be distorted by lymph nodes enlarged due to malignant disease. A film of the mediastinum at this time would demonstrate the main lymphatic through the chest, the thoracic duct. We find this only rarely of value in patient management decisions.

The following day films of the abdomen and pelvis are taken to show the opacified nodes with oblique views to project the nodes away from underlying bones. At the same time intravenous urography is undertaken to show the relationship of the opacified nodes to the kidneys and ureters.

THE COMPLICATIONS OF LYMPHOGRAPHY

The complications of lymphography are important:

1. Allergic reactions to Patent Blue Violet, local analgesic and the iodine containing Ultrafluid Lipiodol occur occasionally. These range from oedema at the injection site to generalized urticaria, laryngeal oedema and profound hypotension. However, severe reactions are rare and emergency drugs must always be available whenever the procedure is carried out.
2. Patients should be warned that the blue dye will gradually be uniformly absorbed causing a dusky complexion. The dye is excreted through the urine which will be green or blue for forty-eight hours. The blue stain on the feet is usually hardly visible after six weeks but may linger for several months.
3. Calf pain may occur if the injection is carried out too quickly.
4. A slight pyrexia and 'flu'-like feeling are common on the evening of the procedure but clear by the next day.
5. Some of the injected oil always finds its way into the pulmonary capillaries. Some of this oil will pass into the pulmonary alveoli over two or three days reducing pulmonary function for this time. While this usually causes no significant problem it is obviously more important in patients with pre-existing lung disease. General anaesthesia should be avoided during the week following a lymphogram.
6. Lymphography is not undertaken for six weeks following radio-

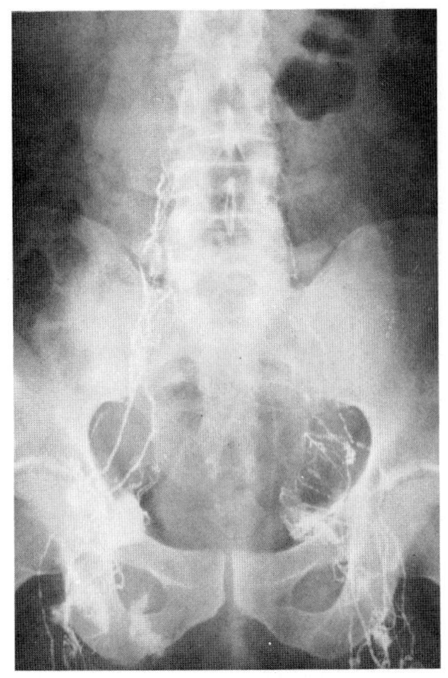

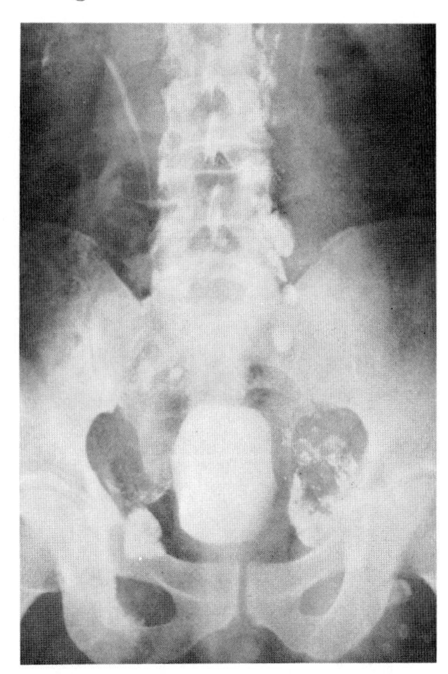

Figure 5.10(a) The lymphatic channels are displaced away from the lateral walls of the pelvis on both sides. (b) Carcinoma of bladder, visible as irregularity low on the left, with massive lymph node metastases on both sides of pelvis.

therapy to the chest as the pulmonary capillaries will fail to trap the iodized oil which will be distributed in the systemic circulation and may cause infarction in whatever organ it reaches.

INTERPRETATION OF A LYMPHOGRAM

Interpretation of a lymphogram can be divided into two parts, evidence of disease shown by the lymphatic channels (the lymphangiogram phase) and in the lymph nodes themselves (the lymphadenogram). Replacement of lymphoid tissue within a node by a metastasis may cause obstruction to the lymphatic vessels running to that node. Alternative pathways known as collateral channels will carry lymph around the obstruction. This may occur in a small local area or on a much wider scale. Stasis may be seen in obstructed lymphatics. Normal lymphatics may be displaced by a tumour mass (Figs. 5.10(a) and (b)).

Lymph node abnormalities are commonly demonstrated in the lymphomas and a number of metastatic diseases. These include tumours arising in the pelvis from bladder, prostate, cervix and body of uterus, ovary, testis and renal tumours and sarcomas of the limbs and retroperitoneum.

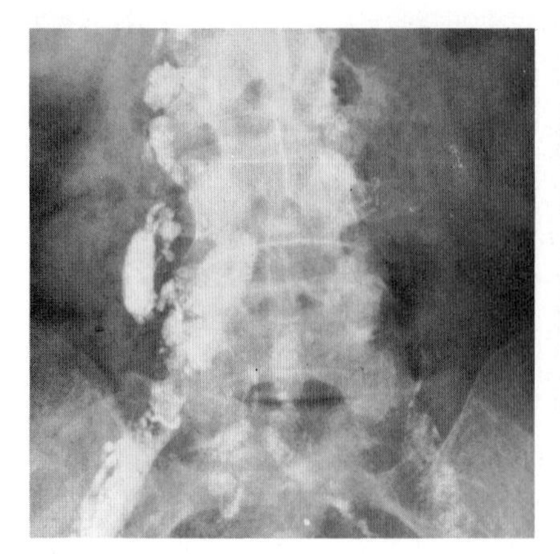

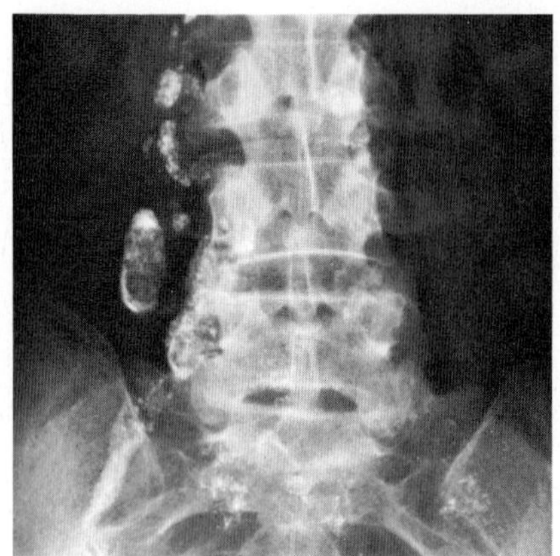

Figure 5.11(a) Normal lymph node in patient with melanoma of right leg. (b) Eight weeks later an obvious lymph node metastasis has developed.

Normal lymph node tissue will be seen as opacified areas ranging from 2–3 mm circles to ovals up to 3·5 cm in length. The normal node has a homogeneous granular interior with an intact clear linear outline (Fig. 5.11(a)). Metastases cause dark filling defects within lymph nodes, often at the periphery (Fig. 5.11(b)). As the metastasis enlarges it will replace the lymphoid tissue until only a crescent of opacified node may be seen (Fig. 5.12). Eventually the lymph node may be completely replaced by tumour so that it does not opacify with contrast medium at all. We then have to make decisions about its presence by the effects on tissues around, that is the lymphatics, other lymph nodes, the ureters and kidneys. A filling defect within a node may need to be followed up by further films of the abdomen at four and eight weeks for evidence that the defect is actually growing before a decision can be made that it really represents tumour. Filling defects may be seen in a normal node which has been doing its regular work of combating infection. These filling defects do not increase in size.

The lymphomas cause a loss of the homogeneous granular texture of the involved nodes, which usually enlarge, often enormously. The pattern within the node becomes foamy (Fig. 5.13). Filling defects may be seen throughout the whole node but the clear-cut margin is usually retained. It is not possible to distinguish the histological types of lymphoma one from the other on their lymphographic appearances.

Follow-up films are taken during the course of the patient's illness to demonstrate the response to therapy and to search for evidence of recurrence.

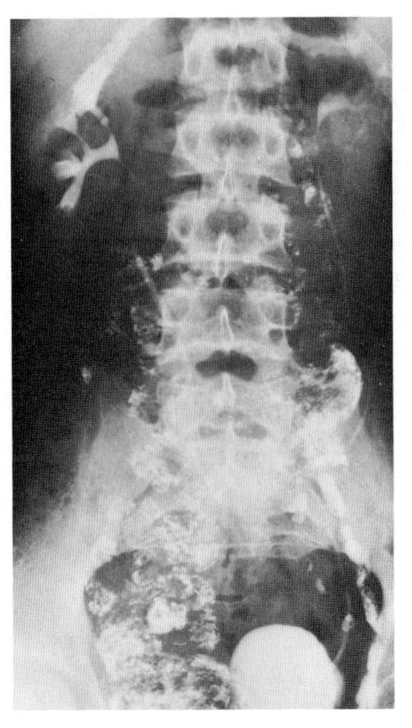

Figure 5.12 Lymphogram and urography in patient with gross lymph node metastases from teratoma of testis, displacing the bladder.

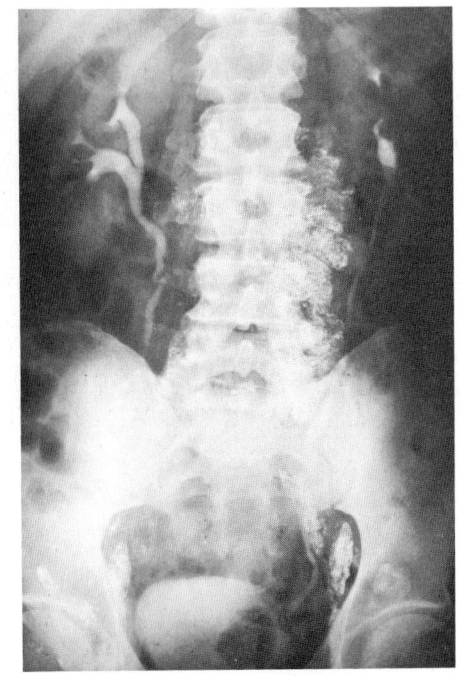

Figure 5.13 Foamy lymph nodes in a lymphoma causing rotation of the left kidney.

The Alimentary Tract

TUMOURS OF THE LARYNGOPHARYNX

Tumours of the laryngopharynx are common among the elderly. A lateral radiograph of the neck may reveal the soft tissue mass of a tumour. Comparison of films taken during inspiration and while the patient sings 'eeee' will show if tumour infiltration restricts mobility of the epiglottis and hyoid. Tomography is invaluable in demonstrating lesions of the vocal chords and the degree of tumour extension into the subglottic angle, below the true chord, an area invisible to the endoscopist (Fig. 5.14). Extension of the laryngeal tumour laterally into the pyriform fossa may be shown on the tomograms, but barium swallow is often more useful. This is the technique of choice for intrinsic pharyngeal tumours. The patient swallows undiluted barium emulsion while films of the throat are taken at the rate of two per second. Pharyngeal tumours are recognized as mass lesions protruding into the normally

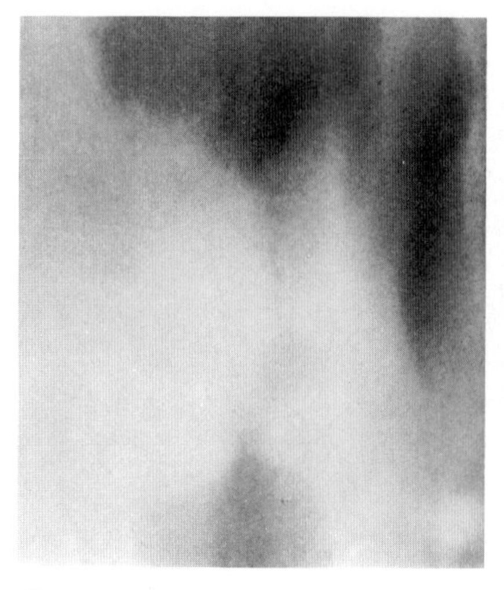

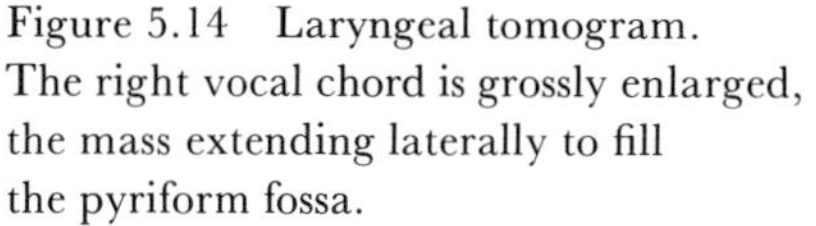

Figure 5.14 Laryngeal tomogram. The right vocal chord is grossly enlarged, the mass extending laterally to fill the pyriform fossa.

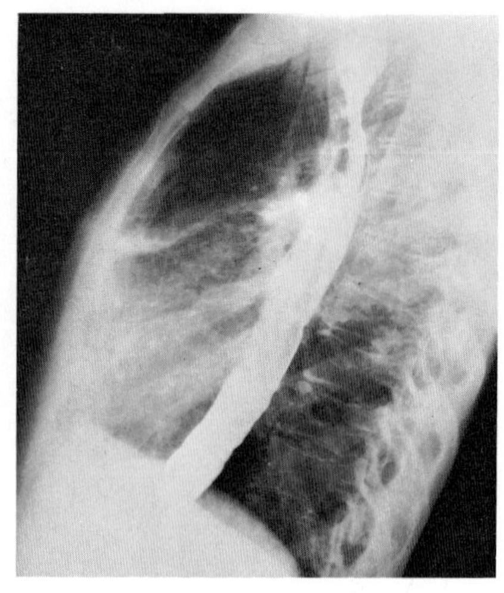

Figure 5.15 Barium swallow shows a carcinomatous stricture in the upper third of oesophagus.

air-filled passages or as constant irregular narrowing. Many patients with pharyngeal carcinomas find it difficult to swallow without some liquid passing through the larynx into the bronchi. If this is likely to occur a contrast medium, such as Dionosil, which will cause no adverse reaction in the lungs should be used and the volume swallowed restricted.

OESOPHAGEAL NEOPLASMS

Oesophageal neoplasms are investigated in a very similar way, but rapid filming is not necessary. These tumours usually cause a narrow segment with irregular margins, which considerably hinders the onward descent of the barium (Fig. 5.15). Food debris may be trapped above the stricture and cause a complete block. The oesophagus above the tumour dilates and the food and fluid which collect there may spill over into the airway causing basal pneumonitis and changes on the chest X-ray. The radiologist tries to demonstrate the vertical limits of the tumour and evidence of extraoesophageal spread as a guide to treatment planning. Invasion of the oesophagus by a mediastinal tumour or lymph nodes enlarged by metastases may give very similar appearances to a primary oesophageal cancer. Following radiotherapy the radiological evidence of an oesophageal neoplastic stricture may become much less obvious.

GASTRIC NEOPLASM

The barium meal is the most important single investigation for patients thought to have a gastric neoplasm. Gastroscopy, which is more of an ordeal for the patient, can add useful information and allows biopsy to be undertaken. The two techniques are complementary.

Double contrast examinations of the stomach have gained in popularity among radiologists in recent years largely due to development of the technique in Japan where there is a high incidence of gastric cancer. This investigation requires the patient to fast overnight. 0·4 ml of Glucagon is given intravenously to temporarily arrest gastric peristalsis. The patient then swallows forty very small Baritop tablets, which release carbon dioxide, and about five mouthfuls of undiluted barium. One or two minutes must now be allowed for gas to come off the tablets and during this interval the patient is rolled from side to side to coat the stomach with the barium. In this way films can be obtained which show the fine pattern of the gastric mucosa and any destruction of this pattern by early carcinoma.

Usually the tumour is fairly advanced before the patient presents, in which case a mass is discovered which is often ulcerated. The tumour may spread extensively in the submucosal layer causing a rigid stomach much reduced in size (linitis plastica) (Fig. 5.16). Not all tumours of the stomach are carcinomas, lymphomas and secondary deposits usually from melanoma, pancreas or breast are sometimes seen.

MALIGNANT LESIONS OF THE LARGE AND SMALL BOWEL

Malignant lesions of the large and small bowel may show evidence on plain abdominal radiographs of intestinal obstruction, perforation or tumour calcification. Primary malignant neoplasms of the small intestine are rare but involvement by secondary deposits through direct invasion, haematogenous spread or seeding onto the peritoneum covering the bowel is more commonly seen. These abnormalities are shown on the barium follow-through examination. This is usually carried out after a barium meal when the patient drinks a further 300 ml of undiluted barium emulsion. Films of the whole abdomen are taken at intervals as successive loops of intestine are filled. The radiologist will screen the abdomen from time-to-time and observe the mobility and pliability of the intestine on the television.

Direct invasion by an adjacent tumour causes rigidity and irregularity of the bowel wall. This is most commonly seen in the duodenum due to carcinoma of the head of the pancreas. The lumen of the invaded

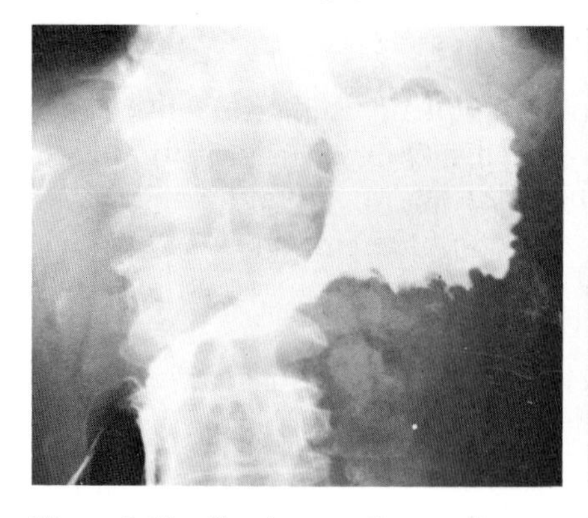

Figure 5.16 Carcinoma of stomach. Linitis plastica with gross reduction in stomach volume.

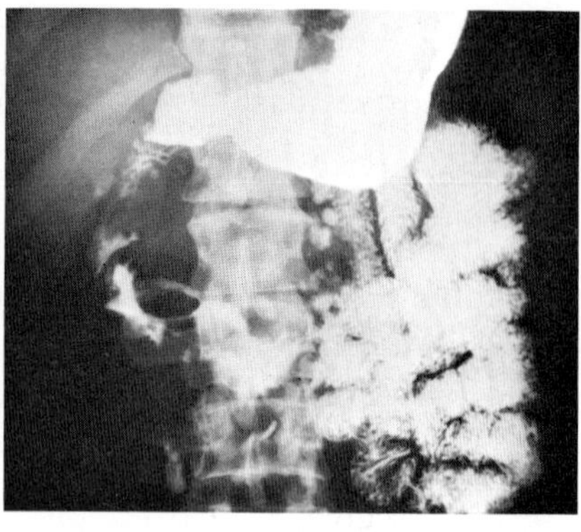

Figure 5.17 The duodenum is grossly distorted due to invasion by an adjacent teratomatous mass.

bowel becomes narrowed and eventually obstructed (Fig. 5.17). Secondary deposits lying within or on the intestinal wall cause multiple rounded filling defects. This is commonly seen in malignant melanoma and carcinomas of the stomach and pancreas (Fig. 5.18). Primary carcinomas of the small intestine cause short strictures with irregular walls and end surfaces which protrude into the normal adjacent bowel.

The lymphomas may cause displacement of bowel loops by lymph node masses, infiltration of the bowel wall with strictures and filling defects and occasionally a malabsorption pattern of dilated loops and segmentation of the barium column.

Tumours of the large bowel are one of the most common presenting forms of malignancy. Growths arising in the anal canal and rectum will usually be diagnosed by digital examination or sigmoidoscopy. Recently colonoscopy has become reliable in allowing sight and biopsy of tumours throughout the large bowel. However, barium enema remains the most important investigation in the detection of large bowel cancer. Its value lies in showing the position and extent of the tumour, excluding the possibility of another tumour further along the colon, and demonstration of other diseases such as diverticulosis which may complicate resection.

A high standard of examination will only be achieved if there has been adequate evacuation of faeces from the bowel. Many of the patients we see are too ill to stand the vigorous preparation appropriate to other colonic diseases. Satisfactory results are usually obtained by giving an oral Senokot preparation, X-Prep, the day before the procedure. Occasionally a cleansing enema will be needed in addition.

Tumours of the colon and rectum are usually carcinomas, but

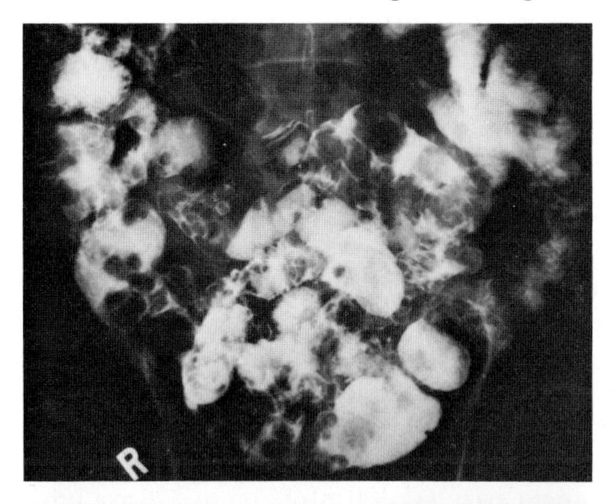

Figure 5.18
Barium follow-through showing multiple rounded defects due to melanoma metastases.

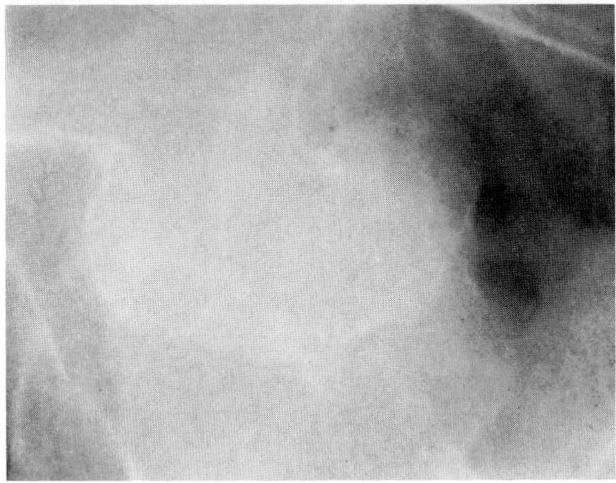

Figure 5.19
Barium enema. A fleshy carcinoma hangs from the roof of the sigmoid colon.

lymphomas and sarcomas are occasionally seen. A number of appearances are found:

1. A fleshy filling defect growing into the bowel lumen with destruction of the overlying mucosa (Fig. 5.19).
2. An irregular stricture with overhanging ends.
3. An ulcerated mass.
4. A fronded villous tumour often occupying a large area.
5. An area of rigidity due to 'linitis plastica' in which tumour tissue spreads in the submucosal layer leaving the mucosa intact.

Before surgery, intravenous urography is undertaken to detect ureteric involvement by local invasion (Fig. 5.20).

Three months after the removal of any gastrointestinal tumour, a follow-up barium examination should be undertaken to provide a base-line against which to assess evidence of recurrence.

The Urinary Tract

KIDNEY TUMOURS

Kidney tumours commonly cause haematuria, a mass in the loin and pain. However, the patient may present with symptoms which do not directly call attention to the urinary tract such as anaemia, fever or evidence of bone, lung, liver or brain metastases. Whenever a renal tumour is suspected, intravenous urography should be undertaken. Fluids are restricted for six hours before the examination. It is wise to enquire about allergies before contrast medium is injected. A plain abdominal film is taken and this may show a mass arising from the kidney, sometimes containing flecks of calcification. A dose of contrast medium suitable to the patient's size, 60–100 ml of Conray 420 in adults, is injected intravenously, and radiographs of the renal areas exposed at intervals. Under normal circumstances the contrast medium causes a uniform increase in the opacity of the renal parenchymal tissue maximal at one minute after the injection. This fades as the contrast medium passes into and demonstrates the pelvicalyceal system and ureter. Tomograms may be taken to eliminate the obscuring effect of overlying bowel gas and faeces.

Superficial renal tumours may be shown as a bulge in the outline of the kidney and more deeply placed neoplasms as a generalized enlargement of a pole or the whole of the kidney. The calyces and renal pelvis may be displaced by the tumour and the new positions they adopt will depend on the site and size of the tumour mass (Fig. 5.21). This may extend into and completely obstruct the renal pelvis or renal vein in which case no contrast medium will be excreted from that kidney, there will be a 'non-functioning kidney'.

A number of benign conditions can produce similar urographic appearances making it necessary to undertake further investigations to confirm the presence of a neoplasm. Ultrasound is extremely accurate in differentiating cysts from solid tumours.

Angiography is undertaken to confirm the malignant nature of a renal mass and to show that a similar condition is not present in the other kidney. An angiographic catheter is introduced, under local analgesia, into the femoral artery and advanced up the aorta to the origin of the renal arteries. An injection of contrast medium may be made into the aorta to show both renal vessels and those supplying the perinephric tissues, or the catheter may be passed into the renal artery itself. A number of films are exposed during the few seconds after the injection. Normal renal arteries are smooth walled and branch in an

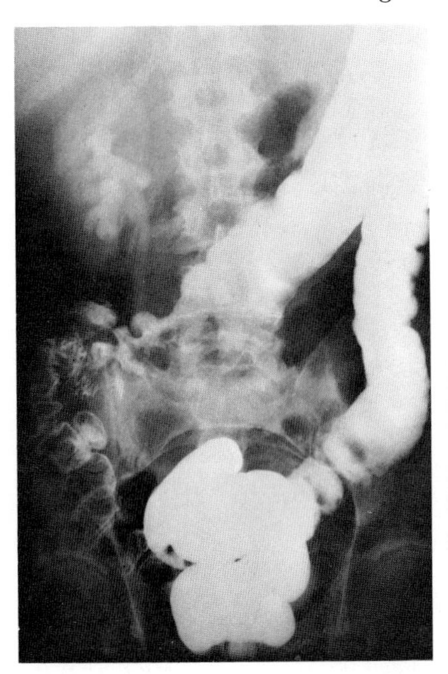

Figure 5.20 Obstruction to the right ureter by recurrent carcinoma of transverse colon following previous hemicolectomy.

Figure 5.21 Urography shows a large calcified kidney tumour, a Wilms's, in a child.

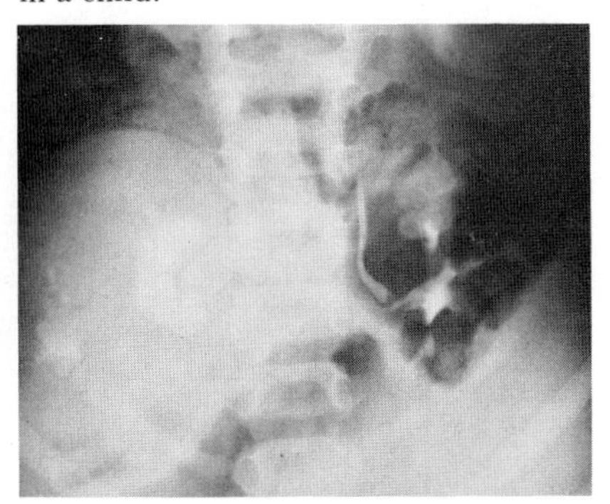

orderly way, tapering towards the periphery. In renal cancer the vessels branch irregularly, show abrupt calibre changes, arteriovenous communications and venous pooling. It is important for the surgeon to know if the renal vein and inferior vena cava contain tumour. An accurate demonstration of this is obtained by injecting contrast medium, through catheters threaded up the femoral veins, to opacify the inferior vena cava. Lymphography should be undertaken before surgery to enable the surgeon to plan the operation to remove any nodes shown to contain metastases.

TUMOURS OF THE MUCOSA

Tumours of the mucosa lining the calyces, renal pelvis and ureter appear as filling defects within the opacified drainage tract at urography. Should the renal pelvis or ureter be completely obstructed the kidney will be non-functioning and urography will not demonstrate the lesion. In this case retrograde urography, in which a catheter is passed up the ureter, allows the lower limit of the tumour to be shown. The upper limit of the tumour can be shown by antegrade pyelography (Fig. 5.22). The patient lies prone on the X-ray table and a needle is advanced, under local analgesia, into the renal pelvis so that contrast medium can be injected. This also provides an opportunity to obtain a specimen of urine for cytology. Tumours of the urothelium lining the

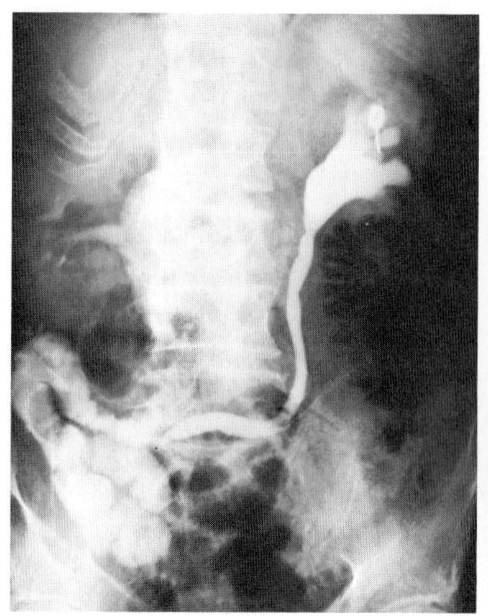

Figure 5.22 Antegrade pyelography demonstrates the drainage tract of a non-functioning kidney following cystectomy and ileal conduit construction.

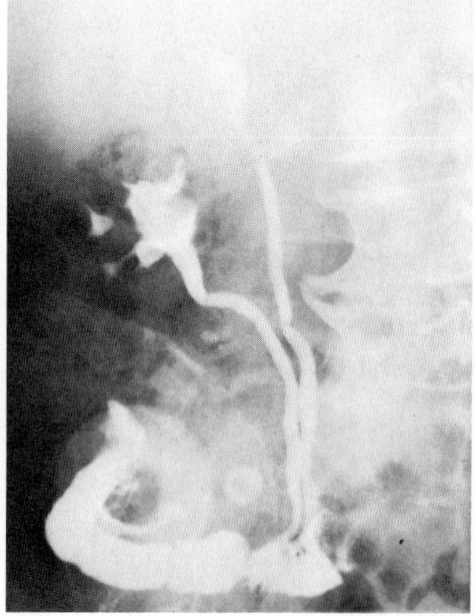

Figure 5.23 Loopogram shows the ileal conduit and both ureters to the right kidney. Further tumour has formed in the lower right renal pelvis. The left ureter is completely obstructed by tumour at its junction with the ileum.

urinary drainage tracts are often multiple so that the patient may have previously undergone cystectomy, and replacement by an ileal conduit, for a similar tumour. In this event the loopogram is a useful method of showing the drainage tracts (Fig. 5.23). A 14F Foley catheter is passed through the stoma of the ileal bladder and the 5 ml balloon inflated. Up to 40 ml of Conray 280 is injected through the catheter to opacify the ileal loop and reflux up the ureters. Recurrent tumour will be revealed as filling defects or complete obstruction.

TUMOURS OF THE BLADDER

Tumours of the bladder may be shown during intravenous urography but cystoscopy is a more valuable way of assessing the primary tumour. Urography is important to show the absence of similar tumours in the upper urinary tracts and to show if the tumour is obstructing the ureter. Lymphography is essential before treatment is planned since metastases may be present in the pelvic and para-aortic nodes.

Radiology does not have an important role in the detection of prostatic neoplasms. But, skeletal survey, chest radiographs and lymphography to show metastases and their response to treatment are of great value. Urography is undertaken in patients with prostatic disease to assess the obstructing effect of the tumour on the upper urinary tracts.

Soft Tissues

MAMMOGRAPHY

Mammography holds an important place in the detection of breast cancer. Two processes are in common use. The Xerox system produces blue and white prints with excellent detail but at a high radiation dose. X-ray film used with intensifying screens can show good detail at a much lower radiation dose to the patient.

Mammography has two roles: the screening of asymptomatic women and the demonstration of known breast disease possibly as a preliminary to treatment. The screening role is dealt with in Chapter 8. Xerox mammography is an accurate method of detecting carcinoma of the breast but it becomes even more reliable when combined with clinical, thermographic and cytologic assessment of the patient. Tumours are recognized by one or more of the following features.

1. An opacity, usually with ill-defined or irregular margins and commonly spiculated.
2. Minute calcifications may be present in groups within or extending beyond the opacity (Fig. 5.24).
3. Skin thickening or retraction may be present including nipple retraction.
4. Increased vascularity compared with the other breast.
5. Enlarged lymph nodes may be seen in the axilla.

It is important to examine both breasts carefully since bilateral tumours may be present simultaneously, not always with obvious clinical features. Before radical surgery is considered a chest X-ray, skeletal survey and isotope scan are obtained to exclude distant metastases. The operative specimen is X-rayed to help the pathologist in selecting the appropriate portion for histology.

Malignant tumours of the other soft tissues include sarcomas of fibrous tissue, fat, skeletal muscle, synovium and blood vessels. These will be identified as a mass interrupting or displacing normal tissue planes. Adjacent bone may be eroded. It may be difficult to differentiate one soft tissue sarcoma from the others. Synoviomas, however, may be

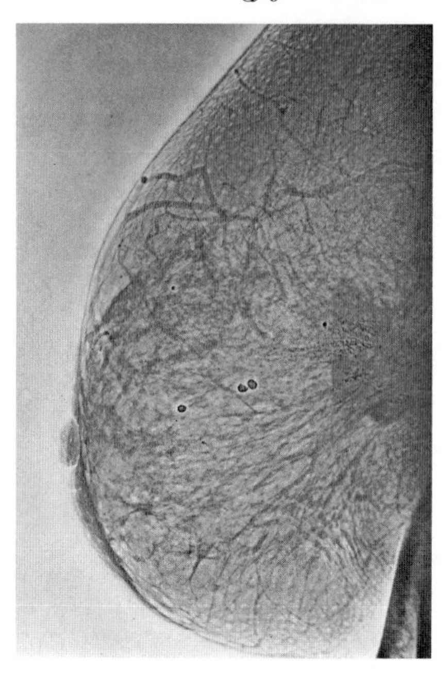

Figure 5.24 Xeromammogram showing a large spiculated carcinoma with microcalcification deep in the breast.

calcified and liposarcomas are more radiolucent than the normal soft tissues around (Fig. 5.25). Angiography may be used to define the limits of these sarcomas, to confirm their malignant nature and to help in choosing a suitable site for biopsy (Fig. 5.26).

Skeletal System

Cancer commonly involves the skeletal system. Metastatic spread to bone from tumours arising in the breast, prostate and bronchus is much more frequent than neoplasis arising primarily within bone. About 20 per cent of autopsies on patients dying of all malignant diseases will reveal bone deposits. Most metastases are found in the axial skeleton, that is the skull, spine, ribs and pelvis or the proximal ends of the humeri and femora. A screening test, the skeletal survey, entails radiographing all of these areas to detect asymptomatic deposits. This survey is repeated from time to time to reveal deposits as they form and to show their response to therapy. Spread to these sites is by the haemotogenous route, the deposits commencing in the medulla of the bone. As the trabeculae in this region are sparse the deposit may reach some size before a change occurs in the bone which is detectable by radiography. Dense overlying cortical bone obscures medullary metastases making early diagnosis less likely. Because of these difficulties it is important to

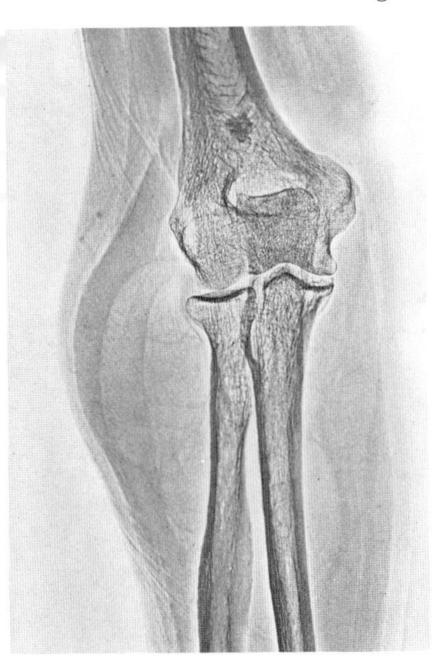

Figure 5.25 Soft tissue xerox print reveals a low density liposarcoma encircling the upper ends of radius and ulna.

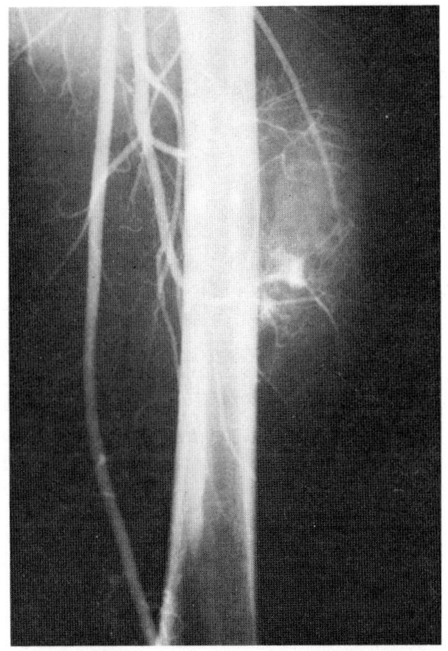

Figure 5.26 Femoral angiogram shows a tumour blush in an angio-sarcoma lateral and eroding the femur. 'Malignant vessels' are present.

correlate the findings of physical examination, biochemical tests, isotopic and radiographic surveys when considering if bone involvement is present.

Most metastases to bone cause osteolysis. The lucent areas produced by the deposits are typically very poorly defined in outline and multiple. Pathological fractures through such lesions are frequent in the vertebral bodies, pubic rami and femoral and humeral necks. An osteoblastic, bone forming, response is seen around some metastases, particularly lesions from tumours of the prostate, breast and bladder. These may occur as ill-defined patchy areas of increased bone density but in prostatic disease many vertebrae, the whole pelvis and the ribs may be uniformly dense. Both sorts of deposit, osteolytic and osteoblastic, may arise from the same primary tumour.

PRIMARY MALIGNANT BONE TUMOURS

Of primary malignant bone tumours multiple myeloma is the most common. This disease is characterized by the proliferation of abnormal plasma cells in the marrow which diffusely infiltrate the bones of the

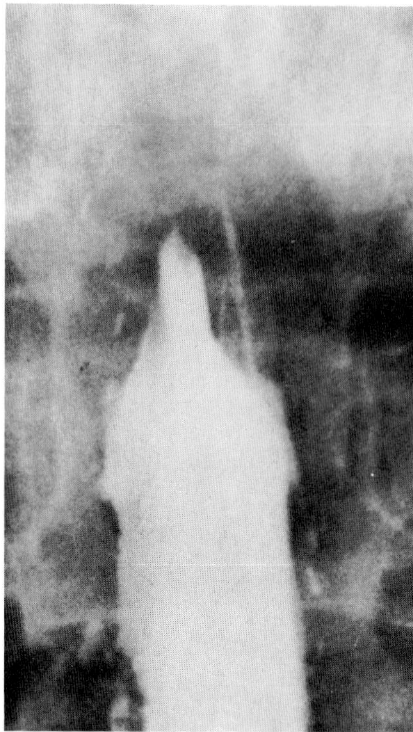

Figure 5.27 Myelography demonstrates the site of complete obstruction in this patient with Hodgkin's disease. Note the dense white vertebra.

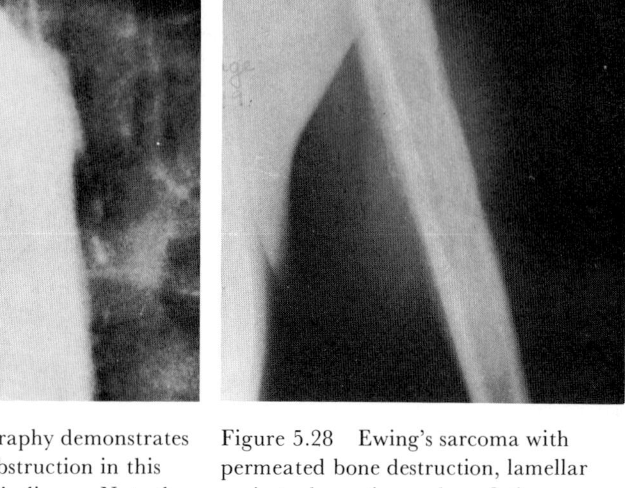

Figure 5.28 Ewing's sarcoma with permeated bone destruction, lamellar periosteal reaction and a soft tissue mass.

axial skeleton causing multiple lucent areas of indistinct outline. The process may be so generalized that the decreased density of the skeleton resembles the senile osteoporosis often present in the age group affected by this condition. Sharply marginated round lesions may be seen in the skull and long bones late in the disease. Large aggressive myeloma deposits accompanied by a soft tissue mass are often seen in the ribs. Collapse of vertebral bodies is common in myelomatosis and extension of tumour tissue from such a lesion may compress the spinal cord or nerve roots causing neurological symptoms. The same situation may arise in metastatic disease, the lymphomas and leukaemias. The extent of compressing tumour may be shown by myelography. 9 ml of Myodil is introduced into the subarachnoid space at lumbar puncture. The patient is securely harnessed on an X-ray table which is tipped to allow the contrast medium to flow between the sacral and cervical regions. The column of Myodil will be displaced by tumour and there may be complete obstruction (Fig. 5.27). Pictures are taken to record the extent of the lesion and localize it prior to laminectomy. In neuroradiological practice it is usual to remove Myodil at the end of the procedure. It may be an advantage in oncology patients to leave the Myodil *in situ* so that it may be rescreened to show the response of the tumour to therapy.

The diagnosis of primary malignant bone tumours of the connective tissues found within bones depends on close co-operation between the clinician, radiologist and pathologist. Just as the pathologist will always require to see the radiographs before interpreting the histology of a bone lesion, the radiologist must have careful regard to the clinical findings. Primary malignant bone tumours cause destruction of the surrounding normal bone. The pattern in which this occurs gives some indication of the aggressiveness of the tumour. A well-defined area of destruction with a sharp outline indicates a slow rate of growth. The sarcomas are revealed by multiple poorly delineated areas of destruction extending into the surrounding bone with no definite indication of where the tumour ends and normal bone starts, this is 'permeated bone destruction'. The tumour may extend beyond the confines of the bone causing a soft tissue mass which displaces normal tissue planes. As the periosteum is stripped up by the tumour, lamellae or spicules of new bone will be formed (Fig. 5.28). This is typical of Ewing's sarcomas and osteosarcomas but less of a feature in chondrosarcomas, reticulum cell sarcomas and fibrosarcomas.

Lymphography will be positive in one-third of bone sarcomas at presentation. When reticulum cell sarcoma within bone is shown histologically, a lymphogram is mandatory, since the bone lesion may be part of a generalized histiocytic lymphoma.

References

Bagshawe, K. D. (1975) *Medical Oncology. Medical Aspects of Malignant Disease.* Blackwell Scientific Publications.

Goldman, Myer (1966) *A Nurse's Guide to the X-Ray Department.* Livingstone Nursing Texts.

Steckel, R. J. and Kagan, A. R. (1976) *Diagnosis and Staging of Cancer. A Radiologic Approach.* W. B. Saunders.

Sutton, D. (1975) *Textbook of Radiology.* Churchill Livingstone.

Wright, F. W. (1973) *The Radiological Diagnosis of Lung and Mediastinal Tumours.* Butterworths.

Chapter 6

Radioisotope Imaging in Oncology

DAVID J. MANNING
H.D.S.R., D.N.M., S.R.R.
Department of Nuclear Medicine and Ultrasound
Royal Marsden Hospital
Surrey

and

V. RALPH McCREADY
M.Sc., M.R.C.P., D.M.R.D., F.R.C.R.
Department of Nuclear Medicine and Ultrasound
Royal Marsden Hospital
Surrey

Introduction

Originally it was thought that the place of radioisotopes in cancer would be mainly for its treatment. Indeed, the first radioisotope to be used clinically, namely ^{131}I, was and still is extremely valuable in the treatment of functioning thyroid carcinoma. One of the first patients to be treated in the UK for such a cancer in 1948 is still alive with grandchildren. However, over the intervening years relatively little progress has been made in the use of radioisotopes for therapeutic purposes. In about 1960 a primitive scanning system was developed to take pictures of the radioactive sources used for radiotherapy. It was the advent of an isotope generator system which could produce short-lived isotopes continuously in the hospital which revolutionized the use of radionuclides in medical diagnosis. These short-lived isotopes enabled high levels of radioactivity to be given to the patients (which produced good pictures) while keeping the radiation dose down to the level given by ordinary diagnostic X-ray procedures. From the patient's point of view the rectilinear scanners made diagnostic imaging a slow process as well as requiring the patient to lie horizontally. During the 1960s the development of the gamma camera enabled the pictures to be taken within minutes or seconds with the patient sitting, standing or lying down. Thus in a few years both the ideal imaging apparatus and radionuclides became generally available.

Although radionuclide techniques can be used to trace most metabolic processes in the body, their main current use lies in the detection of benign and malignant tumours in the various organs. Thus it is appropriate that a book dealing with oncology should devote considerable space to the application of these relatively new and exciting techniques to the detection and follow-up of the treatment of cancer. While it was thought that some of the initial enthusiasm might diminish with time, in fact the reverse has been the case. The emergence of new treatment techniques of cancer especially those involving drugs demand accurate staging and follow-up. The radioisotope methods although lacking in detail are atraumatic and have virtually no morbidity. They are therefore ideal for patients who already have had to undergo many complicated and sometimes painful tests.

Imaging Equipment

The equipment used for imaging radionuclide distributions falls into two main categories, namely scanners and cameras. The rectilinear scanner consists of a detecting system which contains a radiation-sensitive crystal which moves in a series of lines backwards and forwards across the area being studied. In front of the crystal is a lead collimator which permits only those radiations from a small area to be registered by the detector. This 'focuses' in turn on each individual part of the organ under study as the detector moves along.

The radioactivity concentration or uptake is represented by blackening of a photographic film or by the number of dots placed on a sheet of paper. Modern scanners use colour to accentuate small differences in dot density between one area and another. Even if the end-result is rather confusing to the inexperienced, at least it looks pretty! Since by its very nature scanning is rather slow, the latest scanners use one detector in front of another detector behind the patient in an effort to speed up the process. Unfortunately, to fit between the scanning system the patient must lie flat, an uncomfortable position for those with metastases or dyspnoea.

The gamma camera also uses a radiation-sensitive crystal. This time it is very large – somewhere between 280–480 mm in diameter. Thus by placing the patient against this type of detector the radiation coming from all parts of the patient can be seen simultaneously. This greatly speeds up the process of taking the pictures, reducing the time involved often to seconds. The particular advantage of the gamma camera is its ability to image radioactivity moving through the body. One can trace a bolus of radioactivity moving along a vein or through the heart or through the lungs. Such dynamic studies can also be of value in evaluating the function of the kidneys. Nowadays it is usual to link the gamma camera with computer equipment which can display the actual number of counts detected at each part of the crystal's surface at each point in time. It is then possible to plot graphs of the counts collected in each unit of time in a particular area of interest. These time/activity curves are extremely valuable giving a much more objective assessment of the change of radioactivity than is possible by studying sequential pictures. Originally it was hoped that such data analysis equipment could improve the diagnostic quality of the pictures but so far this has not proved to be the case. It may be that redisplaying the gamma camera pictures in colour similar to those from the rectilinear scanner will be an improvement over the present situation.

The most recent development in imaging equipment is that of whole body scanning using either a scanning type detector or a gamma camera which moves over the patient from head to foot. These are used for the whole body surveys carried out to detect metastases in bone, functioning thyroid metastases or the distribution of tumour localizing agents. In fact, it is now quite difficult to decide the correct name for a particular piece of equipment when it looks like a camera but scans over a patient. Hence we use the word imaging rather than scanning, since the picture may be produced in a wide variety of ways.

Radiopharmaceuticals

To image organs or body systems it is essential to have a radiopharmaceutical which will concentrate in the area of interest labelled by a radionuclide which can be easily detected by the imaging equipment. It must be non-toxic and give an acceptably low radiation dose to the patient. Radiopharmaceuticals differ from other medications in that: they are used merely as a tracer and do not produce any pharmacological effects; and they are 'tagged' with a radionuclide which allows them to be detected from outside the body. It is clear that the radionuclide used for labelling must either be the same as one of the elements already in the compound, or, if for technical reasons it must be different, it must not upset the physiology of the system being studied. The more complex radiopharmaceuticals are usually obtained direct from the manufacturer, but those that involve short-lived radionuclides and in-

Table 6.1 *Radionuclides in common use in oncological nuclear medicine*

Radioisotope	*Symbol and relative atomic mass*	*Half-life*	*Typical uses*
Sodium	Na 24	15 hours	Gamma emitter. Investigation of circulatory system
Phosphorus	P 32	14·3 days	Beta source. Intravenous. Therapeutic for Polycythaemia Vera
Chromium	Cr 51	27 days	Gamma emitter. Labelling red blood cells
Iron	Fe 59	4·7 days	Gamma emitter. Blood studies
Iodine	I 131	8 days	Mainly gamma emitter Diagnosis and therapy of thyroid tumour
	I 123	13 hours	Gamma emitter. Thyroid scanning
	I 125	60 days	'*In vitro*' thyroid hormone assays
Gold	Au 198	2·7 days	Instillation, implantation into tissues
Technetium	Tc 99 m	6 hours	Very short physical half-life permits use of high doses with low resulting tissue radiation
Gallium	Ga 67	72 hours	Gamma emitter. Whole body scanning for tumour and inflammatory processes
Indium	In 113 m	100 mins	Gamma emitter. Placental scanning
	In 111	3 days	Gamma emitter, beta emitter. Used with tumour-seeking agents

volve simple preparation are produced in a special area in the hospital. The decay of a radionuclide is measured in terms of its half-life. This is the time it takes for the radioactivity of a sample to decay to half of its original value. In our clinical work we use radionuclides with widely varying half-lives from seconds in the case of $^{81}Kr^{m}$ to sixty days in the case of ^{85}Sr. In general, we prefer the half-life to be about twice the time required from injection to completion of the examination.

The most frequently used radioisotope in current use is undoubtedly $^{99}Tc^{m}$. This has the conveniently short half-life of six hours giving a low radiation dose to the patient and emits a gamma-ray of 140 KeV, ideal for use with imaging equipment. It is produced by the decay of ^{99}Mo (half-life sixty-nine hours). This parent radionuclide is made up into a generator system which permits the $^{99}Tc^{m}$ to be separated from it by washing through the column with saline. The eluate of technetium in its 'raw' state can then be used to label a variety of materials including the red blood cells, colloidal particles for investigation of the liver, phosphates for bone imaging or it may simply be injected into the bloodstream to image the thyroid, brain or salivary glands. Similar generators exist for the production of $^{87}Sr^{m}$, ^{132}I, $^{113}In^{m}$, all of which have special advantages in particular situations.

Although most tests are carried out with $^{99}Tc^{m}$ compounds, some radionuclides with short half-lives required for special tests need to be produced in or near the hospital. A few hospitals now have cyclotrons in use. These devices are used to provide radiation both for therapy and for the production of radionuclides. Until recently ^{18}F was the ideal isotope for bone imaging. This cyclotron-produced isotope has a half-life of two hours greatly reducing the radiation dose compared to the strontium-85 used previously. The two hour half-life means that its use is limited to those hospitals within a radius of two hours around the cyclotron. More recently (relatively) cheaper cyclotrons have become available which will enable a larger number of hospitals to use them. This will enable the radionuclides of carbon, nitrogen and oxygen, which all have very short half-lives, to be more generally available. Their clinical value has yet to be established.

Thyroid Imaging

Since the thyroid gland utilizes iodine in the synthesis of the thyroid hormone thyroxine, radioiodine is taken up into the normal gland. The ability to trace iodine metabolism with radioactivity, in conjunction with the early availability of the iodine radioisotopes, contributed in no small way to the generalized acceptance of radionuclides in medical diagnosis. Radionuclides can be used for tests involving samples or patients. For example, hormone production by the thyroid can be accurately assessed by laboratory '*in vitro*' techniques on samples which do not involve the administration of radioactive materials to the patient. If the radioiodine or radiopertechnetate is given to the patient it concentrates in the thyroid gland. Thyroid imaging is useful in showing the functional status of each part of the gland. Areas with increased function show increased radioactivity. Likewise normal functioning thyroid tissue outside the region of the gland also concentrates the radioiodine. This can be very valuable in deciding whether lumps in the neck or tongue are thyroidal in origin.

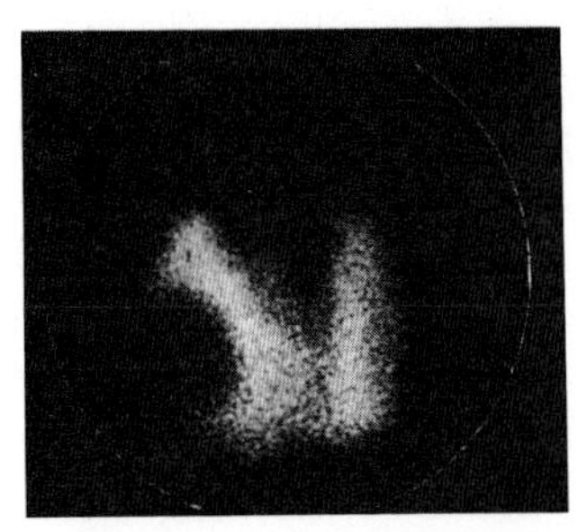

Figure 6.1 Gamma camera scintigram of thyroid thirty minutes after injection of 2 mCi $^{99}Tc^{m}$ pertechnetate. The left lobe is normal but the right lobe shows a large 'cold' area which proved to be carcinoma.

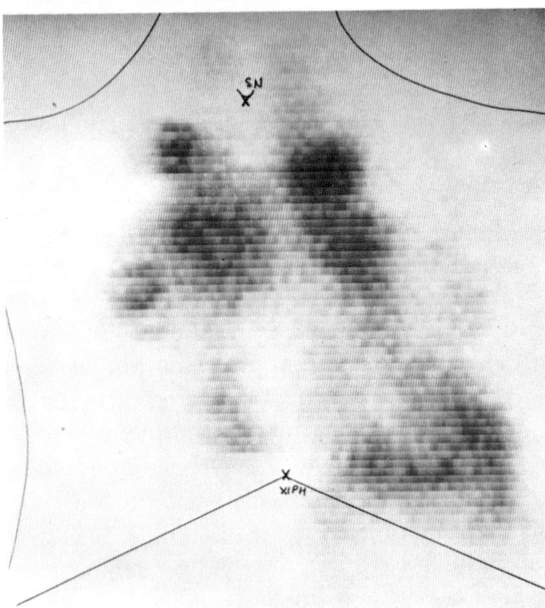

Figure 6.2 Rectilinear scan of chest four days after a 150 mCi therapeutic dose of ^{131}I. The thyroid has been previously ablated and the high radioactivity in the chest is due to functional metastases from a primary follicular thyroid carcinoma.

The most commonly used radionuclide for thyroid scanning is ^{131}I, which is readily available in capsule form. A 20 μCi oral dose is followed twenty-four hours later by a simple scan of the neck area. Alternatively, if an uptake measurement is not required $^{99}Tc^{m}$ as pertechnetate may be given intravenously followed by a scan after thirty minutes. Hyperfunctioning nodules in the thyroid gland appear as 'hot' areas reflecting increased radioiodine or pertechnetate concentration. 'Cold' nonfunctioning areas or lumps are seen as regions of diminished uptake. Generally a 'hot' area virtually excludes a carcinoma. A 'cold' area can be due to a carcinoma, a cyst or thyroiditis. Figure 6.1 shows a typical thyroid image with a 'cold' area in this case due to a carcinoma. In cases of well-differentiated papillary or follicular carcinoma of the thyroid, distant metastases sometimes function sufficiently to show radiodine concentration. Because the thyroid cancer functions with low efficiency a large activity of ^{131}I is required to permit whole body scanning to follow the course of treatment of the tumour. Figure 6.2 is a chest scan of a patient with iodine concentration in metastases from follicular thyroid carcinoma. Thyroid scanning with radioiodine requires a certain amount of patient preparation. Because the actual quantity of iodine in the radioactive solution administered is very small it is important that it represents a sizable fraction in the body's iodine pool. For this reason the patient is instructed to avoid iodine-containing foods or medicine (including X-ray contrast media) for at least forty-eight hours prior to scanning, since these can saturate the body with iodine. Although in general the mangement of patients after diagnostic scanning requires only simple hygiene, in the case of thyroid carcinoma diagnosis and therapy quite large activities of ^{131}I may be involved requiring special precautions.

Liver and Spleen Imaging

Liver imaging is now a routine part of the assessment and follow-up of patients with malignant disease. The examination is simple, fast and non-invasive and combined with ultrasonic B-scanning provides a relatively accurate method of discovering space-occupying lesions within the liver. For imaging purposes the liver may be considered as being composed of two quite different compartments: the reticuloendothelial system (RES) and the biliary system. The phagocytic properties of the reticuloendothelial system are used to demonstrate the morphology or structure of the liver. Radiopharmaceuticals which are metabolized by the liver are used to demonstrate the biliary system.

When colloid particles are intravenously injected they are phagocytosed by the reticuloendothelial system. Figure 6.3 shows a normal liver scintigram. This system is present in liver (Kupffer cells) but is also found in the spleen and bone marrow. It is easy to label colloids with radionuclides such as $^{99}Tc^m$ or $^{113}In^m$ and to map their distribution after intravenous injection. The size of the particle determines where predominantly the deposition will occur. Very small particles concentrate in the liver while larger ones are localized mainly in the liver or spleen. In patients with normal livers colloid is removed from the blood very rapidly within a few minutes of injection, but where there is severe dysfunction it may be better to delay the scan for rather longer until there is maximum uptake in the liver substance. The rate of clearance of colloid from the blood has in fact been used by some workers as a test of the function of the reticuloendothelial system in Hodgkin's disease.

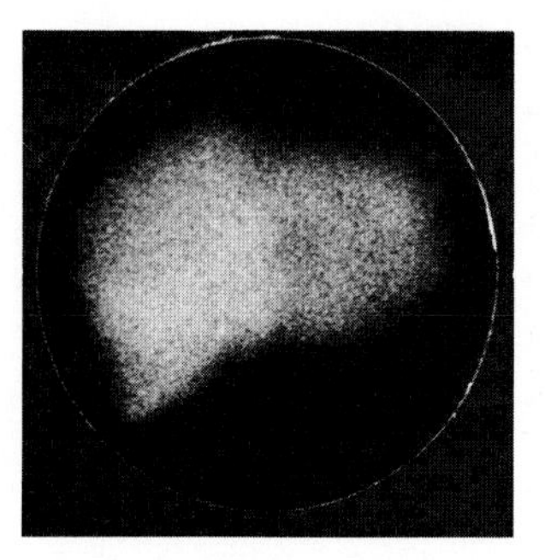

Figure 6.3 A normal liver scintigram thirty minutes after intravenous injection of 4 mCi $^{99}Tc^{m}$ sulphur colloid. Anterior view.

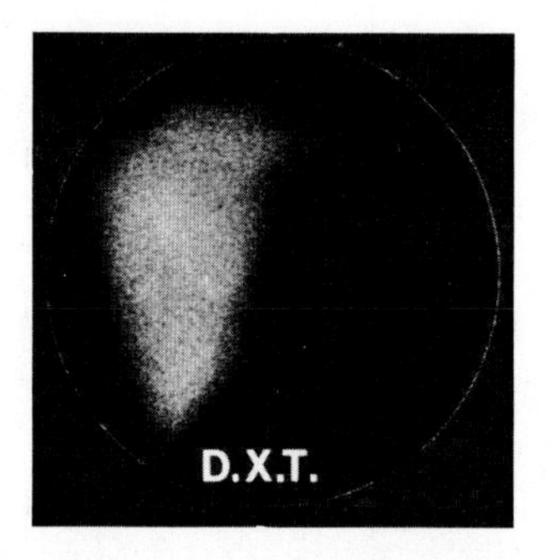

Figure 6.4 Liver scintigram, anterior view, showing very marked reduced uptake in the left lobe as a result of radiotherapy to the para-aortic lymph nodes in a Hodgkin's patient.

The liver scan represents, then, an image of the distribution of the reticuloendothelial system. Most space-occupying lesions such as cysts, tumours, or abscesses do not have Kupffer cells and are therefore seen as a 'cold' non-radioactive area. False positives can be seen due to anything altering the reticuloendothelial system content, for example following deep X-ray therapy (Fig. 6.4). Due to respiratory movement of the liver and the fact that the tumour or lesion is non-radioactive in the radioactive background, the smallest lesion detectable is probably in the region of 2 cm diameter. Despite this, however, the liver scan is a valuable diagnostic aid when account is taken of the type of disease being studied. Metastases from breast carcinoma and Hodgkin's disease can be difficult to find. Some of these diseases often produce a large number of small deposits spread diffusely throughout the liver. This gives an image with a generalized non-specific patchy uptake. It is likely that liver abnormalities in such cases will be evident clinically or biochemically before a radioactive image will reveal them. Conversely, carcinomas of the gut and bronchus often produce fewer but larger metastases which are frequently seen by radioactive techniques before they become evident in any other way.

Figure 6.5 shows a liver scintigram with cold areas due to metastases from colonic carcinoma. The accuracy of detection in liver image taken in isolation is therefore dependent on the disease under investigation.

The biliary system of the liver can be studied by means of various agents labelled with ^{131}I, ^{123}I, $^{99}Tc^{m}$. The most frequently used radiopharmaceutical in current use is $^{99}Tc^{m}$ – H.I.D.A. After intravenous injection the excretion can be followed by sequential scans of the upper

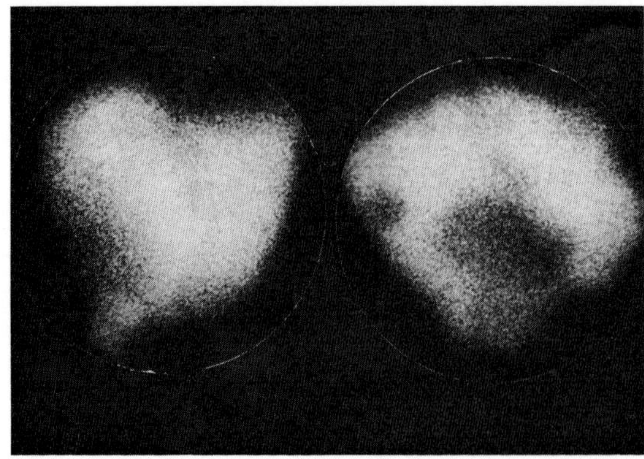

Figure 6.5 Anterior and right lateral views of liver after 4 mCi $^{99}Tc^{m}$ sulphur colloid injection. The liver has two large space-occupying lesions which are metastases from a primary large bowel carcinoma.

abdomen. In the normal subject it passes into the hepatic ducts, is concentrated in the gall bladder and cleared into the duodenum within twenty minutes of administration. Where the problem is one of differentiating between obstructive or non-obstructive jaundice, this investigation is very helpful and it can also indicate the level at which obstruction arises. This is true even when bilirubin levels are too high for successful X-ray cholangiography.

The usefulness of spleen scanning in malignant disease is mainly restricted to estimation of size, shape and position. This information is valuable in helping to decide the cause of lumps in the upper abdomen. Unfortunately, spleen size in itself is not a good indicator of spleen involvement by cancer, since spleen enlargement may be related to the immunological status of the patient. Rarely can one successfully image space-occupying lesions in the spleen due to malignant disease.

Brain Imaging

The radioisotope brain scan is extremely valuable as a screening procedure in patients with suspected intracranial lesions. It is fast and safe and provides a means of selecting patients for more invasive tests such as cerebral arteriography or the expensive X-ray computerized axial tomography (CAT) scans. The accuracy of the investigation is high and a negative brain scan can be regarded as more significant than, say, a negative liver scan. However, the examination must be read in conjunction with the clinical signs and symptoms. Some small lesions and abnormalities in the posterior fossa are difficult to detect. Its further use is in the follow-up and assessment of patients who have undergone surgery and/or radiotherapy.

The concentration of the radiopharmaceutical in or around intracranial lesions depends on the breakdown of the blood–brain barrier. This applies to both primary and secondary neoplasms as well as vascular lesions such as infarcts, abscesses or subdural haematomas. The most frequently used radiopharmaceutical is $^{99}Tc^{m}$ pertechnetate given intravenously. This is distributed throughout the body water and is excluded from the normal brain. Any derangement of the blood–brain barrier, however, results in an accumulation of the radionuclide in the oedema surrounding the lesion. Detection of a tumour depends on the difference in uptake between the lesion and surrounding tissues. For this reason there is high diagnostic accuracy in supratentorial lesions where there is less interfering background activity. Other useful radiopharmaceuticals include $^{99}Tc^{m}$ DTPA, ^{169}Yt DTPA or $^{113}In^{m}$ DTPA, all of which are metal chelates and concentrate in brain lesions by the same mechanism as $^{99}Tc^{m}$ pertechnetate.

The apparatus used for imaging, either gamma camera or rectilinear scanner, has little effect on the accuracy of the examination. The pictures produced by the scanner are more impressive and there may be some advantage in using a rectilinear scanner in cases where a life-sized image might help with radiotherapy planning, but for most patients, the speed and ease of a gamma camera make it the equipment of choice. An advantage of the gamma camera is its ability to image the passage of the radionuclide through the brain. This is usually done by linking the gamma camera to a computer to enable time–flow curves to be constructed. Patient preparation for brain scans is minimal; a 200 mg oral dose of potassium perchlorate being given one hour before the isotope. This has the dual purpose of effectively blocking the thyroid gland and discharging the choroid plexus which would otherwise accumulate $^{99}Tc^{m}$ pertechnetate and interfere with the detection of overlying lesions. In very rare instances atropine may be given to prevent uptake in the salivary glands and paranasal sinuses. This would be used, however, only in cases where high background activity from these sources was obscuring a clinically strongly suspected lesion.

The rate of detection of primary brain tumours varies with histology. Meningiomas are easily demonstrated partly because of their superficial position and partly on account of their high vascularity. The amount of isotope taken into gliomas on the other hand depends on the grading of the tumour: the well differentiated taking in less than the poorly differentiated (Fig. 6.6). It is accepted that a grade I glioma for example may be completely undetectable isotopically. Craniopharyngiomas are now seen in 70–80 per cent of cases (De Land) which, for these cystic lesions, represents a high detection rate. Cerebral infarcts also vary in how clearly they are visualized by radioisotope

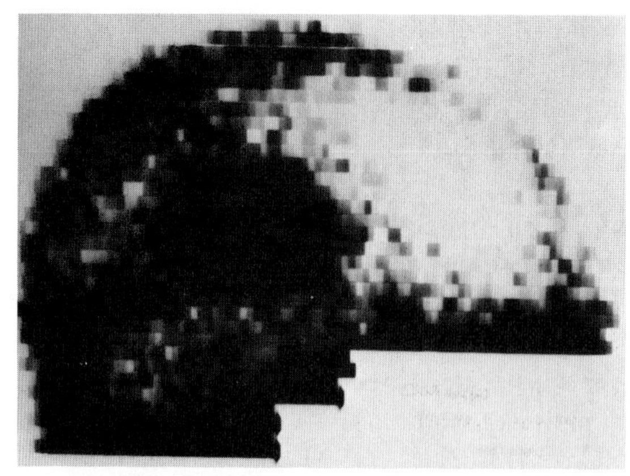

Figure 6.6 Rectilinear brain scan, right lateral view $^{99}Tc^{m}$ pertechnetate. The patient has a temporoparietal astrocytoma IV.

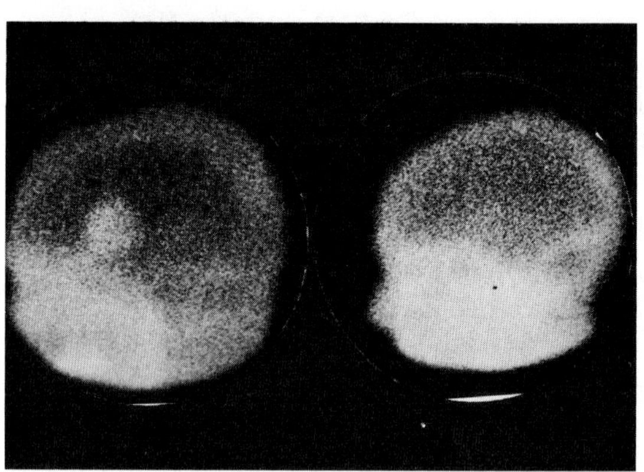

Figure 6.7 Brain scintigrams of (right) a normal patient and (left) a cerebral metastasis from a carcinoma of bronchus.

imaging. The important factors affecting visualization are the presence or otherwise of haemorrhage and the time since the onset of symptoms. Haemorrhagic infarctions are better detected overall and optimally at about ten days after the vascular accident (Fig. 6.8). Those which do not involve bleeding, however, have a lower detection rate and are usually seen rather later after the event. These lesions, almost always follow the lines of distribution of the larger cerebral vessels – especially the middle cerebral artery – which helps in their differentiation isotopically, from tumours.

Metastatic space-occupying lesions have variable characteristics. It is mainly those deposits which cause surrounding oedema which are the best shown on scans. A typical scintigram of a patient with metastases from a lung carcinoma is seen in Fig. 6.7. Very small metastases, and those causing little local reaction may go undetected. This means that a negative brain scan cannot be depended upon to exclude metastases. It is possible that after radiotherapy and drugs to reduce cerebral oedema, a lesion ceases to concentrate isotope. The difficulty in such

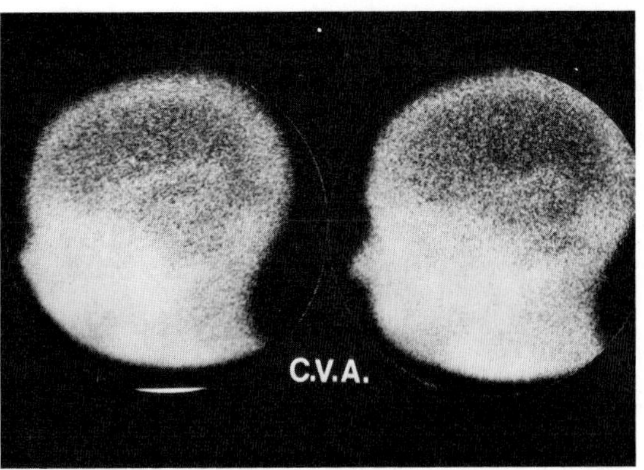

Figure 6.8 Left lateral views of brain taken with a gamma camera after 10 mCi of $^{99}Tc^{m}$ pertechnetate. These scintigrams show a resolving lesion following a CVA. The left scan was ten days and the right scan five weeks after the incident. Note that the area of increased activity follows the line of the middle cerebral artery.

cases is not only one of detection but of determining whether the deposit has been destroyed or if the oedema has simply resolved.

Overall, then, brain scanning may be described as an excellent simple test for the presence of intracranial lesions. As discussed, the accuracy of detection depends on histology and position, but generally lesions above the tentorium are seen in 70–80 per cent of cases.

Skeletal Imaging

A frequent and distressing complication of neoplastic disease is the development of bony metastases. There is a very wide variation in the incidence of bony involvement by different tumours. Seminomas of the testes, for example, rarely metastasize to bone whereas in carcinoma of the breast this complication can occur in up to 75 per cent of cases depending upon the stage when they are scanned. An obvious and often most frequently used diagnostic aid for discovering bone lesions is undoubtedly the radiographic skeletal survey. This is not, however, a particularly sensitive method for early detection because for bony tumours to become apparent on X-ray there has to be a considerable amount of bone destruction. This destruction may amount to 50 per cent of a vertebral body before the lesion will be seen radiologically. Such gross changes are clearly very late on in the spread of malignant disease. Radioisotope bone scans not only detect deposits at a much earlier stage than X-rays but can identify lesions which have yet to become apparent clinically. It is of enormous importance in carcinoma of the breast to obtain early bone scans. In this tumour, even when at a clinically early stage, 15 per cent of patients have isotope evidence of metastases which, when followed up, later produce symptoms at these sites (Fig. 6.9). Radioisotope bone surveys therefore enable the disease

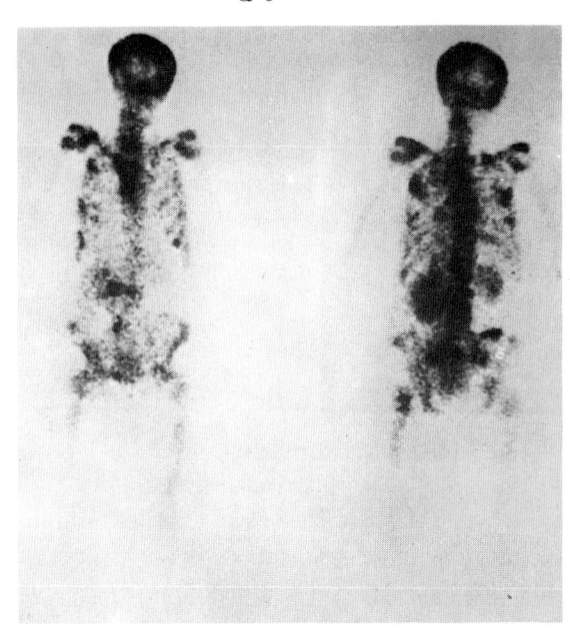

Figure 6.9 Anterior (left) and posterior of whole skeleton four hours after technetium polyphosphate 10 mCi. There are multiple areas of increased activity in the ribs, pelvis, spine and hips consistent with metastatic breast carcinoma.

to be staged more accurately and more appropriate treatment to be given.

Radioactive imaging agents localize in normal bone but concentrate preferentially in areas with increased mineral turnover. Unlike X-rays which demonstrate differences in the mass of bone present, radiopharmaceutical concentration is independent of the amount of osseous material and relies only on biochemical changes taking place. Essentially bone scintigraphy presents a picture of a physiological process whereas radiology gives one of anatomical change. Increased bone mineral turnover can be caused by a number of pathological conditions other than malignant disease. The bone images therefore should be carefully interpreted in conjunction with clinical history and X-ray findings. This is particularly true in older patients where Paget's disease or degenerative changes in joints may be seen as areas with increased radioactivity on the scan. Healing fractures or inflammatory processes such as osteomyelitis can also be mistakenly interpreted as metastatic deposits if the scintigram is seen in isolation. Other sites of quite normal increased activity are at the growing ends of long bones or in empty tooth sockets after recent extraction.

The radiopharmaceuticals which have transformed bone scanning are the $^{99}Tc^{m}$-labelled phosphate compounds. Technetium-99m has ideal characteristics (see above), for nuclear imaging but is not a bone-seeker in the pertechnetate form eluted direct from a generator. If, however, it is used as a complex such as disodium pyrophosphate, sodium polyphosphate or monofluorophosphate it becomes a highly specific tracer for bone studies. When injected intravenously, it is cleared from the blood within three hours and presents a picture with a very high bone to soft tissue ratio of radioactivity. This ratio depends largely on the efficiency of clearance by the kidneys as well as mineral content of bone. Therefore in patients with renal impairment or very marked osteomalacia the skeletal scan may be of lower quality than usual. However, in most patients the phosphate compounds show the normal skeleton in relatively great detail enabling precise localization of the position of abnormalities. As they are cleared by the kidneys $^{99}Tc^{m}$ phosphate compounds accumulate in the bladder, and tend to obscure lesions of the lower pelvic girdle. Patients are therefore requested to empty their bladder immediately before an image of the pelvis is started.

In summary, bone imaging with $^{99}Tc^{m}$-labelled phosphates is an essential part of the work-up of a wide variety of patients with malignant disease. Simple, inexpensive and atraumatic, it should ideally be performed in patients with any neoplasm where there is clinical or even radiological uncertainty of metastatic involvement of the skeleton.

Tumour-seeking Agents

There are a number of radioactive materials which are used as non-specific tumour localizing agents. If the radioisotope tracer has a suitable half-life and emits gamma rays of detectable energies then scanning techniques can be used to visualize the extent of a malignant process. Unfortunately, there is no one radiopharmaceutical which can be used for all situations and it is a matter of some argument which is the best agent for a particular tumour.

One of the earliest tumour-seeking agents was ^{32}P. Although this nuclide was not ideal for scanning, because of its pure β-particle emission, it was used to assess the extent of and to diagnose melanomas of the eye. The rapid proliferation of the tumour cells took up more radiophosphorus than neighbouring normal tissue. Current tumour-localizing agents probably rely on the same principles but their radiation characteristics make them more suitable for imaging.

It was discovered by chance in the later 1960s that ^{67}Ga accumulated in Hodgkin's tissue. Since then it has been used to investigate a number of malignancies but in many cases results have been disappointing. By far its greatest value is in carcinoma of the bronchus, Hodgkin's disease and seminoma, where detection rates for lesions are as high as 90 per

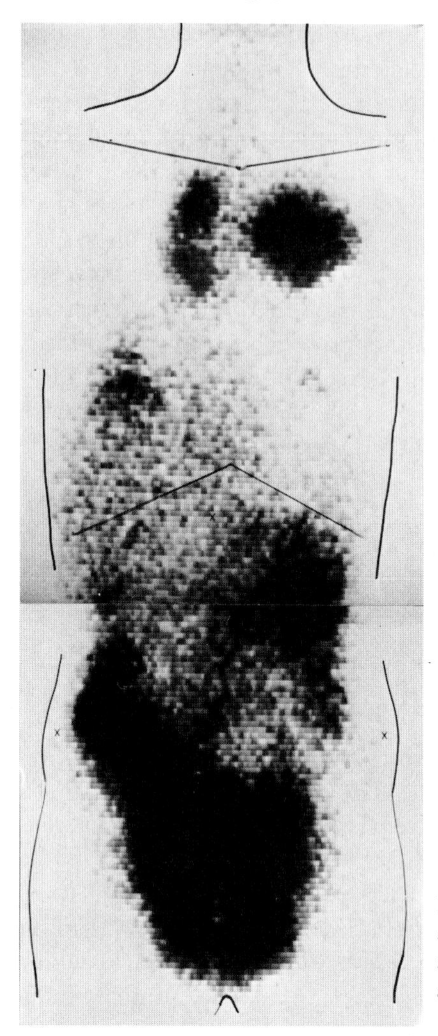

Figure 6.10 Rectilinear scan two days after 2 mCi of ^{67}Ga citrate. There are large areas of tumour concentration in the chest and abdomen from a primary seminoma of testes.

cent. Figure 6.10 is a typical scan of the chest and abdomen in a patient with a seminoma of testes. It is still unclear how gallium localizes in malignant tissue but one explanation is that tumour cells ingest plasma proteins which are ^{67}Ga-labelled. These proteins are then catabolized, leaving behind the label which becomes attached to the lysosomes. This process can also occur in inflammatory lesions such as sarcoidosis and tuberculosis. Gallium scanning, therefore, cannot be used as a diagnostic screening test but is useful rather in the staging of known neoplastic disease. Effort, too, is being put into discovering the effects of radiation and chemotherapy treatment on the uptake of gallium into tumour. If the degree of uptake represents a true picture of tumour activity then ^{67}Ga could be confidently used in the assessment of each patient during and on the completion of treatment.

Several antitumour agents have been labelled in an attempt to produce better localizing agents. Examples of these are ^{111}In bleomycin, ^{57}Co bleomycin and ^{195}Pt^{m} *cis*-dichlorodiaminine (DDP). Of these, ^{111}In bleomycin appears to be the most useful although ^{67}Ga appears to be superior in cases of carcinoma of the bronchus. One major advantage of the labelled antimitotic drugs is that they are cleared by urinary excretion and do not, like gallium, accumulate in the bowel. There is, therefore, no need for preparation of the abdomen before imaging with these agents.

The amino acid analogue selenomethionine has been used with some success in differentiating between malignant and benign space-occupying lesions in the liver. A normal colloid liver scan will display any lesion as a cold radioactive area. If there is some doubt as to whether this is due to a benign cyst or a solid tumour a repeat scan using ^{75}Se-methionine is indicated. The selenomethionine will often be selectively taken up into malignant tissue but will have a similar distribution to colloid if the lesion is cystic.

Radiation Protection

Mention should be made here of the possible radiation hazards to both the patient and those in close contact with him. From the patient's point of view the radiation dose he receives during a diagnostic nuclear medicine test is, occasionally, much less than for conventional X-ray examinations of the same organ. For the most part, however, the radiation doses are very similar to those in radiology, and for this reason those precautions and considerations which apply when patients are to be X-rayed also apply in isotope scanning. Specifically women of child-bearing age have their tests arranged in the ten days after their menstrual period, thus avoiding the exposure of an early pregnancy.

For those who come into contact with patients who have received radioisotopes for diagnosis the radiation risks are small indeed. Being occupationally exposed to radiation, physicists, radiographers and radiologists are allowed to receive what is considered to be a 'safe' quantity of radiation, namely the Maximum Permissible Dose.

Nurses, physiotherapists and technicians who are not in continuous and exclusive contact with such patients are limited to receiving only one-third of this figure. If in addition one realizes that only rarely do radiographers receive more than 5 per cent of their permitted dose, it becomes clear that the radiation hazards in this speciality are minute in the extreme and are only fractionally above the hazards from natural background radiation.

Slightly higher risks are involved when patients receive therapeutic doses of radioisotopes and in these cases the 'time and distance' principle comes into effect. With regular monitoring from the nuclear medicine department personnel are instructed 'how long and how close' they are allowed near the patients until his radioactivity has reached a negligibly low level.

Conclusion

Whereas treatment of cancer with radioisotopes has been less successful than predicted (with the notable exception of thyroid cancer), their use for diagnosis has exceeded even the most optimistic predictions. Their main limitation is in the minimum size of lesion which may be visualized. However, their potential strength is in the ability to trace metabolic processes *in vivo* by external monitoring yet without upsetting the physiology of the system being studied. There have been real advances in the quality of the imaging apparatus over the last few years. It is hard to see how it can be developed much further. The most likely developments now lie in the field of radiopharmacy where more disease-specific compounds are being researched. The very small lesions which can be detected with radioiodine in thyroid cancer give great encouragement to continue the struggle to find disease-specific radiopharmaceuticals.

The original reasons for being enthusiastic about radioisotope imaging techniques are still valid. The tests require minimum trauma to the patients – usually a simple injection. They are relatively fast and yield information obtainable by other methods only with considerable effort and some degree of pain or morbidity. The use of the term radioactivity evokes considerable fear in the patient's mind. It is worth impressing on him the low radiation dose involved and the fact that the doctors and radiographers and physics staff deal with many patients having such tests over many years with complete safety.

References

Gottschalk, A. and Potchen, E. J. (1976) *Diagnostic Nuclear Medicine.* Baltimore: Williams & Wilkins.

De Land, F. (1975) in *Nuclear Medicine.* Wagner (ed.). New York: HP Publishing Co. Inc.

McCready, V. R. (1972) *Seminars in Nuclear Medicine*, **2**, No. 4, p. 108.

Maynard, C. D. (1969) *Clinical Nuclear Medicine.* Philadelphia: Lea & Febiger.

Merrick, M. V. Bone scanning, *British Journal of Radiology*, **48**, No 569, pp. 327–51.

Oldendorf, W. H. (1972) *Clinical uses of Radionuclides: Critical Comparison with Other Techniques.* AEC Symposium series 27, pp. 25–52.

Paterson, A. H. G. and McCready, V. R. Tumour imaging radiopharmaceuticals, *British Journal of Radiology*, **48**, No 571, pp. 520–31.

Pochin, E. E. *British Journal of Radiology*, **49**, No 583, pp. 577–9.

Code of Practice for the Protection of Persons Against Ionizing Radiations from Medical and Dental Use. H.M.S.O.

Chapter 7

Diagnostic Cytology

P. A. TROTT
M.B., B.Chir., M.R.C.Path.
Consultant Pathologist in Cytology
Royal Marsden Hospital
London

Introduction

Cancer is a manifestation of exaggerated cell growth and cytology is the study of the cells contained in a tumour to establish its diagnosis. Diagnostic cytology is a comparatively new subdivision of pathology and can justly claim to be one of its fastest growing branches. The main impetus to its development came from the work of Dr G. N. Papanicolaou, a Greek gynaecologist working in Colorado, USA, during the 1940s. Following work on the changes observed in cells exfoliated from the rat vagina during the oestrous cycle, he promoted the idea of the possibility of the detection of cancer of the neck of the womb at an early curable stage from the identification of abnormal cells scraped from the uterine cervix. Nowadays, large community programmes are established in many countries to screen healthy women for the early diagnosis of cervical cancer using Dr Papanicolaou's techniques. During the 1930s Dudgeon and Bamforth, two pathologists working at St Thomas's Hospital in London, examined cells shed from the cut surface of freshly removed malignant tumours and demonstrated the ability to diagnose cancer from the appearance of the cells alone. These workers together with Wrigley then proceeded to examine sputum from cases of suspected lung cancer and showed that fragments of tumour and individual carcinoma cells could be recognized and the diagnosis confirmed.

The modern cytology laboratory examines tissue from almost all organs of the body. The cells are obtained in one of two ways, either exfoliated from an epithelial surface such as covers the cervix, or aspirated using a narrow needle from lumps that are palpable or visible by radiological techniques. Cancer cells are less adherent than benign ones and hence exfoliation is facilitated. The majority of malignancies are epithelial cancers (carcinomas) and the surface cells readily exfoliate into the lumen or cavity. For instance, cells from carcinoma of the lung are often found in sputum in compact clusters together with mucus and inflammatory debris suggesting that malignant cells shed into a bronchial tube cause a block that on forced expectoration is coughed up. The identification of carcinoma cells in the sputum reveals the diagnosis. Similarly, malignant cells from tumours of the gastrointestinal tract can be collected with the aid of fibre-optic instruments that enable a gastroenterologist to see inside almost the whole length of the gastrointestinal tract. In this way, the lesions suspicious of carcinoma can be gently washed and the dislodged cells removed for examination by a cytopathologist. Cells from tumours not directly involving epithelial surfaces can be removed by needle aspiration. This technique has been used extensively in Scandinavia and other European countries for about fifteen years but has only recently been tried in the United Kingdom. The best results are obtained in the more accessible tumours such as the breast, although prostatic carcinoma for which a specially designed needle is used, can be diagnosed by aspiration through the rectum. In centres having a neurosurgical unit, brain tumours and other lesions can be diagnosed by smearing tissue removed at operation onto a slide and examining it microscopically in the operating theatre, a technique which is faster than conventional rapid processing techniques for histopathological examination.

Laboratory Preparation of Material

Material for cytodiagnosis comes to the laboratory either already smeared on a glass slide or as a fluid in liquid state like urine, or more gelatinous in consistency, such as sputum. It is the duty of the laboratory technician to process the material in such a way as to transfer the cells it contains on to slides where they can be stained and examined under the microscope. While the cells are suspended in fluid, they are liable to degenerate and so appear abnormal when examined. Therefore, the nurse or porter must ensure that specimens of this kind reach the laboratory as soon as possible after they are produced unless a preservative is used when extreme urgency is no longer required. For example, urine is often collected in factories from workers who are at risk of developing bladder cancer because of exposure years before to certain carcinogens. The urine is collected in plastic bottles containing a glycol or similar preservative which enables the specimen to be sent through the post without deterioration of the cells. Serous cavity fluids often contain sanguinous material and to avoid the risk of clotting the fluid is collected into citrate anticoagulant.

Once in the laboratory, the more liquid fluids such as urine, serous fluids and gastric washings, are spun in a centrifuge and the supernatant discarded. The deposit contains the cells and these are transferred onto a glass slide, either with a loop or fine-bore pipette. For fluids of small volume, 10 ml or less, Shandon Elliott have designed an ingenious centrifuge called a 'Cytospin' that centrifuges and deposits the cells onto a small area in the centre of a microscope slide, thus ensuring that all the cells are collected and may be examined easily. This machine is particularly useful for the examination and preparation of cells in cerebrospinal fluid and fluids from serous cavities.

The cells are stained in one of two ways. The first of these consists of a modification of the haematoxylin and eosin method used in histopathology laboratories called the Papanicolaou method. The second is the Romanowski technique which is the basic stain used for blood cells in the haematology department. Both methods have advantages and disadvantages and their proponents will argue strongly in their favour. The point is, however, that the Papanicolaou method requires the cells to be fixed in spirit while they are still wet, whereas the Romanowski technique can only be used satisfactorily on cells that have been air dried. Thus the doctor, nurse or technician taking the smear or processing the fluid, must be aware what staining method will be used before the smear is taken or the fluid processed. Failure to plunge a slide into fixative within a few seconds of making a smear will render the cells unsuitable for cytodiagnosis because of cellular distortion. On the other hand, smears that will be air dried must be made thinly with another slide or coverslip at an angle of 45° so that the cells will not overlap and to enable them to dry as rapidly as possible.

General Criteria of Malignancy and Guidelines for Reporting

Cytology technicians in training are usually taught the 'criteria of malignancy'. This is a list of the abnormal features of cells, none of which by itself is characteristic of malignancy, but considered together they enable the observer to decide whether or not a cell or cluster of cells is malignant. The criteria of malignancy, however, vary from tissue to tissue so that the organ from which the cells originate must be known in order to make an accurate diagnosis. Nevertheless, as a general guideline, this list will be found useful:

1. Enlargement and prominence of the nucleus;
2. Irregularity of nuclear shape;
3. Inequality of the size of the nuclei in cell groups;
4. Increase in the amount of chromatin in the nuclei;
5. Rearrangement of the chromatin pattern;
6. Prominent nucleoli;
7. Enlargement of the cell generally;
8. Inequality of the size of cells;
9. Abnormal staining reactions;
10. Formation of groups and clusters.

The list consists mainly of abnormalities of the nucleus and the Papanicolaou method stain is specifically designed to demonstrate changes in the nucleus especially in preinvasive carcinoma *in situ* of the uterine cervix.

Technicians in cytology laboratories are encouraged to write reports about the cells they examine. When reporting the results of a cytological examination important considerations must be borne in mind. These involve the purpose of the cytological examination and whether it is as a detection study or a diagnostic one. For instance, the examination of cervical smears from healthy asymptomatic women is a detection procedure, whereas sputum examined from patients with a cough and perhaps haemoptysis is a diagnostic procedure in order to diagnose bronchial carcinoma. So far as the report is concerned, different emphasis must be applied when abnormal cells, suspicious but not characteristic of malignancy, are observed. In the case of cervical cytology these suspicions must be reported in order to alert the referring clinician or general practitioner that there may be an abnormality and an early repeat smear taken. On the other hand, when slightly abnormal cells are seen in a sputum specimen their presence should be recorded but not reported as it is of little use to a clinician to be told that cells are merely suspicious of carcinoma. Further tests will be performed to establish a diagnosis as the patient is under surveillance on account of his symptoms.

The reports issued by a laboratory must be concise and unambiguous. They are the outward and visible sign of the efficiency of the department and therefore the standard of typing and clean appearance of the report are almost as important as the meaning of the words it contains. Cytology reports should be in three sections, describing, first, the nature of the material examined, be it sputum, breast aspirate, or peritoneal fluid. Second, the microscopic appearances of the cells including an indication of the quantity and quality of the material must be included, and third, a conclusion consisting of a single word, e.g. carcinoma or abscess, completes the report. Thus a busy clinician can see at a glance from the first section where the specimen came from and he can see the conclusion by looking at the brief third section of the report. More detailed information can be read at leisure from the middle section.

Gynaecological Cytology

Cancer of the cervix uteri and to a lesser extent of the endometrium, can be diagnosed by examining cells removed from the cervix using a wooden spatula. Cervical carcinoma begins in the epithelium covering the external part of the uterine cervix on the so-called transformation zone at the junction of the squamous (flat cell) epithelium, and the columnar (cuboidal cell) epithelium that extends upwards to line the inside of the uterus. It is known from work done on experimental animals that cancer results from a genetic abnormality of a single cell which divides to form a 'clone' of potential cancer cells that eventually spread beyond the epithelium and invade vital organs and kill the host. In the case of cervical cancer, the early stage of this process can take between five and fifteen years, during which time the abnormal cells are confined to the epithelium and can be detected by the microscopic examination of cells scraped from the cervix.

This method of diagnosis was established by Dr Papanicolaou and his colleagues who showed as early as 1928 that cancer cells could be detected in a vaginal smear. In 1943 Papanicolaou and Traut published their classic paper entitled 'The Diagnosis of Uterine Cancer by the Vaginal Smear' and showed that the intraepithelial stage of the disease could be detected even in asymptomatic women. Thus it was hoped and indeed confidently predicted that such a method of detection would eliminate cancer of the cervix which kills about 2,500 women annually in England and Wales. The facts are, however, that despite extensive and comprehensive screening programmes in several centres throughout the world, the disease is still tragically apparent, although in reduced incidence. There are two main reasons for the failure of cervical cytology programmes to prevent cervical cancer entirely. First, there are undoubtedly some cases of cervical cancer that are very aggressive and have an extremely short preclinical or intraepithelial stage and only the examination of cervical smears at very frequent intervals, for instance every three months, would detect such cases. Such a programme is of course impractical in terms of deployment of the medical manpower required to examine populations of women frequently. Cases of the more aggressive rapidly growing variant of cervical cancer are probably rare, but the second and more important cause of failure of screening programmes lies in the very nature of the disease itself that commonly affects the women least likely to offer themselves for examination. Cervical cancer strikes the lower, poorer social classes, those with children rather than those without and those who are promiscuous rather than women with less prolific sexual habits. Therefore, women with little money, confined to their homes by several children and with little intelligence are most likely to develop cervical cancer and least likely to attend for a cervical smear.

The most extensive screening programme in the world is in the Province of British Columbia, Canada and their recent claim is to have examined more than 80 per cent of the female population. Over the years the figures show a substantial fall in the incidence of cervical cancer as well as the mortality rate from the disease. However, it must be stated that statisticians remain unimpressed by these figures and point out that the incidence of cervical cancer throughout the world has been falling ever since the turn of the century. In strict statistical terms the usefulness and effect of cervical cytology screening programmes can only be proven by a controlled epidemiological trial whereby the incidence of cervical cancer can be compared in two matched populations, one of which has been screened and the other not. Such a programme, which denies the test to a group of women, will not be sanctioned because of ethical considerations, so that (as the statisticians point out) a properly designed experiment will never be undertaken. However, those involved in the field of cytodiagnosis, including gynaecologists, are convinced that cervical cytology prevents cervical cancer and the more extensive the cover to the population, the fewer cases will occur. Convincing figures to illustrate this come from the work of Dr McGreggor in Aberdeen, who has screened 90 per cent of the population through the help of the general practitioners. Clinical cervical cancer in that city in screened women is an extremely rare occurrence.

The cells shed from the cervix with an intraepithelial carcinoma *in situ* are larger than normal ones and have irregular nuclei that show increased affinity for the haematoxylin stain. Thus they catch the trained eye of the cytotechnologist when the slide is examined with the medium objective of a microscope (Fig. 7.1). Other features are important too when assessing the appearance of abnormal cells and

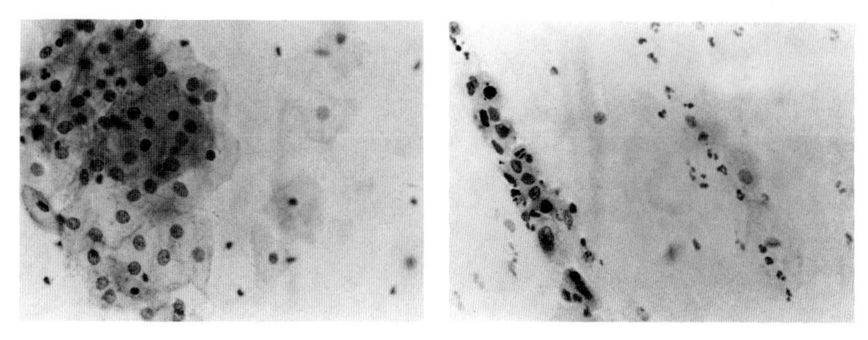

Figure 7.1(a) Normal cervical epithelial cells compared to (b) those from carcinoma *in situ*.

lesser degrees of abnormality, involving more superficial layer cells, indicate an unstable epithelium that must be watched by the clinician and smears taken at regular intervals to detect any progression to a more serious lesion. The fully developed intraepithelial carcinoma *in situ* of the cervix (Fig. 7.2) is cured by surgical excision, either by hysterectomy in older women or, in women still planning to have a family, by cone biopsy. This involves removing a pyramidal-shaped piece of cervix which includes the transformation zone but not the internal os so that the cervix remains competent if pregnancy occurs. The cone biopsy is examined by a histopathologist and the extent of the lesion assessed.

Carcinoma of the endometrium can be detected in older women in whom clusters of adenocarcinoma cells are found in the vaginal pool specimen. Some centres have designed special aspiration pipettes that directly remove cells from the endometrium and so enable the diagnosis to be made more easily.

Sputum Cytology

Cells coughed up from the bronchial tubes in patients with bronchial carcinoma often show characteristic changes that enable the diagnosis of cancer to be proved. Patients with this disease usually have a productive cough so that good quality samples are not difficult to obtain. The best specimen is an early morning one when secretions are present that have been accumulating in the bronchial tubes during the night. Patients are asked to spit the first deep cough specimen into a plastic pot directly after waking in the morning. Sometimes only saliva is produced and in these cases and in other patients who have difficulty in producing sputum, a few pats on the back by a nurse with the patient leaning over the side of the bed, or better still, following percussion by a

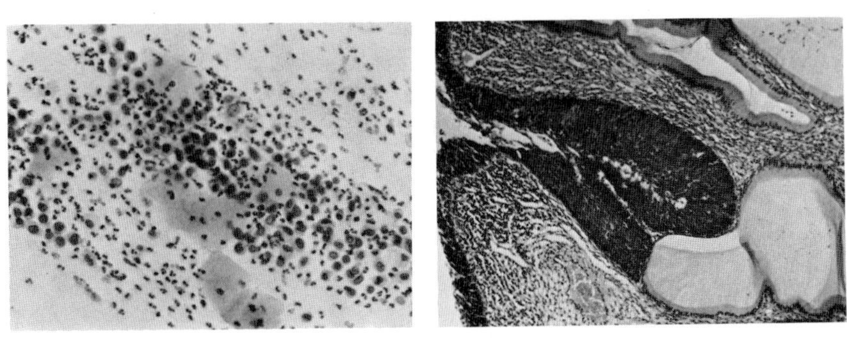

Figure 7.2(a) Cells shed from carcinoma *in situ*; (b) removed in a cone biopsy.

physiotherapist, can often encourage the patient to produce a good quality specimen.

The specimen must be taken fresh directly to the laboratory where it is examined by a cytotechnician who will recognize abnormal colour and changes in consistency in the sample that may contain the carcinoma cells. Watery, salivary material can be rejected as unsuitable, but the sample must be examined under a good light and in a vacuum extractor to minimize the chances of bacterial contamination. Sputum tinged with blood or yellow purulent areas should be selected for examination avoiding mucus if possible. The material is transferred to a labelled glass slide with a pair of forceps or wooden stick and spread evenly. Usually three slides are made which are then plunged into alcoholic fixative before they have dried and stained by the Papanicolaou method. In some laboratories sputum is stained with methylene blue and examined before it has dried. The disadvantage of this technique is that no permanent preparations can be made for subsequent examination, but it is a simple stain that enables the diagnosis to be made in a few minutes.

Carcinoma cells in sputum often group together in clusters or streaks and they are often mixed with inflammatory cells. Four types of malignant cells can be recognized. These are squamous carcinoma, 'oat cell' carcinoma, adenocarcinoma and undifferentiated cells. The squamous cells are the most easily seen and they are the commonest. They have an elongated shape, usually a central, heavily stained nucleus with an irregular edge to it (Fig. 7.3) and some may have brightly pink-staining cytoplasm that reveals its ability to become keratinized. Indeed, keratinized squamous carcinoma of the bronchus may appear as irregular shapes of brightly pink- or orange-staining material in which no nucleus can be identified. These appearances are characteristic.

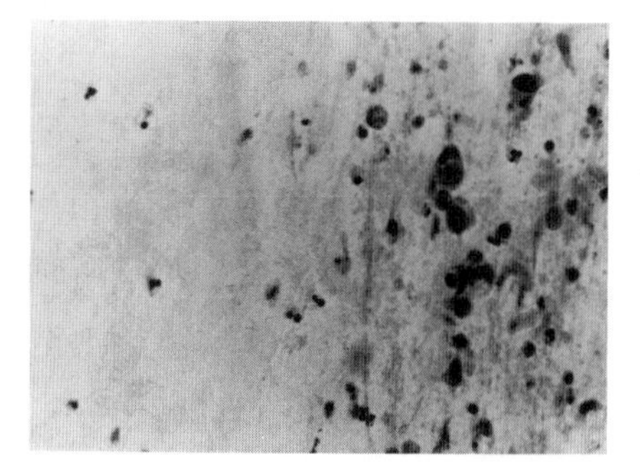

Figure 7.3 Streak of squamous carcinoma cells.

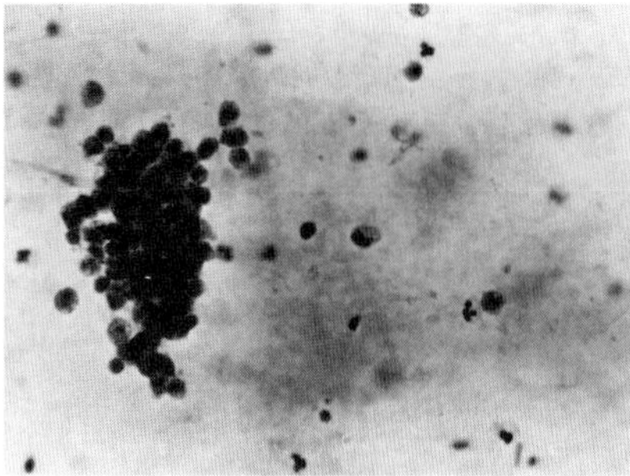

Figure 7.4 Cluster of 'oat cell' carcinoma cells.

'Oat cell' carcinoma of the bronchus is a very interesting tumour that has a characteristic histological pattern, resembling ears of oats packed together. The exfoliated cells and those seen in pleural effusions and metastases in other sites, consist of round small nuclei with scanty cytoplasm that are closely packed together having a characteristic pinkish colour and consistency when stained by the Romanowski technique. They appear in sputum as small cells in rows or clusters about twice the size of lymphocytes, with the edge of one nucleus indenting the edge of its neighbour (Fig. 7.4). The tumours themselves are the subject of much research in recent years, as not uncommonly they secrete a hormone such as cortisone, antidiuretic hormone or serotonin and it is the effects of the hormone that give the patient his symptoms. This phenomenon is known as 'inappropriate' hormone secretion.

Undifferentiated malignant cells usually turn out to be poorly differentiated carcinomas on histological examination. They appear in the sputum as small round or oval cells of varying shapes and sizes, often clustered and sometimes showing bizarre nuclear shapes (Fig. 7.5). These cells, like those from 'oat cell' carcinoma, can be difficult to find and experienced cytotechnicians may overlook them on cursory examination of the stained slides. Cells from these cases are often buried in mucopurulent material and when one group is identified, many more may become apparent.

Adenocarcinoma cells are the least common of the four varieties and these tumours may be primary bronchial carcinomas or metastases. The primary tumours are often situated at the periphery of the lung fields and so are unlikely to be shed into the more central bronchi, but when they do they are characteristic. They always occur in round cohesive clusters with eccentric nuclei containing prominent nucleoli (Fig. 7.6) and often with cytoplasmic vacuolation. Tumours of the

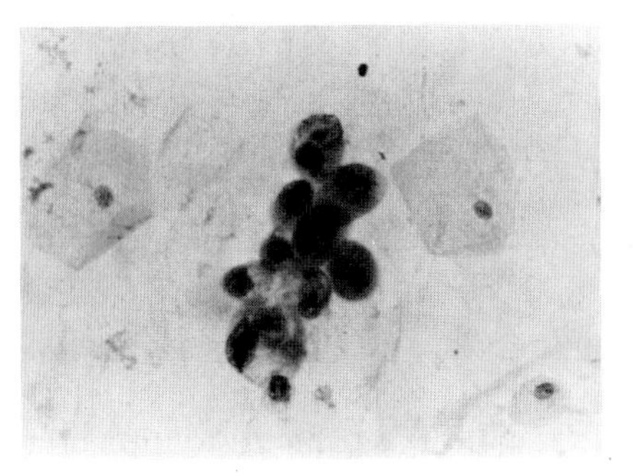

Figure 7.5 Cluster of undifferentiated malignant cells.

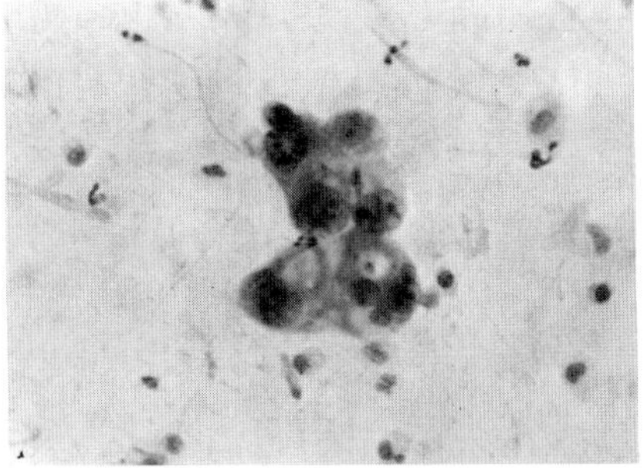

Figure 7.6 Adenocarcinoma cells with vacuolated cytoplasm.

kidney, gastrointestinal tract and breast commonly spread to the lung fields. The cells from these tumours usually resemble adenocarcinoma and those from a renal cell carcinoma sometimes having a characteristic 'clear cell' appearance from the abundant vacuolated cytoplasm. In this way the cytologist may give valuable assistance to the clinician in his hunt to pin-point the site of a primary tumour.

Many reports have indicated the value of sputum cytology in the diagnosis of lung cancer and these emphasize the importance of avoiding the false positive diagnosis. Indeed, the prognosis of this disease is so poor that the cytopathologist must understand that his report of cancer cells identified is often the signal for the clinician to give up other investigations and start radical forms of treatment, usually radiotherapy or chemotherapy. Consequently, some cytopathologists are reluctant to give a definite positive diagnosis of cancer and the report of 'highly suspicious of carcinoma' is used. The important thing, however, is for there to be a close liaison between cytopathologists and clinicians so that between them the correct diagnosis is reached.

Serous Cavity Fluids

The heart, lungs and viscera are allowed to move freely because they are covered by a thin membrane that is reflected onto surrounding structures. This membrane, therefore, lines an enclosed potential space that in the healthy state contains a small amount of thin lubricating fluid. These spaces, the pericardial cavity, the pleural cavity and the peritoneal cavity, are the sites of accumulation of fluid in many diseases of adjacent and distant organs, including malignant ones.

The lining membrane of all these cavities is composed of a single layer of cuboidal cells called mesothelium and in any disease resulting in accumulation of fluid, these cells proliferate and shed into the adjacent fluid. Once detached they slowly begin to deteriorate and the cytoplasm swells and they become phagocytic, i.e. they are facultative histiocytes. Examination of mesothelial cells exfoliated into a serous cavity fluid will, therefore, show a range of appearances extending from a small compact well-stained cell with an eccentric round nucleus via larger cells with foamy cytoplasm and indented nuclei to one that looks obviously degenerate in the final stage of cell death. It is this variety of appearances of benign reactive cells that can be so difficult to interpret when examining fluids that may also contain malignant cells.

In benign conditions two processes may result in the accumulation of fluid in serous cavities. A transudate is the result of a failure to function of the heart or kidney or the result of local mechanical obstruction whereby fluid is forced into available space. Fluid in these cases contains few cells and very little protein. Exudates on the other hand are protein rich and result from a locally aggravating disease in which the mesothelial membrane actively secretes fluid and a variety of inflammatory cells are also exuded. Pneumonia of any kind may cause pleurisy and the cells exfoliated into the pleural cavity may include neutrophils, plasma cells and histiocytes. Pulmonary infarcts are often associated with large numbers of mesothelial cells in the pleural fluid, whereas they are very scanty in effusion in cases of tuberculosis. In two diseases, disseminated lupus erythematosis (DLE) and rheumatoid arthritis, distinctive features are present that enable a definitive diagnosis to be made. In DLE the neutrophils contain a large opaque structureless body which stains pale purple in the Romanowski stain and which is the remnant of a nucleus denatured by a distinctive gamma globulin found in the serum of patients with this disease. In rheumatoid arthritis the presence of multinucleated histiocytes, cell debris and fibrin will be diagnostic.

In malignant effusions the characteristic cells will be observed and a few associated features are usually present. These are the presence of red blood cells and lymphocytes. The vast majority of malignant effusions contain blood either revealed by a reddish tinge visible to the naked eye or as red blood cells seen microscopically. Lymphocytes, on the other hand, are less common but when present surrounding single or small groups of large irregular cells (Fig. 7.7) often help clinch the diagnosis.

The malignant cells themselves conform generally to the criteria of malignancy enumerated in the first part of this chapter. However, there is considerable variation according to cell type and those cases where differentiation from degenerating mesothelial cells is difficult

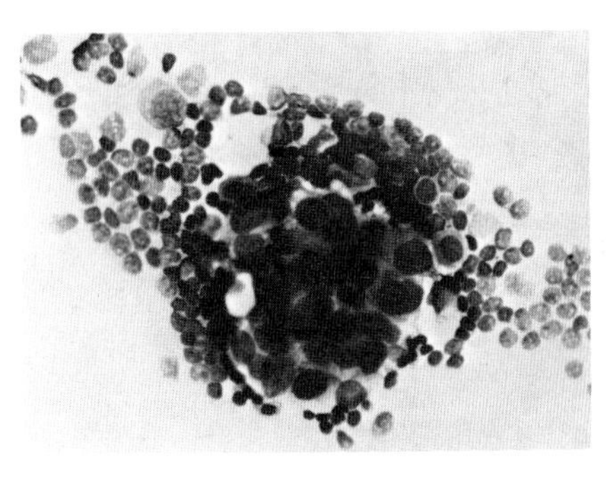

Figure 7.7 Group of metastatic breast carcinoma cells in pleural fluid surrounded by lymphocytes.

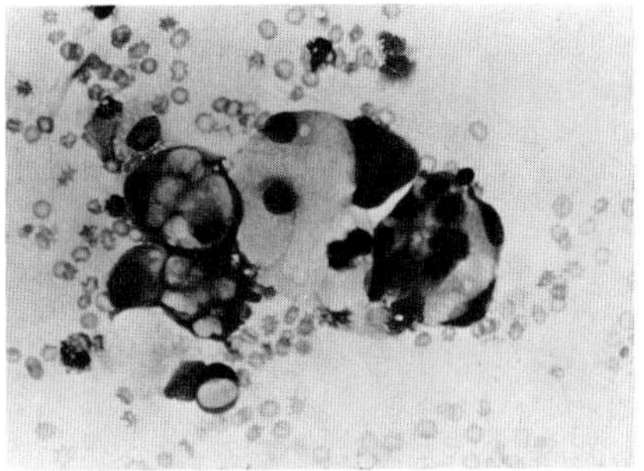

Figure 7.8 Metastatic ovarian carcinoma cells with blown out cytoplasm.

can be particular problems. It is a useful guide that mesothelial cells or histiocytes are nearly always present in malignant effusions and unless one can distinguish a different cell type the appearance of which does not seem to merge with the mesothelial cell series, it is safest to consider malignant cells absent. Some of the most bizarre-shaped cells seen in the cytology laboratory are found in fluids from patients with carcinoma of the ovary that have invaded the peritoneal cavity. Clusters of cells with huge nuclei are found often with mitotic figures present and with blown out cytoplasm (Fig. 7.8) that will stain positive for mucus.

Ovarian cancer usually invades the peritoneal cavity during its malignant progression and this is the commonest tumour to do so. Carcinoma of the breast often invades the pleural cavity and these cells are frequently difficult to distinguish from mesothelial cells. They are usually small and in clusters with irregular nuclei having a sharp affinity for the nuclear stains and surrounded by a rim of cytoplasm that is too little for the size of the cell.

Squamous carcinoma cells from a bronchial cancer are rarely seen but the elongated shape of the cell and its large size makes it easily identified. Maligant melanoma is a tumour containing brown pigment that may present many years after removal of a skin mole. The clinical diagnosis may be difficult but sometimes the pigment is obvious not only in the malignant cells but also in smaller particles in mesothelial cells performing their histiocytic function (Fig. 7.9). As in other sites 'oat cells' are distinctive although easily overlooked by the inexperienced cytotechnician. Similar to their appearance in sputum, they are small and round with scanty cytoplasm but with a very characteristic nucleus which shows a finely divided appearance of the chromatin when stained by the Papanicolaou and Romanowski techniques.

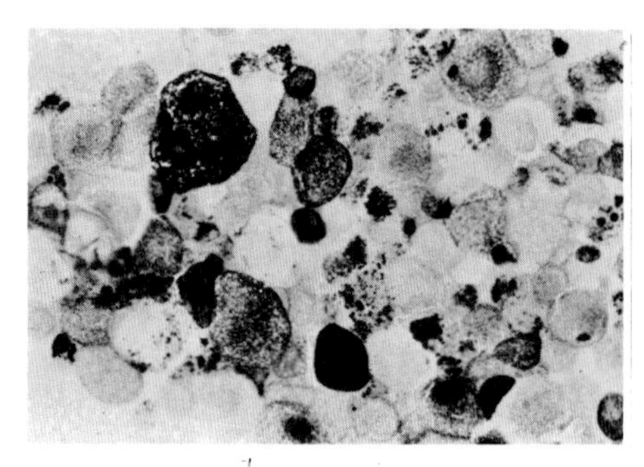

Figure 7.9 Melanin pigment in malignant melanoma cells and mesothelial cells.

Needle Aspiration Cytology

Cells can be aspirated from all palpable tumours using a thin bore hypodermic needle. This is a well-established method for releasing fluid from cysts from the breast and the fluid can be spun down and the cells in the deposit examined. More applicable to cancer diagnosis however, is the aspiration of solid tumours when juice within the lump is extracted and smeared directly on a microscope slide and stained. This technique has been used extensively in Scandinavia and other European countries, but in Britain and the USA more often a piece of the tumour is removed under general anaesthetic and a histopathological diagnosis obtained from examination of the tumour pattern. This procedure, called a diagnostic biopsy, has disadvantages apart from the risk of general anaesthesia. Admission to hospital must be arranged and many patients will need to make arrangements for the care of children and other dependants. Once in hospital, the ward staff, theatre staff and anaesthetist will be involved even before the surgeon performs the operation. Needle aspiration performed in out-patient clinics avoids this expensive use of medical resources and manpower.

A diagnostic biopsy is more helpful compared to needle aspiration in terms of classifying tumours and the accurate establishment of the cell type and many comparative studies have demonstrated this. However, in many clinical situations the ease with which fine needle aspiration can be performed outweighs the disadvantages of a slight reduction of the diagnostic accuracy. For example, in the management of the patient with a lump in the breast, a tissue diagnosis of cancer can be obtained by fine needle aspiration in about eight out of ten malignant tumours, thus avoiding the need for rapid 'frozen' section when the patient is under anaesthetic. When breast carcinoma is confirmed in this way in the out-patient department the patient can be prepared psychologically

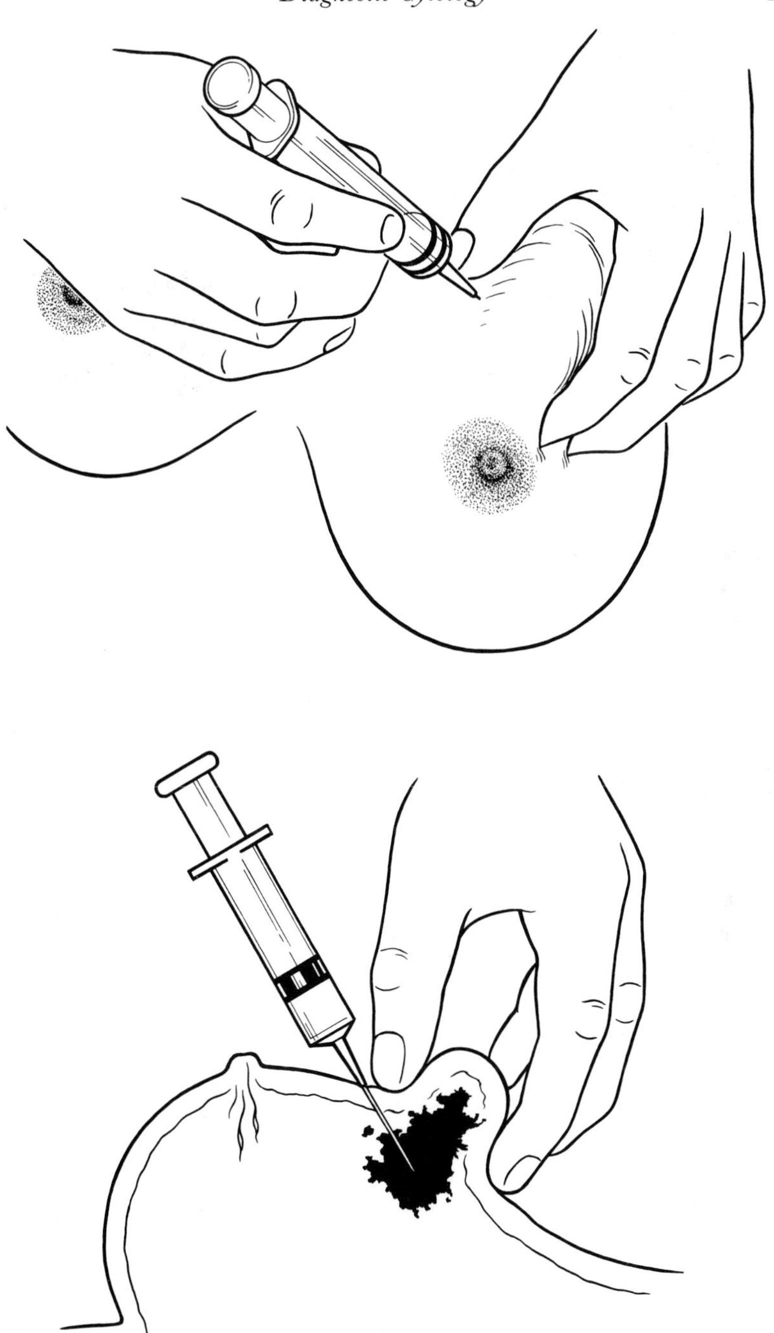

Figure 7.10 Procedure for aspirating cells from solid breast lumps. (a) The tumour is gripped firmly and the needle inserted. In (b) the tip of the needle is shown in the centre of the tumour.

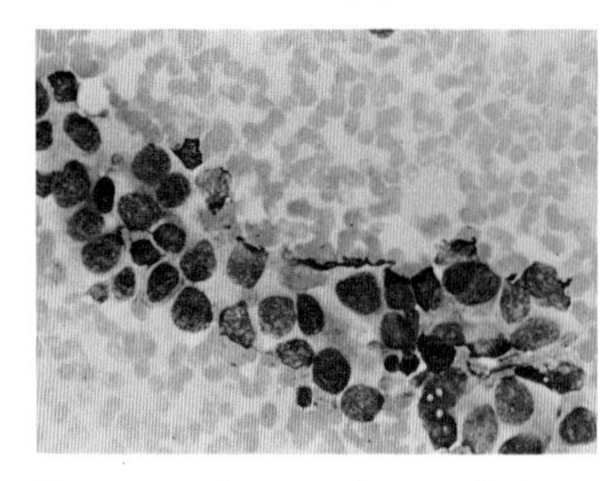

Figure 7.11 Breast carcinoma cells showing abnormal chromatin patterns and nuclear irregularity. Compare with Fig. 7.12.

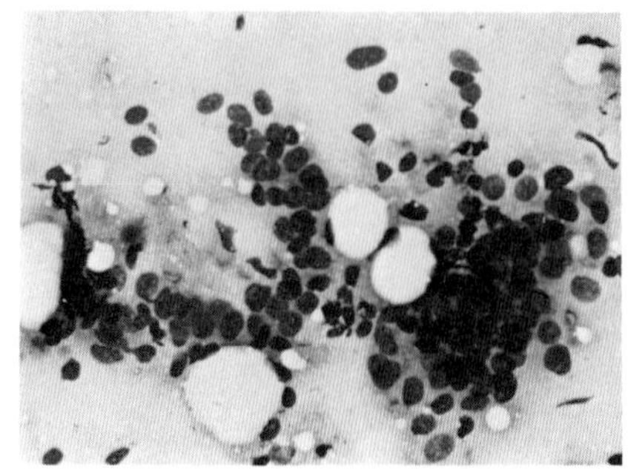

Figure 7.12 Benign breast cells from a fibroadenoma. Compare with Fig. 7.11.

for radical surgery if that is to be the treatment, and she can be investigated for metastatic disease with the certain knowledge of the correct diagnosis.

The method of aspiration is vitally important because without an adequate number of cells properly spread and stained, no diagnosis can be made. Twenty-one- and twenty-three-gauge needles are adequate for most subcutaneous lumps including breast tumours, the larger needle aspirating more cells but being slightly more painful for the patient. In right-handed people it is best to fix the lump firmly between the index finger and thumb of the left hand (Fig. 7.10), having prepared clean slides and having fixative handy. Using a 10 or 20 ml syringe, the needle is inserted into the centre of the tumour and the tip moved about within it, all the time aspirating very forcefully with the barrel of the syringe pulled out as far as possible. Different areas of the centre of the tumour should be aspirated in this way for about a minute and the syringe barrel released before removing the needle. Most of the aspirated tumour juice will be inside the needle and must then be spread thinly like a blood film to be air dried or rather more thickly if it is to be wet fixed.

The aspirated carcinoma cells have large nuclei that vary in size and shape and have irregular borders (Fig. 7.11). One general property of neoplastic cells is useful in making the diagnosis and this is the dissociated or dispersed appearance of the individual cells that have lost their ability to adhere and stick together. Aspirated cells from a benign fibroadenoma can also appear large and irregular but the clustering effect of the duct cells is diagnostic (Fig. 7.12).

Needle aspirates from solid tumours in other organs can provide useful clinical information. For example, lymph nodes in the neck, axilla or groin are the site of metastatic malignant tumours and they are easily accessible for needle aspiration. In this context aspiration can save a considerable amount of diagnostic investigation in those cases where the tissue diagnosis is established by histopathological examination of the primary tumour and cells of a similar type are aspirated from a lymph node. Similarly in subcutaneous tumours suspected of being metastases, needle aspiration will provide confirmation.

Urine

Bladder cancer will exfoliate cells into the urine and provided they are sufficiently abnormal in appearance, they can be identified. The difficulty with attempting to diagnose bladder cancer by urinary cytology is that the commonest type of bladder tumour is composed of slightly irregular cells with even-sized nuclei that may be difficult to differentiate from cells shed into the urine in patients with chronic bladder infection. This type of tumour is composed of fingerlike papillary fronds that protrude into the bladder cavity and provide the origin for the layman's term for this kind of bladder cancer, 'warts on the bladder'. Fortunately, this tumour is slow growing in the majority of cases, unlike the solid variety that does not protrude into the lumen but penetrates the muscle wall, thus providing a solid feel to it on bimanual examination. This tumour is more aggressive than its papillary counterpart and made up of more variable-sized and larger cells easily recognized when searched for in a urine deposit or stained filter.

In recent years, a third type of non-invasive tumour rather similar to intraepithelial carcinoma *in situ* of the cervix has been recognized, known as flat carcinoma or carcinoma *in situ* of the bladder. This lesion predisposes to invasive carcinoma and it is therefore very important to diagnoze it early as recognition may prevent invasion and metastases. Urologists may not recognize this kind of tumour for two reasons; first, because the usual symptom of haematuria is often absent and, second, when the bladder is examined at cystoscopy examination, the flat areas of tumour may resemble an inflammatory cystitis. However, the epithelium of this tumour is very friable and irregular-shaped carcinoma cells are present in large numbers in the urine.

Chapter 8

Screening – The Presymptomatic Diagnosis of Cancer

J. DAVEY
M.B., B.S., D.M.R.T.
Medical Officer in Charge
Early Diagnostic Unit
Royal Marsden Hospital
London

The purpose of screening is to discover those among the apparently well who are suffering from a particular disease. Its value has been questioned in relation to the detection of cancer or other incurable diseases. Differences of opinion have arisen about the existence or definition of an 'early' stage in cancer but it is well established that the prognosis for an individual will depend on such factors as the size and malignancy of the primary tumour and on the extent of spread at the time of the first treatment. Without full epidemiological surveys in controlled population groups it is difficult to prove that patients who have been discovered at a screening clinic to have cancer will have a better prognosis than a similar group presenting in an out-patient clinic. They may fare no better than others in a similar stage, but their outlook may be improved by not waiting until the disease is clinically manifest.

One in five people in Britain die of cancer. Britain has one of the highest instances of breast cancer in the world, and it is important for this and other forms of cancer to be detected at an earlier stage and so reduce this high mortality rate. Diagnostic oncology has always suffered from the fact that a specific diagnostic cancer test comparable to the Wasserman test for syphilis has not been found in spite of an intensive search for specific cancer antigens. Carcinoembryonic antigen, CEA, one of the oncofoetal antigens, gave great hopes in this respect, but the number of localized cancers resulting in significant CEA production are very few. However, it may have a place in the detection of metastatic disease early in its evolution, another important case for screening. Therapy in disseminated disease may be instituted sooner with improved results. Routine screening with CEA would produce even more hazards and distress than an isolated raised sedimentation rate.

The early detection of cancer can be equated with simpler treatment and fewer failures of treatment. The fact that this may not be true for all cancers should be used as a stimulus to improve one method of diagnosis and treatment and not as an argument against sensible and useful detection procedures. Proof of the value of screening programmes requires large numbers of patients with suitable control and several years of follow-up. A controlled screening trial for breast cancer was started in New York by Strax *et al.* and the first reports were available in 1967. This followed the earlier cervical cytology screening clinic report from British Columbia which was started in 1949. Initially both these trials have shown encouraging results and many other screening clinics have been set up as a result of these initial pioneer studies. Screening for lung cancer has also been evaluated and, although the first reports from the mass radiography service in three of the metropolitan regions were encouraging and showed an increase in survival, the size of the group was too small to influence mortality figures and since the outcome of patients with cancer of the lung is so poor screening clinics have not continued for this form of cancer.

This chapter on screening will be mainly referring to cervical and breast cancer screening clinics and it is important in reviewing the value of this type of screening to look at the availability, siting of clinics and patient selection that are used in those that are available in this country at present.

AVAILABILITY

Screening clinics have been available in the United Kingdom for the last fifteen years for cancer of the cervix under the National Health Service. Support for these clinics grew fairly quickly and numerous clinics were set up throughout the country, especially with the local authorities and Family Planning services. However, once the clinics were set up there was an immediate shortage of cytologists and also lack of continued support from patients attending these clinics. Training courses were started for both doctors and technicians and now an adequate service is available provided by the Regional and Area Health Authorities. Support varies according to the area of the country. By 1966 it was thought that enough staff had been trained to screen every woman of thirty-five and over once every five years. Initially the majority of smears were submitted from patients seen at hospital clinics, but after several years appreciable proportions came from local authority clinics and the general practitioner.

It is important to realize that a good cervical screening service must consider the following points:

1. Attract those patients in the high risk group for developing cancer of the cervix, i.e. in the lower socio-economic groups. This is difficult as these patients do not like an appointment system which is necessary for administration.
2. Provide an adequate laboratory service and hospital facilities for dealing with a large volume of smears and treating the women with positive smears when required.
3. Provide a recall service so that women can be alerted when they are due for their next smear.

Breast cancer screening clinics are not available nationally in Great Britain. Following the Strax trial already mentioned, pilot studies were set up by the Department of Health and their initial results supported the claim for the value of breast screening that Strax had shown. However, with limited resources, a national breast screening service is not available and only certain hospitals have facilities for breast screening. Because of the lack of facilities available under the Health Service, certain private women's organizations such as the Women's National Cancer Control Campaign and the private medical insurance firms, for example the BUPA Medical Centre and the Cavendish Medical Centre, started breast screening in 1970. These services have continued to grow and for a modest cost, facilities for breast screening are now available in the Medical Centres in London, Manchester and Glasgow. There is also a newly opened caravan which can operate entirely independently of electrical supplies and can therefore visit offices, factories and companies bringing this service to the people all over the country. A similar caravan screening service is also available for many of the employees of Marks and Spencer, thus screening for cervical and breast cancer is available for the woman at work and abnormalities found are immediately sent to the general practitioner. The cost is small for the company who offers this to their female employees.

SITE OF SCREENING CLINICS

Ideally to be of the most value to the largest number of patients these clinics should be sited in the general practitioner's surgery. However, the cost of equipment used and the lack of facilities available at the general practitioner's surgery, with the exception of some of the newer health centres, make this not economically viable. Family Planning clinics are fairly universally available and facilities for cervical cytology screening are usually available at these clinics. It is suggested therefore that a simple breast clinical examination should be added to the routine when the patients are seen at these clinics, and then the patients are referred to specialist units for the early diagnosis of breast or gynaecological cancer. The latter units should be sited either in district general hospitals or teaching units and perhaps in the newer oncology centres.

PATIENT SELECTION

The failure of the first cervical cytology clinics was due to two reasons: lack of patient support; and lack of cytologists to read the smears that were taken. There was no general organization of these clinics and many closed following an enthusiastic start through lack of patient support. This has not been the experience with breast cancer screening which seems to attract the patients that may be described as the 'worried well'. Although information is gleaned from the national press or the periodical magazines, it is usually due to a friend's experience at one of these clinics that patients come forward and the numbers at most screening clinics have snowballed very rapidly.

With limited financial resources available screening clinics should perhaps be limited to those patients most at risk for developing breast cancer. However, in practice this is difficult to organize as patients who have once attended a screening clinic continue on an annual basis. High risk patient selection therefore is not easy to practise, especially as the identification of high risk groups may be difficult to define.

Education of the medical and nursing profession is essential and the value of screening clinics has been omitted until very recently from the training courses. This is understandable in the present poor economic state, but not enough emphasis has been placed on the value of a simple but efficient clinical examination so that any potential problem patient could be referred to a specialist unit. This would not fulfil the statistically controlled trial requirements of patients being entirely asymptomatic but clinics would be of greater value to a larger number of people than attempting to repeat the statistically satisfactory trials that have already been reported.

CLINIC ORGANIZATION

Ideally these clinics should be walk-in clinics not requiring appointments. This in practice is not feasible and an appointment system must be kept. Unfortunately, this does not appeal to the lower social classes and so is not an effective method of cervical cancer screening among these classes where cancer is most common. Waiting lists for clinic appointments soon become too long and out of hand and, therefore, it is our usual practice to insist on a doctor's letter of introduction for a new patient. This informs the general practitioner of the patient's visit to the clinic and gives the doctor an opportunity of assessing whether the patient is suitable or not for the local screening programme.

Some centres have a form which is completed by the patient prior to her acceptance at a screening clinic. This has proved unsatisfactory because patients, particularly in the higher social classes, soon realize that they will only be accepted if certain conditions exist and they then readily admit to them if this is the condition of acceptance. For example, a family history of breast cancer is an acknowledged high risk group factor and we have discovered that patients will admit to this when it is not in fact true and is probably in their parents-in-law rather than on their own maternal side.

STAFFING

In years gone by it would be assumed that these types of clinic should only be staffed by members of the medical profession. However, with increasing problems, particularly expense, more and more clinics are using nursing and paramedical staff (Fig. 8.1), and perhaps radiographers to read the chest X-ray and mammogram films. The training of the nurse for breast examination and taking of cervical smears takes in the region of two to three months. Combination of this and Family Planning experience is an advantage and has been found to be extremely satisfactory.

At the Early Diagnostic Unit at The Royal Marsden Hospital voluntary workers help with the organization and the running of the clinic. Patients attending are usually free of symptoms and fit people and so it is quite unnecessary to have highly trained nursing staff used in this type of out-patient clinic. The patients attending need reassurance as they are very anxious people and voluntary workers are ideal for this type of work. Future developments at this clinic may introduce nurses as part of the diagnostic team.

Screening Tests

Screening tests used should be acceptable to the patient and non-invasive. They should be reasonable and they should be cost effective

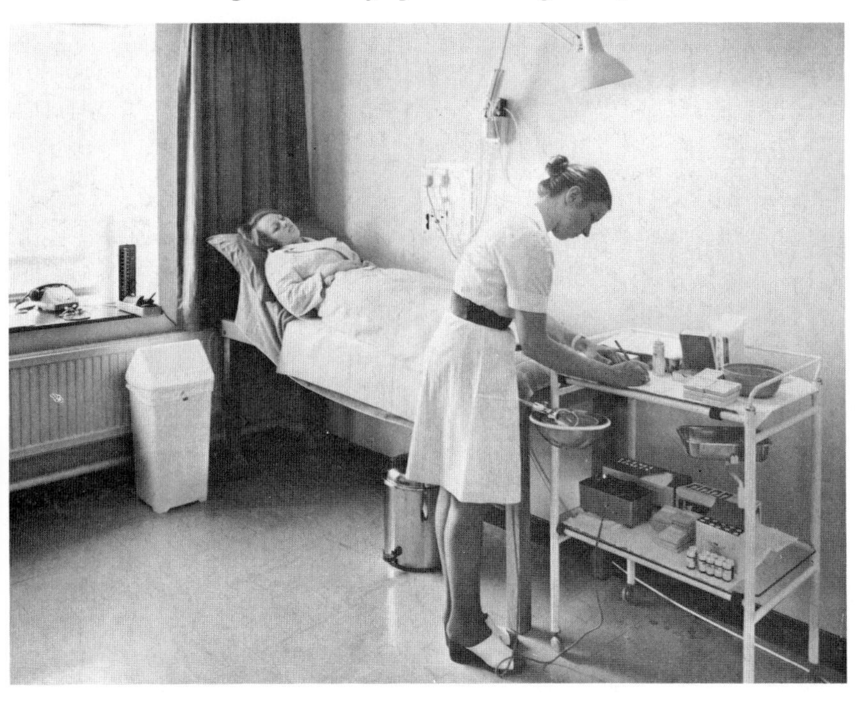

Figure 8.1 Clinical examination by a nurse.

and not time consuming. With reference to breast cancer screening one necessarily thinks of thermography and mammography being the two main tests that are available. Aspiration cytology has recently been added in England, although in Sweden this has been used for many years. A cervical and vaginal cytology technique is described below which is similar to that first used and described by Papanicolaou in 1943. More recently, however, a do-it-yourself Davies kit has been developed and it is particularly useful for those patients living in rural areas, although not in general use in the United Kingdom.

THE TECHNIQUES OF SMEAR TAKING

Several techniques for exradiative cytology are available for obtaining smears from the cervix and vagina. Three types of smear are commonly used and there is a merit in each of them. It is, however, unusual for more than two of these to be used for cancer screening but changes in the sex hormone activity can be shown from the vaginal epithelium scrape smear. It is important to record the type of smear that has been taken and a simple form is used to record the relevant clinical details and menstrual history. One form illustrated here combines the im-

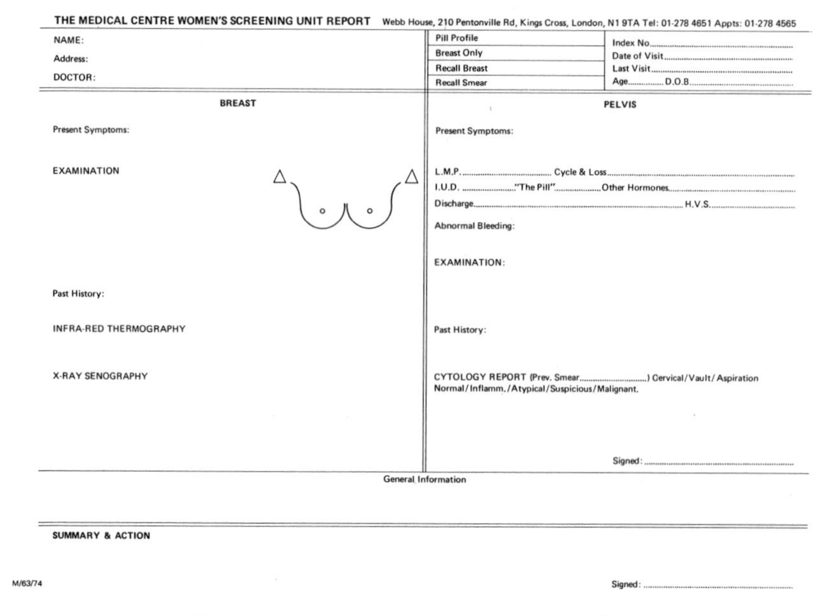
THE MEDICAL CENTRE WOMEN'S SCREENING UNIT REPORT Webb House, 210 Pentonville Rd, Kings Cross, London, N1 9TA Tel: 01-278 4651 Appts: 01-278 4565

NAME:
Address:
DOCTOR:

Pill Profile
Breast Only
Recall Breast
Recall Smear

Index No.
Date of Visit
Last Visit
Age .... D.O.B.

BREAST

Present Symptoms:

EXAMINATION

Past History:

INFRA-RED THERMOGRAPHY

X-RAY SENOGRAPHY

PELVIS

Present Symptoms:

L.M.P. .... Cycle & Loss ....
I.U.D. .... "The Pill" .... Other Hormones ....
Discharge .... H.V.S. ....

Abnormal Bleeding:

EXAMINATION:

Past History:

CYTOLOGY REPORT (Prev. Smear........) Cervical/Vault/Aspiration
Normal/Inflamm./Atypical/Suspicious/Malignant.

Signed: ....

General Information

SUMMARY & ACTION

M/63/74

Signed: ....

Figure 8.2 A woman's screening report form.

portant history details of both the breast and cervical screening and, although complex on first viewing, is quite simple to understand and has the advantage of a summary and action section which is left open to the individual clinician (Fig. 8.2).

THE VAGINAL AND CERVICAL SMEAR

With the patient lying in the lateral or supine position a vaginal speculum is used with good illumination to expose the cervix. A wooden throat spatula, or usually the Ayre spatula specially designed for these smears, is used. Slides are carefully labelled so that vaginal and cervical smears can easily be identified, and the upper third of the lateral vaginal wall is lightly scraped and the material is transferred to a clean glass slide which is immediately fixed with either some form of Cyto-spray or it is dropped into a fixative such as ether–alcohol. A similar smear is taken from the cervix and the ecto-cervix squamo-columnar junction and the material again transferred to a slide which is clearly marked. Care must be taken to include any areas of erosion or abnormal looking areas and a record of clinical findings must be transferred to the form so that any polyps etc. may be recorded. This smear from the cervix is used to detect preclinical carcinoma of the cervix as this is the site of origin of almost all lesions of this type. It is unreliable if endocervical cells are not present. The vaginal scrape smear is the smear of choice for hormonal evaluation but it has little use in the cancer detection process.

VAGINAL ASPIRATION SMEAR

Using the same patient position but no speculum, a bent glass pipette with rubber bulb attached is inserted into the posterior fornix and the aspiration contents are spread on to a slide and fixed as above. This smear is used for detecting carcinomas of the body of the uterus and is often used in combination with a cervical scrape smear in patients over the age of forty who are more likely to have cancer of the body and/or cervix uteri. This method has been modified for the do-it-yourself kits that are available.

Staining of the slides is done in the laboratory and usually the Papanicolaou technique is used. Papanicolaou described five classes for cervical cytology reporting:

Class I	Normal cytology;
Class II	Inflammatory changes and abnormal cells;
Class III	Abnormal cells leading to a suspicion of malignancy;
Class IV	Few malignant cells;
Class V	Many malignant cells.

Quite frequently smears include spermatozoa and are then reported as postcoital. Inflammation is another common finding and two common pathogens are readily identified: *Trichomonas vaginalis* and *Monilia*. Both of these can be readily treated by the practitioner and save the patient local symptoms of vaginal discharge.

Papanicolaou used the term dyskaryosis to describe cells with a normal mature cytoplasm but containing abnormal immature nuclei. These dyskaryotic cells are regarded with suspicion and if abnormal cells persist, a cone biopsy is usually advisable so that areas of early invasive carcinoma can be found. The characteristics of malignant cells are well known but a grossly irregular nuclear membrane is usually seen together with enlargement of the nucleus in relation to the cell volume, the nucleus occupying at least one-third of the cell. Also, there is an irregular chromatin distribution. Other features may exist and the cytoplasm shows some altered staining reaction. (See Chapter 7.)

The results of the cervical and vaginal cytology are always sent to the general practitioner. Where possible it is helpful to alert the patient that all is well and in this way a visit to the general practitioner is avoided.

Information about the time interval before the next smear can also be included in this letter. After two normal smears with a year's gap between, usually a five-year period is recommended before advising further cytology unless symptoms occur earlier.

Breast Screening Tests

CLINICAL AND SELF-EXAMINATION

Facilities for breast cancer screening are at present remarkably few but where nearly 12,000 patients die annually of this condition it is most important that these facilities become more frequently available. In over 80 per cent of cases, breast cancer presents by the patient finding the lump herself. Therefore, the technique and practice of self-examination is very important. Simple leaflets should be available for the patient to take home and instruction given at the visit to the clinic. This will also increase the numbers of interval cancers that present, i.e. those cancers presenting between perhaps annual visits to a screening clinic.

It is helpful to instruct the patient that she should get to know the normal feeling of her own breasts and advise her that this should be carried out on the last day of her period or perhaps the first day of the month if she is not having periods (Fig. 8.3). Films are also available for teaching this self-examination and a model breast with several nodules to show patients what a lump feels like.

A good clinical examination, of course, is important and should always be done before any further test is arranged. Patients should be examined lying supine, the arms extended above the head and a careful examination made of the breasts including the nipple and areola area as well as the axillary tail of the breast. The patient is then asked to turn first on one side, then on the other, keeping the arms extended so that the axillary tail may be further examined. The patient is then asked to sit up in front of a mirror and shown how to examine her breasts and then the axillae and gland areas are felt. The patient is questioned about self-examination and shown how to carry this out if any problem arises. If a localized nodularity or a discrete mass is palpable it is important to record its position and size together with other characteristics immediately. Where possible at this stage, it is not advisable to impart these findings to the patient because unnecessary anxiety arises and the clinical findings are correlated with the other investigations before a diagnosis is made and the patient's next appointment made.

Figure 8.3 Self-examination of the breast:

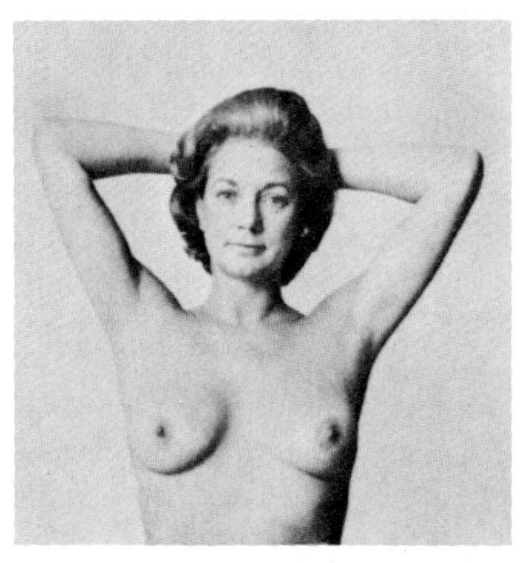

(a) observation in a mirror;

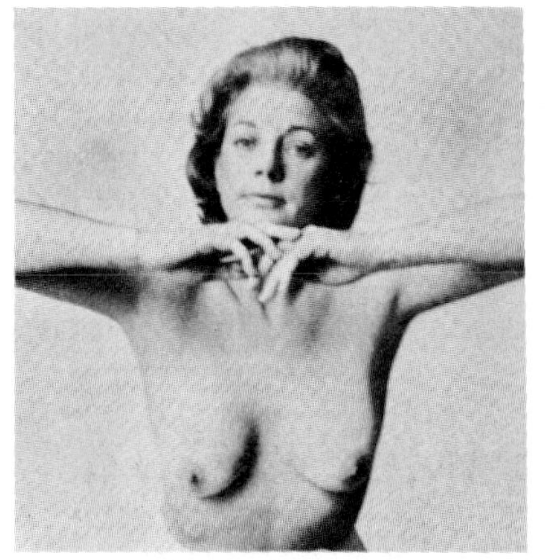

(b) leaning forward to look for dimpling of the skin or retraction of the nipple;

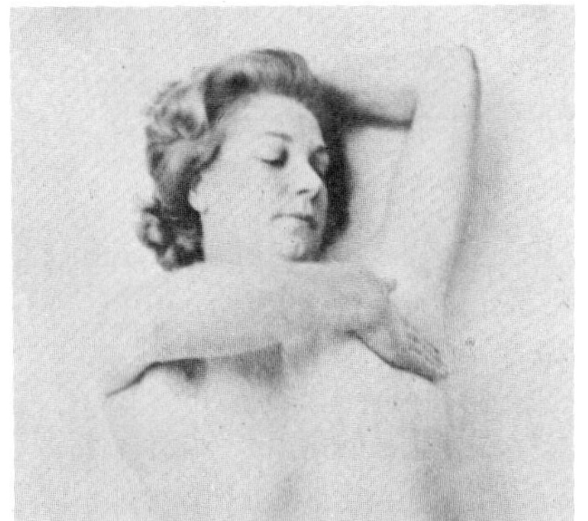

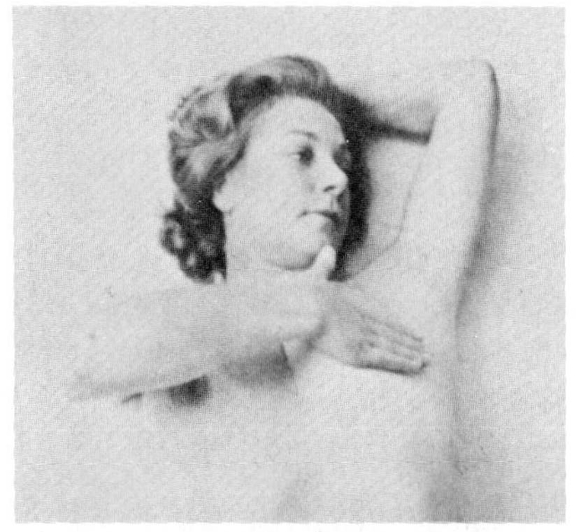

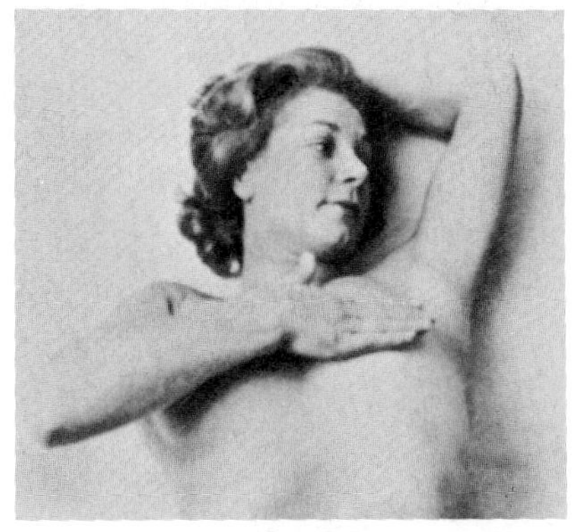

(c) lying down, slide the hand firmly over the breast keeping the fingers stiff like an iron.

THERMOGRAPHY

Thermography has been used in a variety of medical conditions but one of its main contributions has been its use in breast screening clinics. It represents a pictorial recording of infrared radiation emitted from the body, using a heat-sensitive image device, and thus is free of ionizing radiation hazard for the patient. It has been used in the Early Diagnostic Clinic at The Royal Marsden Hospital for over ten years. Although clinical examination remains superior in detection of a breast lump, thermography has been invaluable when used in conjunction with a clinical examination in raising the index of suspicion and thus the diagnostic accuracy in screening clinics. It is an entirely non-invasive technique and an attractive test for the patient, but its limitation is that it is only about 65 per cent accurate in leading to the diagnosis of breast cancer. However, it is constant for a constant hormone state and can be repeatedly used at annual visits.

Theromographic Principles and Technique

Several thermographic scanners are available but the experience described has been gained using the Aga camera 625 or the Rank Thermovision unit. The scanners employ optical mechanical devices to collect the infrared radiation from the body and use a variety of

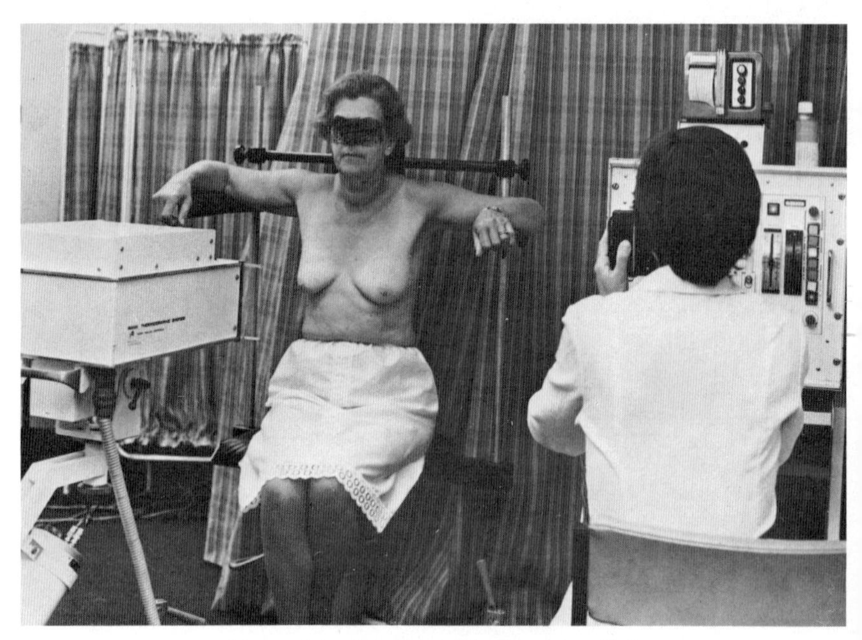

Figure 8.4 The Rank Thermovision Unit.

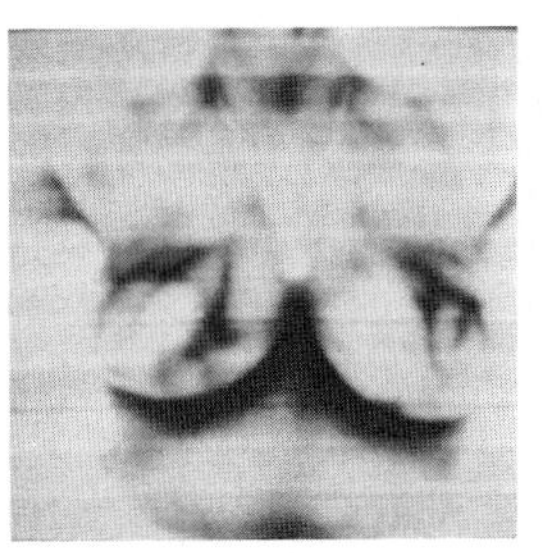

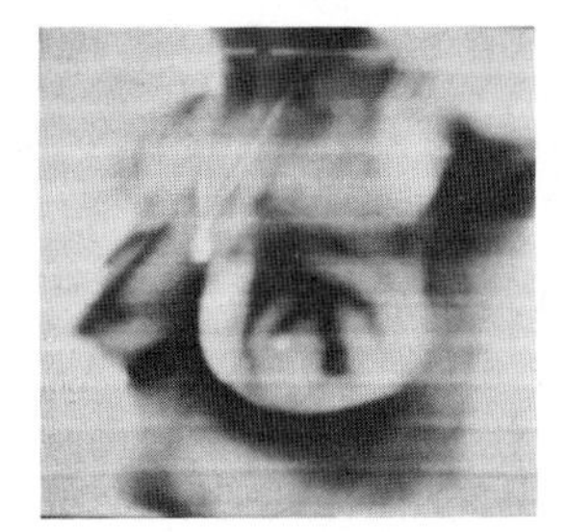

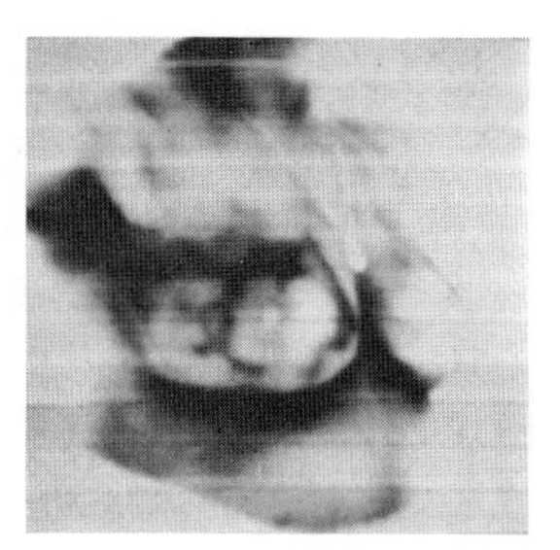

Figure 8.5 Anterior and lateral scans.

detectors with a series of lenses and mirrors to convert this radiant energy into electrical signals. The thermographic image produced may then be viewed on a cathode ray tube and recorded directly on to photographic 35 mm or polaroid film or electrochemical paper. Some twenty years ago Lawson first demonstrated that there is an increased skin temperature over malignant tumours in the female breast when compared with the surrounding skin of between 1–4 °C.

The whole technique is simple and patients are cooled for a minimum of ten minutes in an ambient temperature of 19 °C before the thermograms are recorded. This can be done in a series of air conditioned cooled changing cubicles so that several patients can be cooled at once. Instructions are left in the cubicle telling the patient that they should sit with their arms extended or resting on their heads so that maximum cooling of the axillary tail area can occur, and about fifty patients may be screened in one four-hour session.

As seen in Fig. 8.4, the patient sits in an upright chair with arm supports facing the camera. Three scans are recorded per patient, one anterior and two lateral, as a comparison; the latter may be the most valuable (Fig. 8.5). The use of polaroid films or electrosensitive paper has the added advantage of having scans available for the clinician, if not the thermographer, to see at the time of examination. Some loss in definition occurs and perhaps polaroid film may be more expensive but, again, this depends on the number of patients screened per session.

Normal thermographic patterns with the blacker areas showing thermal activity may be classified into four distinctive pattern types as seen in Fig. 8.6. Unfortunately, about 25 per cent of apparently normal patients produce a mixed pattern type which does not fit into the above classification. It is in this group and those where patches of heat exist normally that errors in reporting accuracy occur. Infrared photography may well help in deciding where the superficial veins lie and is correlated with the thermographic pictures for the venous distribution (Fig. 8.7). Apart from subcutaneous veins, the patterns are also

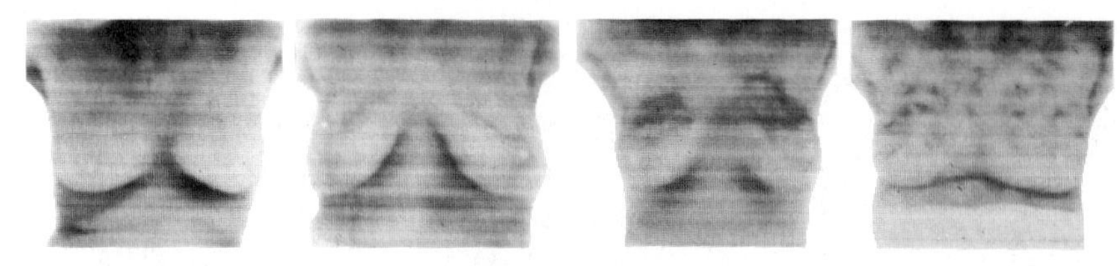

Figure 8.6 Normal thermographic patterns: (a) cold breasts; (b) linear vascularity; (c) generalized vascularity; (d) patchy thermal activity.

altered by recent surgery, changes in hormone state and superficial skin conditions. Pregnancy causes a rapid temperature rise and usually a marked symmetrical vascular pattern; a similar thermogram is shown with lactation (Fig. 8.8). Oral contraceptives can mimic this change, as can the onset of menstruation. After the menopause the temperature is lower, but again the changes are symmetrical.

Temperature differences greater than 1·5 °C are normally considered to be significant and the patterns are classified as abnormal (Fig. 8.9). If no palpable lump is found, the patient could be classified as possibly at risk for developing breast cancer and be screened clinically at regular intervals, and also have X-ray mammography at specified time intervals. The position of thermal activity is also important and activity around the nipple area raises the index of suspicion (Fig. 8.10). Assessment of the thermograms is complex and varies between different centres making correlation between them very difficult. More research is needed into the standardization of techniques and reporting, but the assessment factors used in general are listed below:

1. Thermal asymmetry;
2. Position of asymmetry;
3. Pattern type in relation to age;
4. Maximum temperature difference;
5. Change in thermal pattern between visits.

Results of Thermography

Initially, it was hoped that thermography could be used as a substitute for X-ray mammography, but it soon became apparent that although it was free of radiation hazards it had serious disadvantages in that its accuracy was poor and there were a number of false positives. However, when used with a clinical examination, and preferably preceding it, thermography makes a useful test to raise the index of clinical

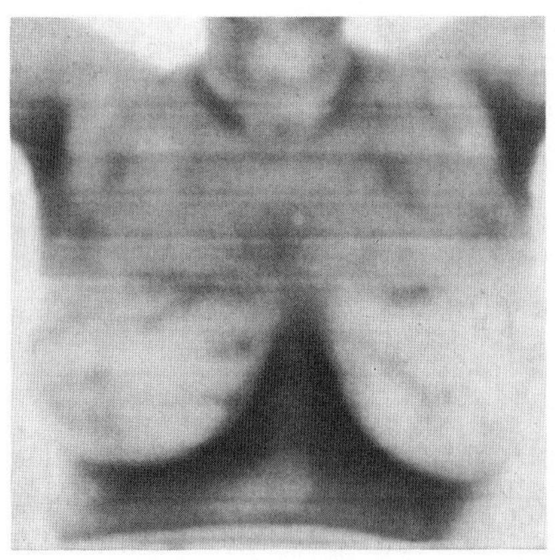

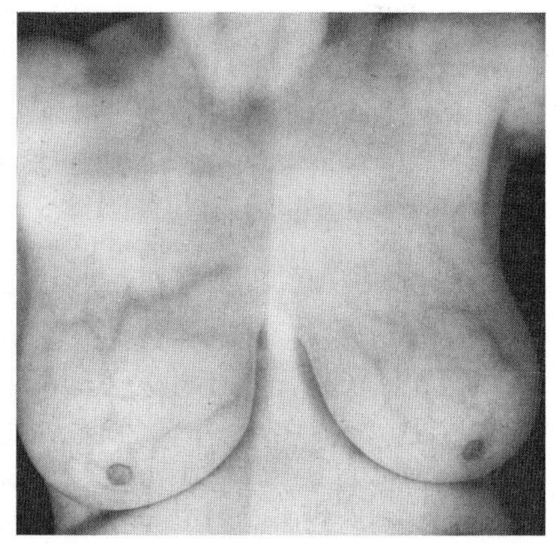

Figure 8.7 Correlation of venous distribution using thermography and infrared photography: (a) thermography; (b) infrared photography.

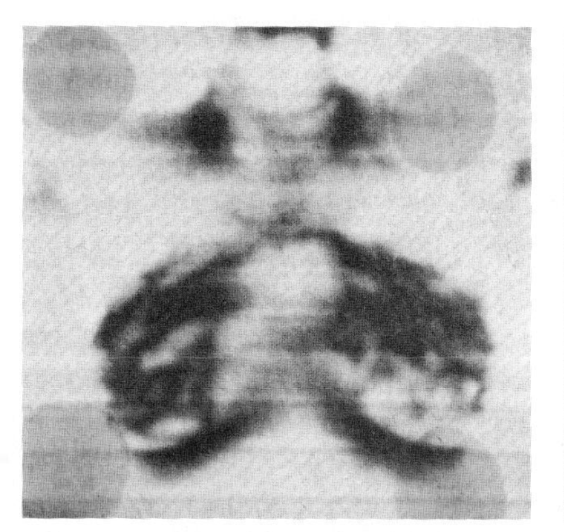

Figure 8.8 Lactating breast thermogram.

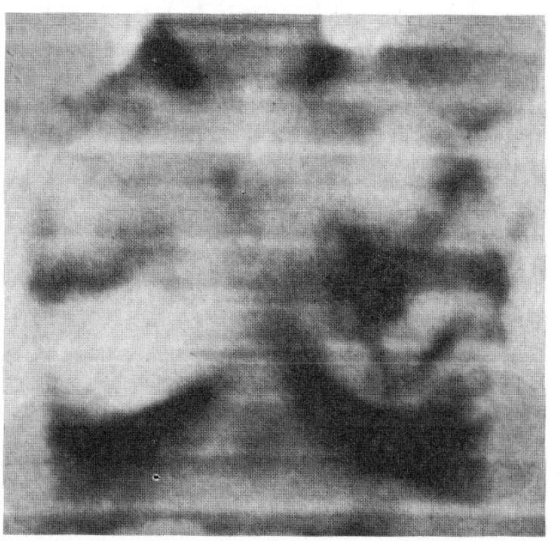

Figure 8.9 Abnormal thermogram left breast.

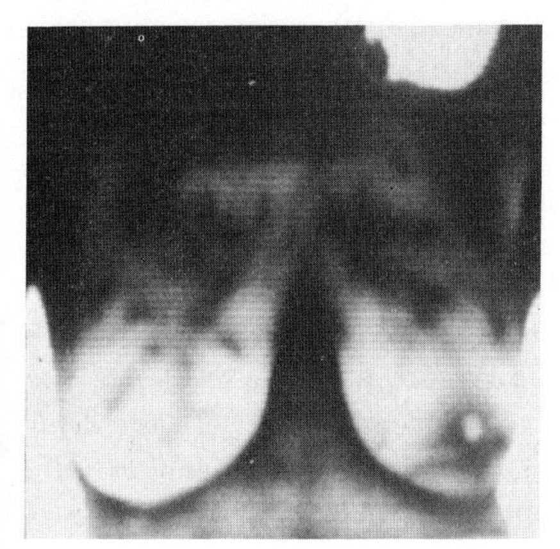

Figure 8.10 Area of thermal activity around left nipple.

suspicion. It is an attractive test for the patient who may feel that clinical examinations are often inadequate and it is a simple technique for either a nurse, technician or radiographer to use. It may also be used to select patients suitable for X-ray mammography, but it must be remembered that clinical examination still remains superior to all techniques available for breast cancer screening, although by using all three modalities the detection rate is increased. About 10 per cent of normal patients have abnormal thermograms and perhaps this group of patients may develop breast cancer in the future. Therefore, these thermograms are used in some centres to show high risk.

In contrast, about 20 per cent of patients with a benign mammary dysplasia are shown to have abnormal thermographic patterns. About 65 per cent of patients found to have cancer have abnormal thermograms and there is some evidence to suggest that thermography may be of value in assessing the prognosis of breast cancer in that a very hot tumour gives a poor prognosis. Although thermography does not always help to distinguish between benign and malignant lumps, it would seem feasible to include thermography in a screening programme for breast cancer providing the disadvantages are recognized and the test is never used alone. The main advantage is to the clinician in that the index of suspicion is raised at the time of examination.

MAMMOGRAPHY

Mammography using conventional film techniques or xeroradiography is now in routine use in many hospitals and screening clinics. Soft tissue X-rays have always been a problem with the low contrast between the various tissues, and specialist equipment is advisable for mammography. Experience described here has been gained from using a senograph machine (Companie Generalie de Radiologie) and a Mammomat unit with a 3-phase generator and a molybdenum rotating anode tube. With the latter equipment the higher output of 250 mA at 28 kV and 100 mA at 50 kV allows a target film distance of 45 cm to be used. Specialist equipment is important because mammography is also difficult because of the anatomy of the breast; the essential technique is to include the part of the breast deep on the chest wall as well as the skin surface. Immobilization of the breast is important with a long exposure time so that movement of the patient is prevented, but with the compression required to produce good pictures this technique can be quite uncomfortable for the patient. Mammography should never be used without a clinical examination of the breast. A problem may well arise in the localization of an impalpable lesion which is revealed by the

X-ray, but on many occasions this may be found on careful re-examination of the breast.

X-ray mammography may or may not be used routinely in screening clinics. In view of the increased density seen in younger patients and the desire to minimize radiation dose to the patient, it is probably best reserved for those patients over the age of forty, especially if it is to be used on an annual visit. However, exceptions occur when definite clinical abnormalities are found or there is a bad family history of cancer of the breast and a base-line X-ray is advisable.

Xeroradiography is based on a photoelectric, rather than a photochemical, imaging process. It is a method of recording the latent image in a beam transmitted through a point by the change of an electrostatic charge in a thin layer of photoconductor such as selenium. Selenium is a good insulator as well and will retain a superficial electric charge for some hours. It becomes electrically conductive when exposed to X-radiation and the surface charge leaks away in the exposed area leaving a charged image of the radiation pattern on the plate. This charged image is developed by exposing it to a powder aerosol in a dark box, for in the light selenium does not act as an insulator. The Rank Xerox system 125 consists of two units – one a conditioner and the other a developer. Each is an independently operated unit from a 13-amp socket. No dark room is required but the units should be situated as near to the X-ray equipment as possible to expedite handling of the plates between the patient and the equipment. The sequence of operation in the 125 system is fully automatic and the plates are not handled at all while in the machines.

When the xerox plate is exposed to X-rays a pattern on discharge corresponding to the various densities in the breast being X-rayed is achieved and a latent image is produced. This is similar to the photochemical effect of X-rays imaging on film emulsion but without the use of silver in any form. With the shortage of silver anticipated in the future and the increase in its price, this is a worthwhile advantage over the use of film. In the developer, after exposure to X-rays, the casette is placed in the machine where the plate is automatically received and transferred to the developer. A cloud of electrically-charged blue powder is sprayed onto the plate and it adheres to the plate in the pattern of discharge that was achieved during the X-ray exposure of the breast so that the latent image is then visible. The plate is then brought into contact with a piece of plastic covered white paper and the powder in it transferred on to the plastic paper. The paper is then heated to fix the image and emerges from a slot at the side of the machine. The whole process takes about ninety seconds. The cost of this process, like

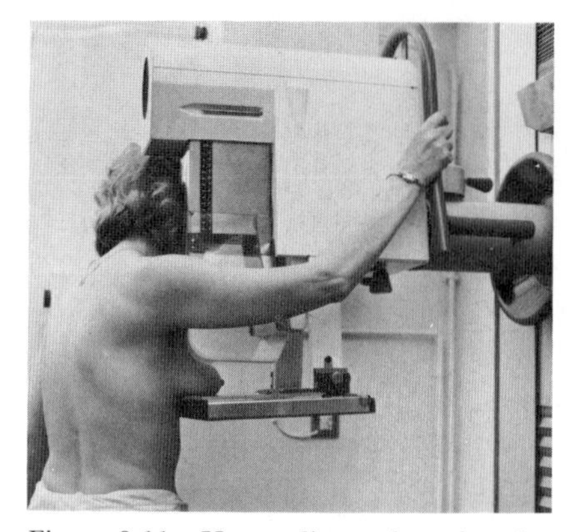

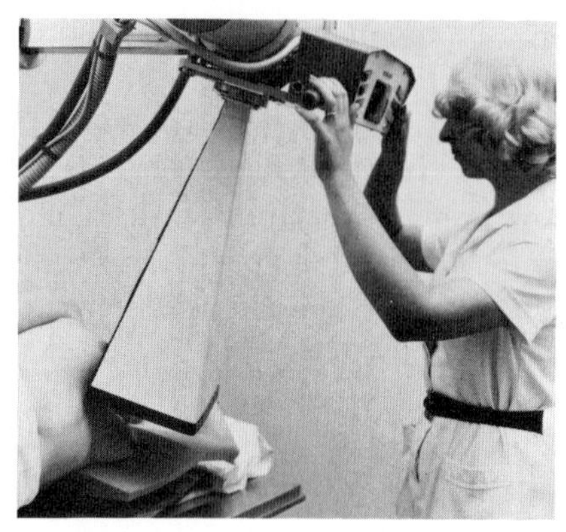

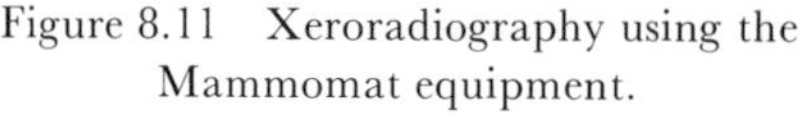

Figure 8.11 Xeroradiography using the Mammomat equipment.

Figure 8.12 The lateral view shown with patient lying down.

the radiation dose, is high. However, changes including display using the negative mode technique (Fig. 8.20), and aluminium filtration have diminished the radiation dose and increased the diagnostic accuracy, especially for screening.

Technique

The technique as in most radiological procedures is vital and approximately ten minutes per patient should be allowed using the specialist X-ray equipment as seen in Fig. 8.11. Usually two views of each breast are obtained and for the cranio-caudal view the patient is generally examined standing and the height of the cassette adjusted to the breast level shown in Fig. 8.11. Particular care is taken to ensure that the whole of the breast is within the radiographic field. The patient leans forward to press her lower rib cage against the edge of the cassette and the breast is so adjusted that the nipple is in profile. Compression has been found to be important in most patients because not only does it reduce the thickness of the breast and shorten the exposure time but it provides better radiographic quality, and also assists materially with immobilization. The cranio-caudal view is seen in Fig. 8.13 and the lateral view in Fig. 8.14(a). The same principles of positioning are applied. Occasionally this view is taken with the patient lying down on the side (Fig. 8.12). This is difficult with the specially designed equipment already described. With these two views localization of a nodule can be limited to a quadrant of the breast. Whether or not the ribs are visible is helpful for the radiologist to make sure that the whole breast is visualized as shown in Fig. 8.14(a). In Fig. 8.14(b) the breast tissue is noted to be very dense. In one centre a single view per breast is taken

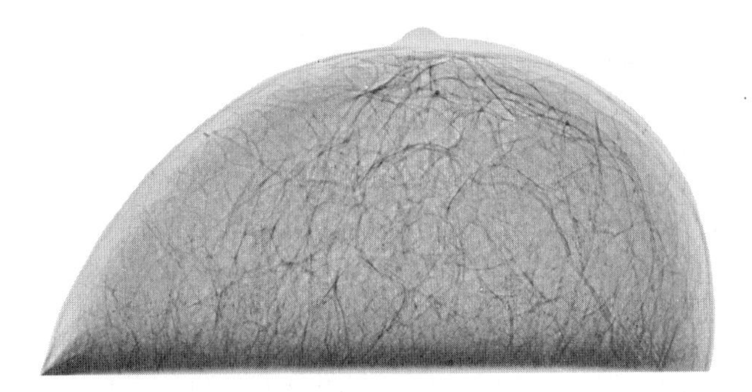

Figure 8.13 A cranio-caudal of a normal breast.

in the oblique projection and this limits radiation dose but necessitates approximately 3 per cent of patients screened to be recalled for further examination. This is particularly difficult for screening patients over wide geographical distribution in a country.

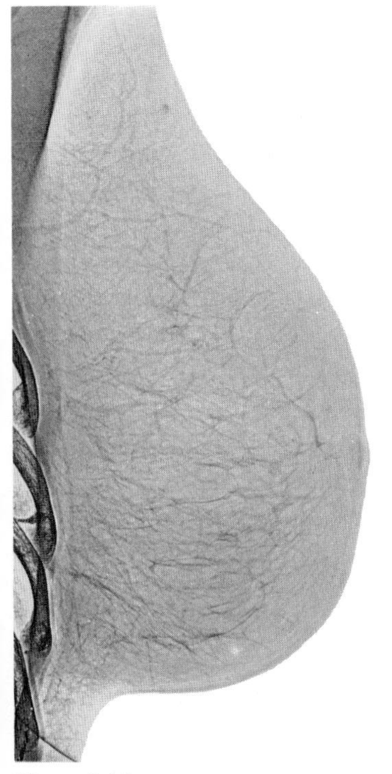

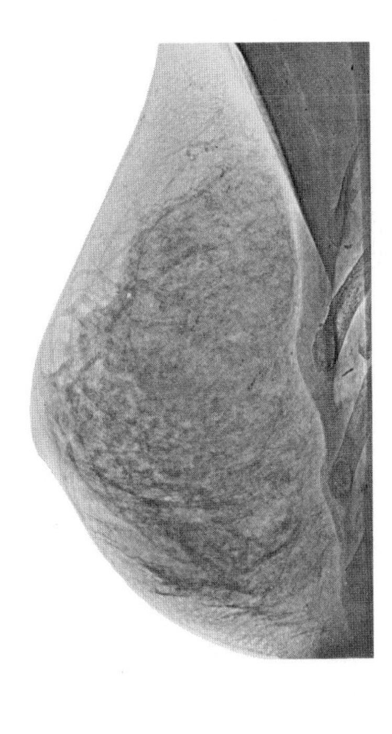

Figure 8.14
(a) A lateral view of a normal breast. (b) a dense breast in a young patient.

Radiographic Features of Cancer of the Breast

These features are listed in Chapter 5 under Mammography. The two most important are, first, opacity which may have an irregular margin (Fig. 8.15) and, second, minute calcifications which may be in groups with or without an accompanying opacity: the characteristics of these small calcifications are important (Fig. 8.16).

An example of a benign and regular opacity which was a cyst is shown in Fig. 8.17 before and after aspiration. A similar opacity is seen in Fig. 8.18 with a single speck of calcification which was a fibro-adenoma. These contrast well with the irregular opacity seen in Fig. 8.19 which also shows some minute calcification and retraction of the nipple. This tumour was found on screening and presented with a clinical examination showing nipple retraction but no obvious mass was palpable until the X-ray had been seen.

Results

The accuracy of mammography is higher than thermography and is in the region of 75 per cent in experienced hands. Difficulties really arise when no mass or density is seen on the X-ray film and there are clusters of minute calcifications which are often seen in association with carcinoma. Methods of localization of these calcifications are available and include injections of methylene blue and the insertion of inactive gold grains prior to biopsy. More recently aspiration cytology under X-ray control has been added to the localization techniques available. An increasing number of breast biopsies are being performed on the basis of abnormal mammograms and problems often arise where there are no definite clinical findings.

Radiation Dose

With improved techniques the dose of radiation should be less than 1 rad per exposure. Purely on theoretical grounds, this dose of radiation could perhaps cause a problem in the future but no definite evidence has been proved so far. Premature distribution of information to the national press has suggested that periodic mammography will produce in the next thirty years or so as many breast cancers as it will save. This report has already discouraged some women from undergoing not only annual screening mammograms but also kept women from having mammography when clinical findings indicated that it was required. It has been estimated that after 100 mammograms per patient you would double the risk of developing breast cancer and then equal the

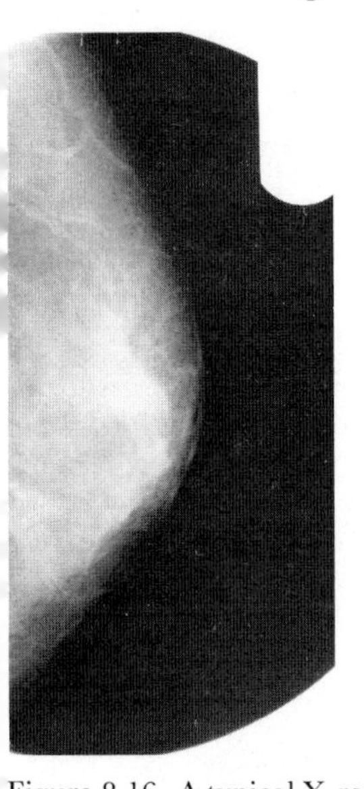

Figure 8.16 A typical X-ray carcinoma with both calcification in and outside the tumour.

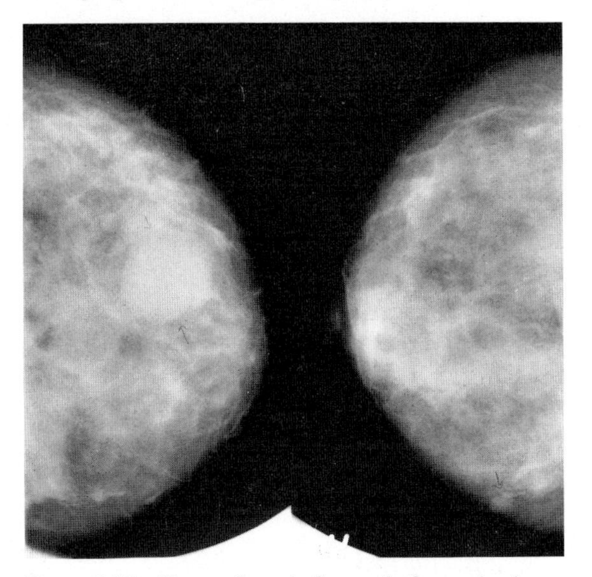

Figure 8.17 X-ray of cyst before and after aspiration.

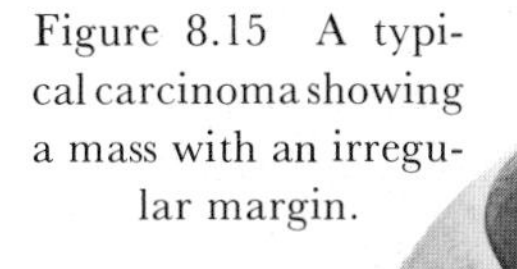

Figure 8.15 A typical carcinoma showing a mass with an irregular margin.

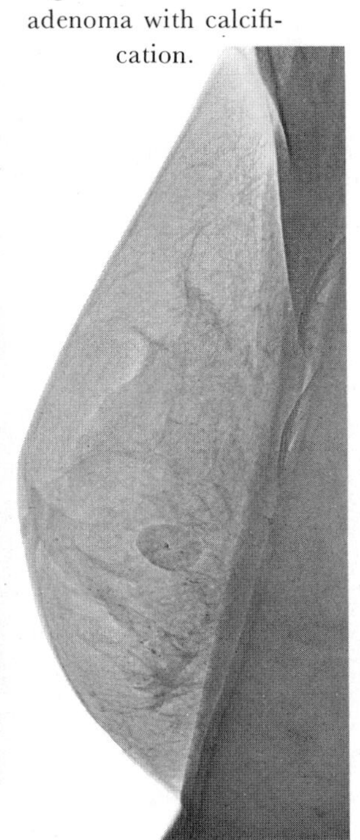

Figure 8.18 A fibroadenoma with calcification.

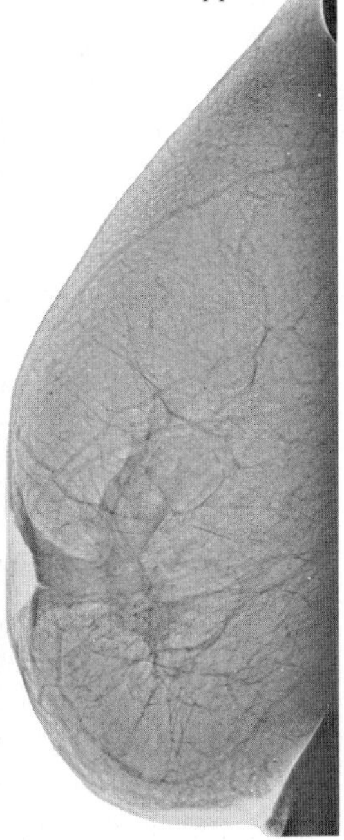

Figure 8.19 A carcinoma lying behind a retracted nipple.

risk in the nulliparous patient, or that you would produce approximately 6 patients with breast cancer per year after 1 million X-rays. However, during that period many hundreds of cancers will have been found that are small enough to have an excellent prognosis and many of these would not have been discovered except by mammography.

When the dose of radiation is kept below 1 rad it can be argued that mammography is safe to use annually but with the thermography and clinical examination, it is probably unnecessary to use this technique at more frequent intervals than perhaps two- or four-yearly unless there is a clinical indication. It is relatively more expensive, although the cost of the equipment is less than thermography. Improvements such as display using the negative mode technique (Fig. 8.20) all contribute to reduction in dose, and these will continue for dose reduction, improved definition and for localization.

ASPIRATION CYTOLOGY

Fine needle aspiration of a breast nodularity or breast nodule is relatively simple and quick to perform. It has been described elsewhere in this book and the trolley that is used is shown in Fig. 8.21. No local anaesthetic is needed and the skin is cleaned with a spirit swab. The needle and syringe is inserted into the area under investigation and the plunger is withdrawn to ensure negative pressure. The needle is withdrawn and reintroduced into the area several times maintaining a negative pressure. The needle is detached from the syringe and about 2 cc of air is introduced into the syringe before it is reattached to the needle and the needle withdrawn. The cells in the needle are spread on to a clean glass labelled slide which may or may not be fixed according to the wish of the cytologist. Aspiration of simple cysts is very rewarding. However, information may now be gleaned using this simple technique for solid tumours so that treatment can be planned adequately before admission.

FREQUENCY OF SCREENING VISITS

The optimum frequency of a patient's visit to a screening clinic whether it be for lung, cervical or breast cancer is not known. Annual visits are probably advisable initially because instruction on self-examination can be checked and encouraged at the patient's second or subsequent visit. At the Early Diagnostic Unit at The Royal Marsden Hospital, it is customary for approximately two-thirds of the patients to return and these patients will then remain on the screening clinic list.

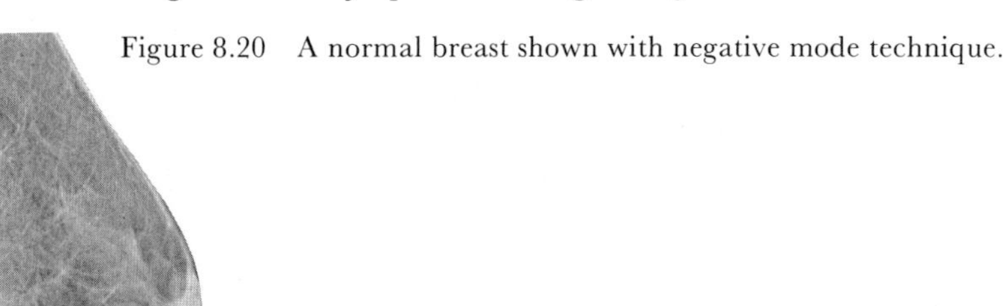

Figure 8.20 A normal breast shown with negative mode technique.

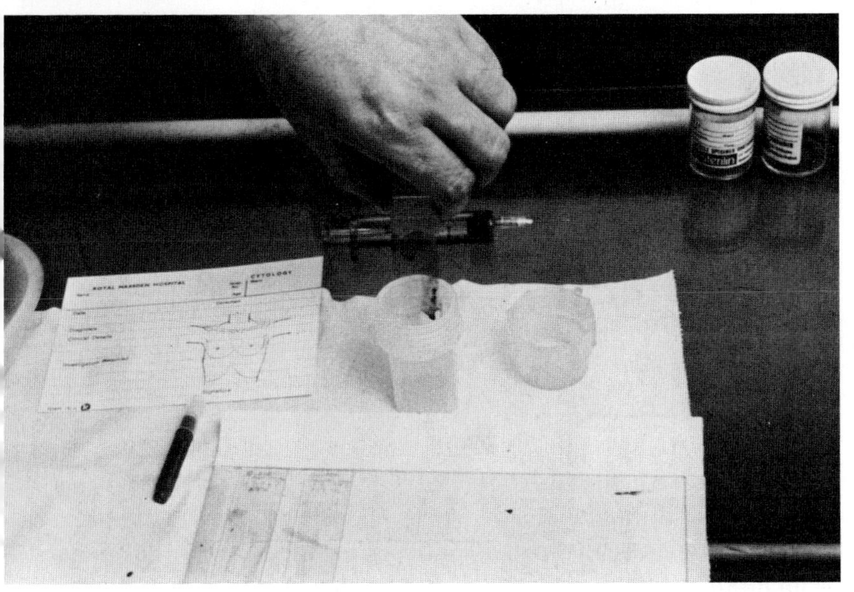

Figure 8.21 Trolley used for breast aspiration cytology.

The Value of Screening

To evaluate screening is very difficult, particularly for malignant disease. Every modality known in medicine is used and therefore great co-operation is involved from all members of the medical and nursing profession. For example, to locate a minute area of suspicious calcification as seen in Fig. 8.22 and specimen X-ray Fig. 8.23, many pathological sections will be cut before it is located by the radiologist and read by the pathologist.

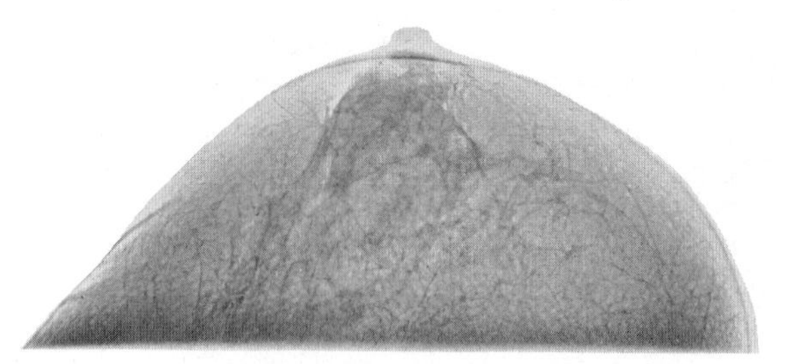

Figure 8.22 Calcification with no associated mass.

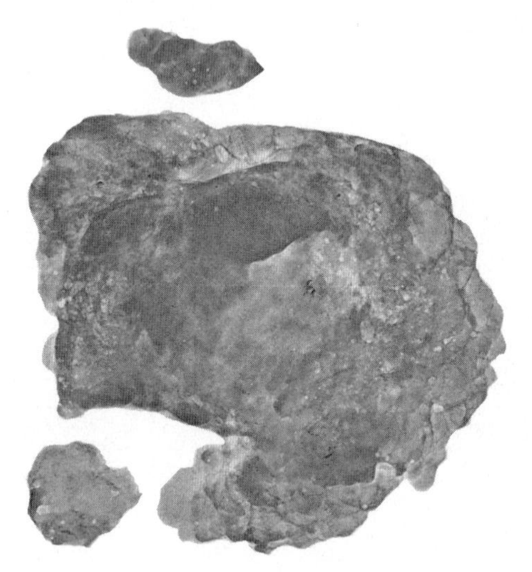

Figure 8.23 Specimen X-ray to localize calcification for the pathologist.

To obtain follow-up information is often very difficult in view of the patients not having their surgery performed where the possible cancer diagnosis was initiated. Where possible, therefore, it is advised that the screening clinic should have a connection with a nearby hospital so as to facilitate early biopsy and evaluate follow-up findings. Not only is interdepartmental co-operation very important but contact with the family, general practitioner, community nursing sister and health visitor are important when a positive finding is suspected.

If there is a possibility of a malignant breast cancer being found it is important to admit the patient for biopsy as soon as possible because all patients attending the screening clinics assume that a biopsy will never happen to them. For breast cancer positive findings occur in just under 1 per cent of 'normal' patients seen, and for cervical cancer in about 0·4 per cent of patients seen. A small yield perhaps but extremely cost effective for the large number of patients who are reassured that they are well following a visit to the screening clinic.

Recently, however, it has been shown that 'prevention was not only better than cure but cheaper'. It is the view of Professor Bagshawe from Charing Cross Hospital that choriocarcinoma is curable. There is a high success rate if the cancer is diagnosed soon after hydatidiform mole following an antecedent pregnancy. Screening of these selected patients can save enormously on cost and benefit the patients. He has demonstrated the cost effectiveness of treating choriocarcinoma at as early a stage as possible as chemotherapy becomes more complex and in-patient costs rise as the prognosis worsens. This gives much encouragement that early diagnosis of presymptomatic cancer is worthwhile and cost effective.

References

Bagshawe, K. D. (1975) *Medical Oncology, Medical Aspects of Malignant Disease.* Blackwell Scientific Publications.

Stoll, Basil (1976) *Risk Factors in Breast Cancer.* William Heinemann Medical Books Ltd.

Skandia International Symposia (1976) *Health Control in Detection of Cancer.*

Strax, Philip (1976) *Mass Screening in Breast Cancer.*

Wachtel, Erica G. (1969) *Exfoliative Cytology in Gynaecological Practice.* Butterworth.

Chapter 9

The Use of Ultrasound in the Diagnosis and Management of Tumours

DAVID OWEN COSGROVE
M.A., B.M., B.Ch., M.R.C.P., M.Sc.
Consultant in Nuclear Medicine
Royal Marsden Hospital
Surrey

Introduction

Ten years ago ultrasonic imaging as a diagnostic tool was regarded as a rather poor relative of radiology, giving less reliable, less useful information which was harder to acquire and so only to be used where X-rays were contraindicated. The restriction of radiology in obstetrics made the development of other techniques urgent and this has become a major application of ultrasound. X-ray toxicity is only rarely a problem in oncological medicine (being confined to the screening of normal populations for early diagnosis of cancer). Had this situation continued there would be no place for a discussion on ultrasound in a volume on oncology.

However, there has been a major change in the basic concepts of clinical ultrasonics which has led to a great increase in its usefulness, essentially because it provides a non-invasive method of examining the soft tissues, which to date remains unique. It is this soft tissue imaging facility, rather than its safety, that has led to an explosive increase in the number of ultrasound machines and diagnostic units. The significance of this may be judged by semi-official estimates that in the next decade, expenditure on new installations is expected to amount to as much as half that made on new radiological equipment (National Science Foundation, 1973), and there is no suggestion that X-ray applications will reduce in extent!

The change in emphasis is the recognition that much valuable information is contained in echoes from the rather poor reflectors that occur within organs. This was lost in the first generation of clinical machines, which gave information only on gross structures such as bone surfaces and major organ boundaries. This has its historical roots in the earliest clinical machines which were closely derived from industrial flaw detectors. These showed up metal fractures by virtue of the fact that they are very powerful sound reflectors. However, this is not a good model for the human body, where the interfaces are mostly much more subtle. It is surprising how much can be gleaned from the images produced by these machines, especially in obstetrics where the surfaces of the foetus in its liquor provide strongly reflecting interfaces. The second generation of machines is designed to detect and process the low level echoes which provide information on the structures within organs at resolutions down to about 1 mm under ideal conditions. They are commonly referred to as grey scale machines; this title only describes the method of display that has been adopted to show the differences between the quiet and the strong echoes. Numerous other advances have been required to allow full realization of the implications of this new concept.

Basic Principles

NATURE OF ULTRASOUND

Sounds are pressure waves, which travel away from the source as alternating zones of compression and rarefaction. The energy contained in these successive zones is transmitted to adjacent particles in the supporting medium, so that there is no bulk movement of particles but only transmission of energy. The process is a three-dimensional version of the radiation of a ripple on the surface of water. It depends on a material conducting medium and thus is unlike electromagnetic radiation (e.g. light, X- and γ-rays). The speed of sound is a characteristic of the medium, being dependent in a rather complex manner on the arrangement of its constituent particles. Roughly speaking it increases with increasing density.

Ultrasound is sound of higher frequency than the upper limit of the audible range (20 kHz, i.e. 20 thousand cycles per second). At frequencies above about 50 kHz it shows two properties that are important in its medical diagnostic applications. First, it will penetrate tissue and, second, it travels in straight lines through homogeneous media. These are two of the fundamental requirements for any imaging tool, together with a third, also possessed by ultrasound, of interacting with tissue.

The property of tissue penetration is frequency dependent. Sound is attenuated approximately logarithmically with frequency, so that about one-third of the incident energy is lost in a centimetre at a frequency of 1 MHz, and twice this at 2 MHz etc. Transferring this to a logarithmic scale there is a loss of 1 dB/cm/MHz. This sets a limit to the upper frequencies that can be employed: in abdominal work 3 MHz is maximal, whereas in the eye up to 20 MHz can be used.

The distribution of the radiated energy from an ultrasound source approximates more and more closely to a pencil beam the higher the frequency used and the larger the sound source. The beam width can be improved further by the use of acoustic lenses, and is an obvious important factor in the ability of the technique to give detailed spatial information.

INTERACTION WITH TISSUE

The fact that ultrasound is attenuated as it penetrates tissue means that its energy is being dissipated by interacting. This takes two forms: that of reflection and that of absorption.

Reflection occurs at interfaces where there is a change in the acoustic impedance, which is the product of sound velocity and density of the medium. Changes in either of these will produce reflection, whose intensity depends on the amount of impedance change. Major velocity changes occur between bone (1,600 mps), soft tissues (1,540 mps) and gases (330 mps), and these are severe enough to produce almost total reflection of the incident sound. Thus such interfaces act as efficient sound mirrors; they are by the same token 'opaque' (or not transonic), and this fact limits the clinical applications of ultrasound in that regions shielded by bone and gas are inaccessible (e.g. the brain and the chest).

For the same reason ultrasound imaging cannot use the silhouette approach, familiar in radiographs, to document the degree of attenuation since there are few regions in the body devoid of intervening bone or gas. Therefore, the echo techniques used in radar and sonar have been adopted. These have the advantage of requiring only a single window to allow examination of large volumes of tissue.

Changes in tissue density are important for the soft tissues, where interfaces between tissue and fluids (e.g. surfaces of blood vessels and amniotic fluid) provide the strong reflections detected by the early diagnostic machines. More subtle density changes occur between cellular and connective tissue (e.g. at vessel walls and in the parenchymal fibrous skeleton within organs) and these probably produce the subtler reflections exploited by the grey scale machines. The whole process is rather similar to the behaviour of visible light passing through heterogeneous but relatively transparent materials, e.g. a glass bottle in a water tank.

Absorption accounts for most of the loss of energy of an incident sound beam. The intimate details of sound energy absorption are poorly understood; they occur as large molecules are vibrated, some of the energy not being transferred in an orderly fashion to the neighbouring molecule. This random vibration is of course heat, and all the incident energy that is not lost as reflected or transmitted sound, finally appears as heat. This mechanism of attenuation is quite unlike that of high energy electromagnetic radiation which deposits most of its energy by causing ionization. Although the total energies absorbed during an ultrasound scan (10^{-2} J/kg) are of the same order as that deposited during a simple radiograph (5×10^{-3} J/kg), the tissue damage is very much less because heat energy is readily dissipated whereas ions initiate damaging chemical reactions.

TOXICITY

Ultrasound at high power intensities is a destructive radiation and this property is used industrially for cleaning and for drilling holes in metals. Damaging effects occur in biological tissues ranging from release of enzymes to disruption of macromolecules and destruction of cell walls. However, these effects only occur at powers of some 10 W/cm^2 (= a pressure of 10 Pa), which is above the maximum peak power employed by pulsed systems; indeed their mean power is about a thousand times lower. At these powers no effects have been observed *in vitro* or *in vivo* in a very comprehensive series of experiments. Similarly, in humans, careful study of infants who have been examined ultrasonically *in utero* failed to show any injurious effects. The lens of the eye is known to be very sensitive to damage by X-irradiation, but again no injury due to ultrasound has been detected (Helman *et al.*, 1970; MacIntosh *et al.*, 1975).

Technology of Ultrasonics

THE TRANSDUCER

Devices that transform energy from one form to another are known as transducers; those for generating ultrasound from electrical signals are piezo-electric crystals. These materials are characterized by very

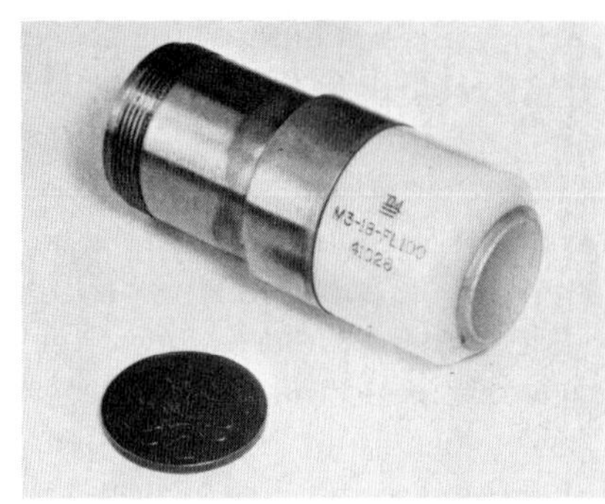

Figure 9.1 Transducer for contact scanning. A 3 MHz transducer focused at 100 mm with an 18 mm aperture (i.e. crystal diameter). The plastic lens (1) on the right covers the front surface of the crystal; the other is in contact with the backing materials in the plastic casing. The metal housing contains the electrical tuning components and the contacts, and can be screwed onto the scanning arm.

asymmetric charge distributions locked within the crystal, originally natural quartz but nowadays usually a ceramic. Application of an electrical charge across the crystal block causes it to change thickness, thus generating a pressure wave, which travels outwards if a conducting medium is present. The effect is similar to a loud-speaker, except that very much higher frequencies can be generated. When stimulated by the application of such a polarizing charge, the crystal will vibrate at a frequency determined by its thickness. Thus it behaves like a bell, where the pitch produced is intrinsic to the instrument, the electrical voltage being analagous to the clapper action (Fig. 9.1).

The piezo-electrical effect is symmetrical in that a mechanical distortion of the crystal will produce a voltage across its electrodes. In this mode the device is a pressure detector; a familiar example is the crystal or ceramic gramophone cartridge. In pulse echo applications the same transducer is used as transmitter and receiver.

The transducer design controls two characteristics of the sound pulse which are very important for the resolution of the scanner. These are the pulse length and the effective beam width. The pulse length is determined by the length of time the crystal continues to ring. Short pulses improve the ability to distinguish successive echoes from closely spaced interfaces, i.e. the axial resolution. The vibration time can be shortened by damping mechanically (heavily absorbent materials are placed on the back of the crystal) and electrically (using resistor and inductor networks). The beam width is largely determined by the frequency of the sound relative to the diameter of the crystal. However, it can be modified by using lenses, usually made of epoxy resin, bonded to the front of the crystal. Such lenses bring the beam to a focus whose position can be selected. The width of the beam at the focus can also be chosen but, unfortunately, if this is made too small then the beam spreads out beyond the focal zone so that the usable region of the beam is restricted. Usually, therefore, weakly focused transducers are chosen for their best compromise of a narrow beam width over a reasonable length.

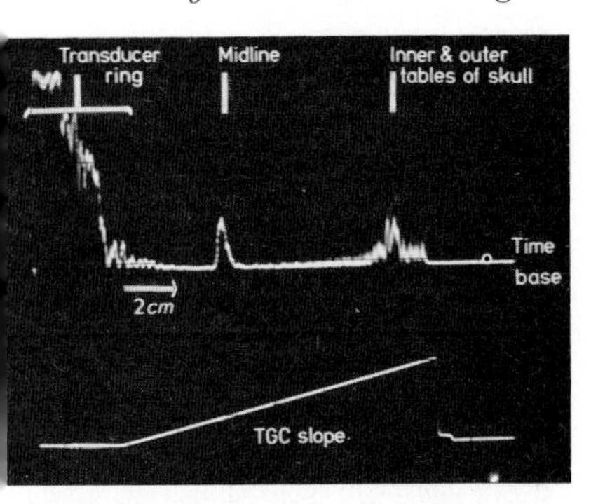

Figure 9.2 'A' scan of the brain. The transducer was coupled to the scalp with acoustic jelly in the above-ear position. The oscilloscope trace is swept from left to right at 1 scale division per 26 microseconds. Upward deflections represent successively echoes returned from the near skull (mingled with the transducer ringing) from the midline structures and from the two tables of the far skull. The TGC slope is also shown.

Improvement in transducer design is one of the major contributing factors to the high resolution of the new generation of ultrasound machines (Kossoff *et al.*, 1964).

THE 'A' SCAN

When a transducer is placed over some part of the body and an ultrasound pulse sent into it, a series of echoes will be returned with varying strengths and varying delays. These generate corresponding voltages in the piezo crystal, which are usually about 1–10 microvolts and appear 13 microseconds after the transmitted pulse for every centimetre of tissue transversed.

$$(1\ \text{s} = 1{,}540\ \text{m, therefore 2 cm, go and return} = 2/1{\cdot}54 \times 10^5 = 13\ \mu\text{s})$$

Following amplification up to about a volt these signals can then drive a cathode ray tube (CRT), sometimes known as an oscilloscope. They are displayed as upward deflections of the spot from its steady left to right sweep (called the 'time base', Fig. 9.2). If the sweep rate is calibrated at 1 cm per 13 microseconds, then a full size trace is produced. Half- and quarter-size displays are simply derived. Similarly, the upward deflections of the spot can be calibrated to show the amplitude of the received echoes. When the sequential echoes are examined, it will be seen that their amplitude reduces rapidly with distance. This is due to the sound being attenuated by the tissue and therefore a compensating amplification must be applied to the signals received to produce a quantitative measure of the real strength of the reflecting interfaces. This is known as the timed gain compensation (TGC, sometimes also called swept gain compensation).

Because the signals so received are displayed as amplitude modulated traces they are known as 'A' scans; the deflections may be translated to

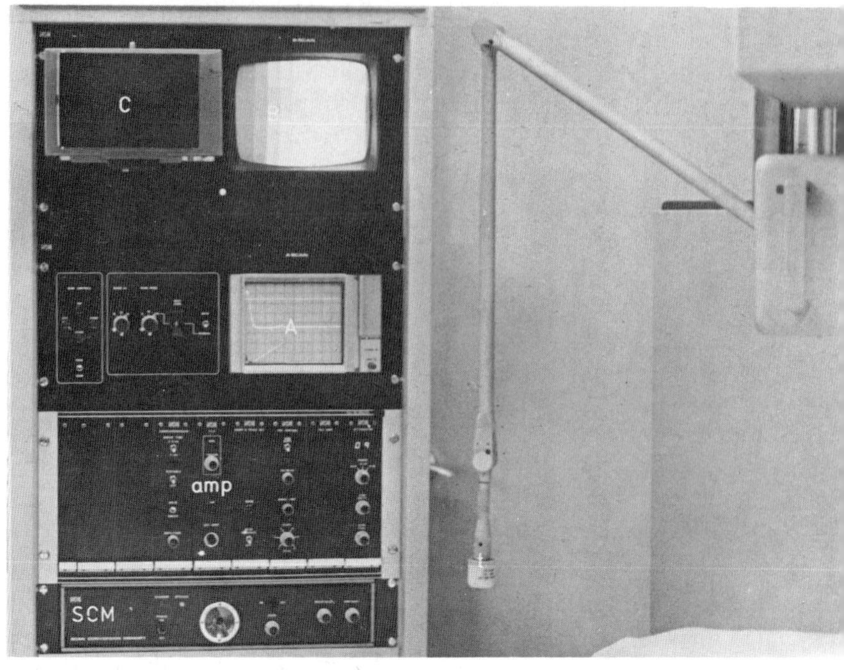

Figure 9.3 A modern 'B' scanner. The transducer is mounted on the flexible arm. Signals are fed to the amplifier system (amp) displayed on the 'A' scan CRT (A) and stored in the scan converter memory (SCM) from which the completed tomogram is read off onto the monitor (B) on which a grey tone sequence was being displayed. The camera (C) photographs a slave oscilloscope carrying the same image as the monitor.

spots whose brightness is proportional to the signal intensity. They are one dimensional, showing range only, so they can be used as a distance measuring device, e.g. for assessing the position of the brain midline structures. The accuracy of these range measurements is very high, 0·1 mm being readily achieved; this is the most accurate measurement produced by any ultrasonic device.

ULTRASOUND TOMOGRAMS

The most important development of the one-dimensional 'A' scans has been the coupling of the transducer to a mechanism for signalling its position to a monitor oscilloscope. This is done by confining the transducer in one plane on an articulated arm to which is attached a set of potentiometers. These produce voltage changes related to the transducer position, which are analysed, usually by a small analogue computer, to generate signals fed to the X and Y plates of the oscilloscope. In this way the start position of the spot can be made to correspond

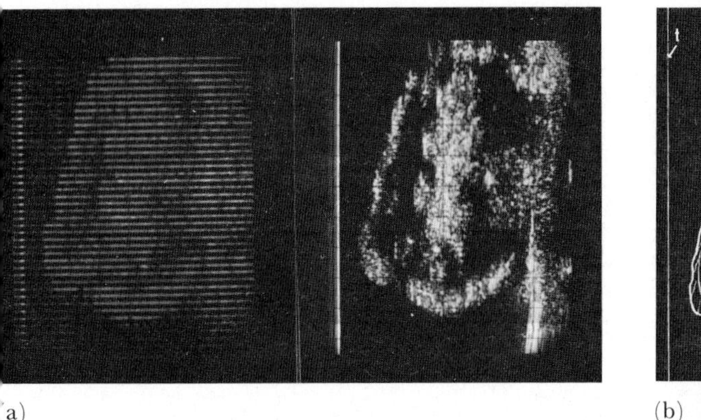

(a)

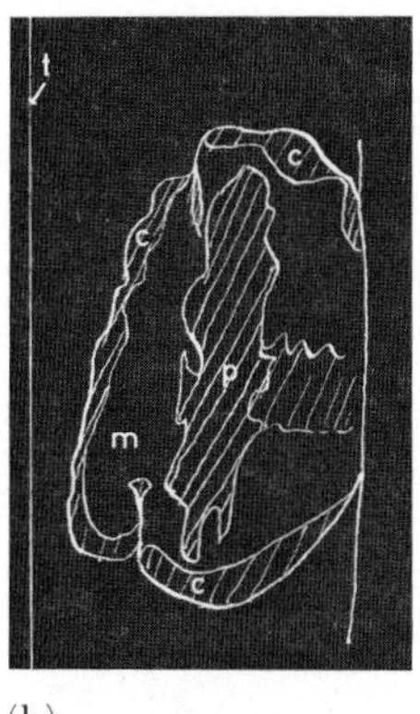

(b)

Figure 9.4 Composition of an ultrasound tomogram. (a) Each line is a brightness modulated one-dimensional trace of the echoes at one location analogous to the 'A' scan of Fig. 9.3. Between each pulse the transducer was moved a small step and the spot position on the oscilloscope was moved with it. The overall is a crude image of a 45-line tomogram through an ox kidney, seen with greater fidelity on the 3,000-line picture (b) (t = transducer ring, c = cortex with lobulations, m = medulla, p = pelvis).

to that of the crystal. Additional angular information on the direction in which the transducer is pointing is obtained from a rotation potentiometer attached to the transducer pivot. This is used to direct the timed traverse (time base) of the spot across the CRT face in an appropriate direction (Fig. 9.3).

Now as the transducer is swept across the target area, the CRT will build up a set of bright spots which are precisely congruous with the echoing interfaces in the organ being scanned (Fig. 9.4).

With this technique tomographic pictures of the echoes from internal organs can be made. It was first applied to the gravid uterus, which is a relatively simple target, with strongly reflecting interfaces. Since it is directional specular echoes that are detected, the sound beam must be directed perpendicularly to the curved surfaces. This means that to obtain complete outlines, a series of views of different orientation have to be combined on a single image. This technique is known as compounding. It allows a complete representation of the curved surfaces that are the rule anatomically, but because of patient movement (pulsations etc.) precise registration of echoes is not possible and the resolution suffers. Where the scattered echoes are important, as in most soft tissue studies, single sweeps are used to obtain the best resolution; these may be arciform (sectors) or linear. Amplification and time gain compensation must be applied as for the A-scans, but a new problem arises in handling the wide dynamic range of the received echoes: the intensity of a strong superficial echo may be as much as a million times

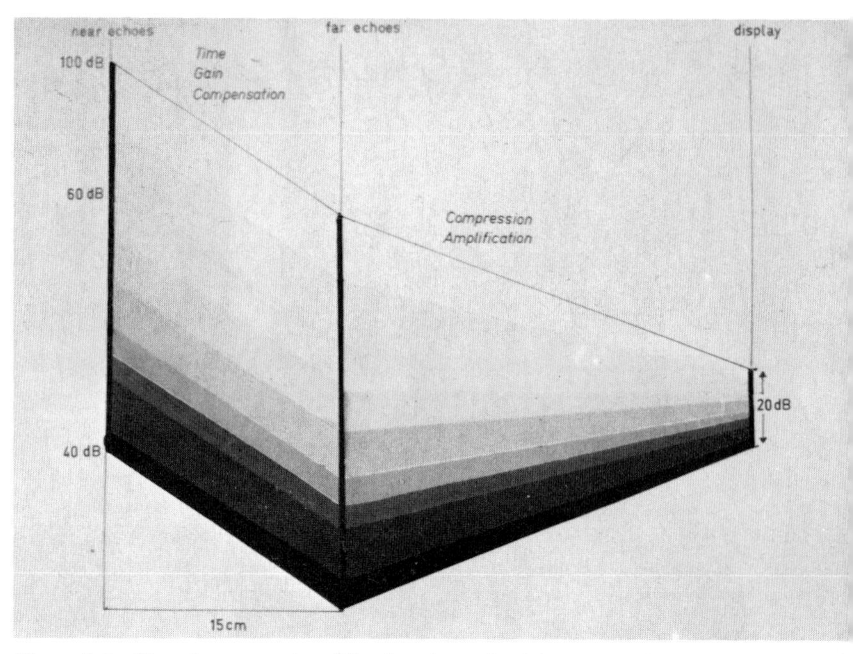

Figure 9.5 Signal compression. The signals received from superficial structures in this example have an intensity range of 60 dB; those from structures at 15 cm depth have the same range, but since these have been attenuated by the intervening tissue, they are some 40 dB reduced in intensity. This gives an overall range of 100 dB (i.e. 100,000 to one ratio!). The TGC compensates for the attenuation but 60 dB must then be compressed to the 10–20 dB that can be displayed on film or television systems.

as strong as the weakest important echoes from an interface at 20 cm depth ($1:10^6$ = 120 dB). Of this some 60 dB is due to attenuation and is corrected by the TGC, but the remainder is the variation in reflectivity of the interfaces, the lower levels being scattered echoes from the parenchyma and the intense echoes arising from the strong specular reflectors, such as bone interfaces or the diaphragm.

This sort of intensity range is enormous, and represents the extremes of the capability of the human eye including its great ability to adapt to light and dark conditions. It vastly exceeds the capabilities of any of the known display systems. Polaroid film for example gives some eight useful levels of grey, i.e. a 16 dB range; transparent film is rather better at 20 dB, and television monitors are capable of 25 dB range.

Obviously massive compression of the signals is required if they are to be displayed simultaneously, as is highly desirable. The most useful method is to apply progressive compression so that the strongest signals are most strongly compressed and the weakest signals, from the poor scatterers of the parenchyma, are allowed to show fully. This has the effect of giving predominance to the weak echoes that are of major interest in soft tissue studies, but it introduces an important degree of distortion into the data. The precise compression pattern is rather arbitrary, and accounts for some of the striking difference in the image quality produced by different makes of grey scale machine (Fig. 9.5). It also affects the ability of a scanner to distinguish some of the subtle changes due to lesions, where a 2 dB alteration in echo intensity may be all that is observed, e.g. in metastases to the liver.

The necessity for displaying a range of grey tones to represent intensity raises another technical problem, that of the display CRT. Conventional, so-called 'bistable' or black and white ultrasonograms are collected onto a storage CRT as the scan is made. These devices hold data as a charge pattern on a matrix of capacitors behind the phosphor of the screen. The charge pattern is written by the normal electron gun, but then the whole screen is flooded with electrons from a second, non-focused, low intensity gun. The information previously stored is thus displayed and held for as long as the charge pattern persists, which may be many hours. The stored image is photographed if a permanent copy is needed.

Storage CRTs are on-off devices, that is they only produce black and white images. Normal CRTs will show degrees of saturation, i.e. greys, just as on a standard television screen, by modulation of the electron beam intensity, but they cannot store data. The dilemma can be solved by using a standard monitor CRT and exposing the recording film throughout the scan time. This has the effect of relieving the CRT of the need for a memory (now taken over by the film) and thus allows its intensity modulation capability to be exploited to produce the required grey scale.

This method, called the open shutter method, is technically simple but in practice rather difficult to use. A new device, the scan converter memory, originally used in television technology for changing television line frequencies, has found application in grey scale ultrasound machines. It operates by storing the accumulated data on a high resolution matrix of capacitors in a vacuum tube that is rather similar to a television camera, except that the information is written in with an electron gun. The memory is in analogue form, i.e. the stored charge changes directly in proportion to the voltage applied to the writing electron gun. The stored data can be read out using another electron beam; it then appears as fluctuating voltages exactly as in a television signal and can be viewed on a standard television monitor. The system is, in effect, a closed circuit television, save that the camera is driven by the ultrasound amplifier and, in addition, it memorizes the data of a scan. In practice this makes the taking of scans much simpler and the scan converter has now almost replaced the open shutter technique (Fig. 9.2).

Another approach to the display of wide amplitude ranges is to convert them to some form of colour display where colours represent sound intensity levels. These have the potential of showing wide dynamic ranges, but in practice have proved disappointing so far.

REAL TIME IMAGING

Real time scanners provide moving two-dimensional images by arranging that the scan is repeated rapidly enough to produce an image free from flicker, i.e. twenty-five times a second. The same principle is used in cinematography and in television. Three approaches have been used.

(*a*) *Mechanical*

A single transducer is moved either as an oscillation or as a continuous rotation. This has been very effective in the eye where a limited field is to be viewed. In other areas these devices tend to be rather clumsy and it has been difficult to design transducers giving adequate resolution.

(*b*) *Multi Element Linear Array*

In this approach several small (*c*. 2 mm) elements are mounted in line to form a transducer 10–20 cm long. The elements are fired in turn so that each produces a single line on a television display to give a rectangular image. This method dispenses with any position sensing apparatus so that the whole device becomes compact and quite portable. However, the resolution is severely limited especially laterally, due to the spacing of the elements (this determines the number of lines per centimetre on the image) and to difficulties in focusing. In addition the whole transducer head is clumsy in use making it difficult to image some of the rather inaccessible but important regions of the abdomen, e.g. the pelvis.

(*c*) *Phased Arrays*

These also employ a linear array of transducers but they are smaller and closely packed into a unit some 4–6 cm long. The elements are fired in groups with accurate delays between them, so that predetermined interference patterns are produced in the resultant sound wave.

Correctly chosen, this produces a narrow focused beam which can be directed at an angle from the ends of the scanning head. This angle may then be swept in an arc to produce a sector scan entirely by electronic means. This method is extremely attractive in principle, obviating all of the problems of the simpler approaches, but it requires rather complicated electronic processes incorporating accurate delay lines, so that to date its theoretical promise has not been realized (Thurstone and Ramm, 1974).

These real time devices will certainly aid the interpretative problems that result from the tomographic nature of the conventional scans, and offer very exciting prospects. Although as yet they do not rival high quality section scanners in resolution, in practice psychological mechanisms relying on the movement displayed increase their diagnostic value so that structures that are readily identified on the real time display may be invisible on the still photographs. This effect is familiar in angiography.

OTHER TYPES OF SIGNAL PROCESSING

Holography is an optical system in which coherent light from a laser is caused to reconstruct wave fronts in a manner that exactly reproduces the optical information from the original object. It produces striking true three-dimensional images in which enormous quantities of data can be presented. Since the organs examined ultrasonically are three dimensional and the amount of data returned is high, the idea of presenting this as holograms is attractive. There are, unfortunately, serious technical and practical difficulties in applying this principle even to small tissue volumes, and the approach seems unlikely to prove valuable in its present form.

The Doppler principle in which the frequency of sound from a moving object is changed according to the direction and rate of movement, has long been used in ultrasonics to detect physiological movements. At present it would seem to have no particular application in oncology, but is mentioned for completeness and because new types of Doppler devices are likely to appear which produce tomograms, and these might have application in this field.

The data contained in echoes from tissue are very complex; current approaches make use only of position and amplitude data. Numerous other changes are imposed on the sound pulse such as velocity changes, phase and frequency shifts, which might contain valuable data. Their extraction and processing require computers at present, so this is a research field, but clinically useful results are anticipated.

Obtaining and Interpreting Scans

'A' SCANS

The application of 'A' scanning for locating the cerebral midline structures is the only one of importance in oncology. The technique requires no patient preparation. A transonic jelly is applied to the scalp above the ear to provide a coupling medium. The transducer is then brought into contact with this jelly, when two groups of echoes are usually seen without further adjustment (Fig. 9.3). The initial group is from the scalp and skull bones at the transducer and the second is the far side of the skull. Subtle adjustment to the angle and position of the transducer are made until the midline echo is detected; this is then photographed and the procedure repeated from the other side of the head. The two midlines are measured back from the opposite inner table of the skull and should lie within 2 mm of each other. Finding the correct position from this may be time consuming since there is only a very restricted window that will align the midline and the far skull planes at right angles to the sound beam.

A development of the method employs a pair of transducers which are used and recorded simultaneously. This eases the location of the midline structures. A further sophistication is offered by the Computer Midliner, a device that senses the collection of an adequate far skull reflection and then samples the major echo about the midline. A large number of readings can be produced rapidly and then plotted as a histogram.

SECTION SCANNING

Water-bath Scanning

When the surface anatomy of the organ under study renders skin contact difficult, coupling of the transducer may be made using a water-bath. Several approaches are possible, the commonest being to use an appropriately shaped plastic bag filled with water. This is then moulded to the skin, with a film of oil to provide contact. The transducer may then be moved in the water either by hand or mechanically. The water bag is rather clumsy in use, but allows organs such as the eye and the breast to be scanned.

Contact Scanning

The transducer is applied directly to the skin with a film of oil as a coupling medium. When high intensity specular echoes are of interest

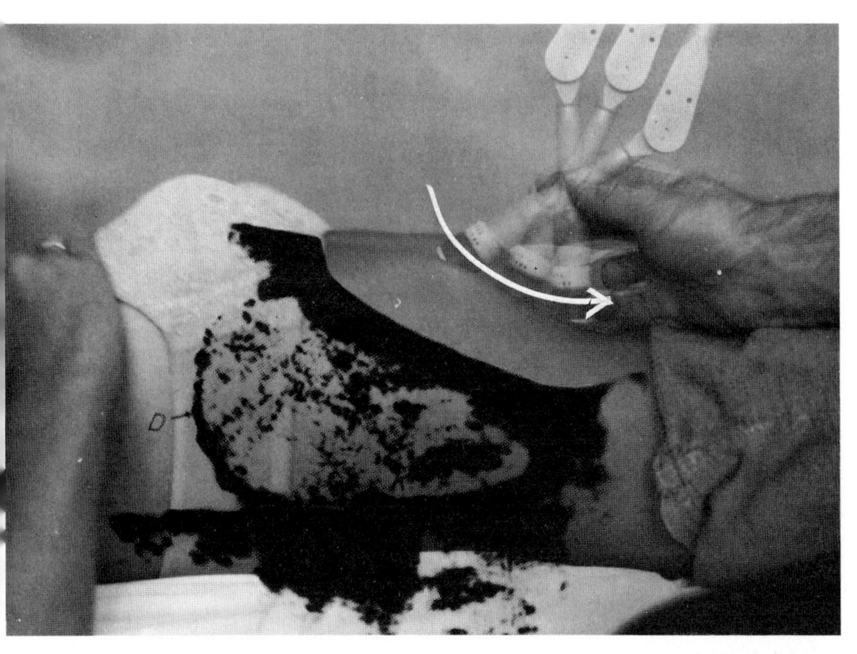

Figure 9.6 Sector scanning of the liver. The transducer is swept in an arc under the costal margin to produce a longitudinal section.

the transducer must be rocked to and fro while it is passed over the region of interest, to maximize the number of times the sound beam strikes the interface at right angles. This technique is known as compound scanning (Figs. 9.16(b), 9.19(b)) and produces good outlines of anatomical structures. However, any errors in the position sensing apparatus blur the image and this is worsened by any movement of the patient during the few seconds taken to make the scan (even if gross movement can be eliminated vascular pulsation inevitably persists). Thus compounding is of most value where scans are required to show organ outlines without internal details.

Simple scanning consists of passing the transducer in a single sweep, e.g. the sector method used to examine the liver (Fig. 9.6). With this technique and high sensitivity machines the dependence upon the angle of incidence of the sound beam is reduced, but nonetheless even strongly reflecting interfaces may produce no echoes if they lie parallel to the sound beam. This may make for difficulties in interpretation, when for example it is difficult to be sure of the limits of a mass adjacent to the liver. Simple scans allow fullest exploitation of fine structure echoes since there is effectively no movement of the interfaces during an examination. Often a combination of compound and sector scanning is required to extract the maximum information from an investigation. In each case as with the water-bath scan a set of tomograms at close intervals is made and the interpretation will depend on viewing these as a group together.

PREPARATION OF THE PATIENT

It is one of the advantages of ultrasound in diagnosis that very little patient preparation is required. There is no discomfort due to scanning unless the very light pressure required is painful as may occur with recent wounds or over abscesses. Sedation is only needed where the patient is extremely uncooperative as may occur occasionally with children, and on the other hand there is no difficulty in scanning patients who are comatose.

For pelvic examinations the bladder must be full, and the rectum and colon empty, so that an aperient the day before is useful together with instruction to the patient to attend with a full bladder. A full examination of the gall bladder includes an estimate of the organ's contractility. An overnight fast ensures that the gall bladder is full and then a fatty meal may be given to stimulate contraction.

In general anatomical examinations colonic gas is a major problem. Usually repeated attempts over a few hours will allow the whole abdomen to be examined, but where a patient is very gassy, aperients or a colonic washout may be helpful.

For ophthalmic examinations the best results are obtained using a plastic water-bag with a cut-out for the eye, the edge being stuck down to the periorbital skin using collodion glue. Where this technique is used, the cornea must be anaesthetized with a few drops of local anaesthetic so that the patient can hold his eye open.

Recent skin wounds make examination difficult because contact is impossible. Very often also the associated oedema produces transonic regions in the subcutaneous tissue which are difficult to interpret. Adherent colostomy bags are an insuperable ultrasonic barrier as are wound dressings and drains.

PRINCIPLES AND PITFALLS IN INTERPRETATION

Apart from the difficulties of taking good scans, a problem that is eased by the facilities of modern machines, the most difficult aspect of interpretation is the confusing anatomical projections which are due to the tomographic nature of the images. The anatomy that appears is quite dissimilar to that conventionally taught, and since each slice is only about 3 mm thick, the relations of vessels and organs is often unexpected and not understandable on one view. For this reason a series of closely spaced views is mandatory and as many as a dozen may be required to cover the abdomen in longitudinal section. In addition, views in two planes at right angles to each other are often needed to clarify confusing images. People learning ultrasonics are usually surprised at the degree of normal variation that must be allowed for, as well as the magnitude of physiological changes, e.g. the diameter of major abdominal vessels may double during a Valsalva manoeuvre.

Knowledge of the suspected abnormalities will allow concentration on the relevant organs. This is important in a technique where the results are proportional to the degree of effort devoted to the examination. An ultrasound investigation is often rather like an extended clinical examination.

Certain machine variables are important in obtaining adequate scans. Obviously an appropriate transducer and correct amplifier settings must be used, but the TGC setting is most critical. If miss-set this may produce artefacts that simulate lesions.

Most of the information on an ultrasound tomogram relates to the intensity of the echoes returned, i.e. the echogenicity of a region; most photographs record the highest intensity echoes as whitest with the darker grey tones for the weaker echoes, but occasionally illustrations will be encountered where this is reversed. The degree of compression required (Fig. 9.5) to produce the grey scale image should always be remembered; effectively much less compression is present on the 'A' scan trace and regions of interest should always be inspected on the 'A' trace. This will give a clearer indication of the level of echoes present. Even on the 'A' scan, however, there are often difficulties in deciding for certain whether a region is truly echo free, especially when small regions are being looked at. This is due to spurious signals from effects such as persistent ringing of the crystal after receipt of a strong echo (e.g. from the surface of a cyst), and to multiple reflections producing repeat signals at regular intervals (e.g. between near and far walls of a cyst or between the transducer and a strong reflector, the sound reverberating to and fro). Such artefacts are often very sensitive to the precise angle and position of the transducer so that changing transducer position will often eliminate or intensify artefacts but leave the true echoes relatively unaffected. These problems are more troublesome with grey scale machines, due to their greater sensitivity.

A certain amount of information is available on a grey scale scan on the rate of attenuation of the sound beam by a particular region of tissue. This appears because the TGC amplifier is set to give an attenuation correction suitable for the average of the tissue traversed. Where the actual attenuation rate diverges from this, then the signals from beyond that region will be low or high in level compared to adjacent tissue, depending upon whether the region has a higher or a lower attenuation rate. The former effect is known as an acoustic shadow, and is commonly seen behind regions of gas and calcified or heavily fibrotic tissue. The reverse effect, a brightup or flare, is seen beyond fluid regions such as the normal gall bladder. In general it may be taken as a fair working rule that the attenuation rate is related to the tissue protein content, so that cystic regions filled for example with necrotic tissue debris will probably not show the TGC induced flare. Essentially the effect relates to the degree of transonicity of the tissue. This should not be confused with the degree of echogenicity which relates to the number and nature of interfaces in the tissue.

Applications of Ultrasound in Oncology

BRAIN

The skull bones prevent useful two-dimensional imaging of the brain. 'A' scan measurements are useful in determining the position of the midline structures in the region of the pineal and just anterior to it (Fig. 9.3). Experienced operators achieve high degrees of accuracy, but there are pitfalls for the less experienced, chiefly misinterpretation of echoes from near midline structures and falsely diagnosing shifts. When the pineal is calcified skull radiographs will give the same measurements more reliably. Neither of these techniques gives any clue as to the cause of a shift: inflammatory and cerebrovascular accidents are as likely as tumours and it should also be noted that since posterior fossa lesions and far frontal disturbances will not usually shift the pineal and third ventricle region of the brain until the disorder is far advanced, these are likely to be missed by both these tests.

In this application computer assisted tomography (the EMI scan) far exceeds ultrasonography in usefulness, but because of its limited availability the simpler technique has a small part to play at present (White, 1975).

OPHTHALMOLOGY

Using a water-bath with the eyelids open high frequency transducers (5–20 MHz) enable very high resolution to be obtained. In the globe

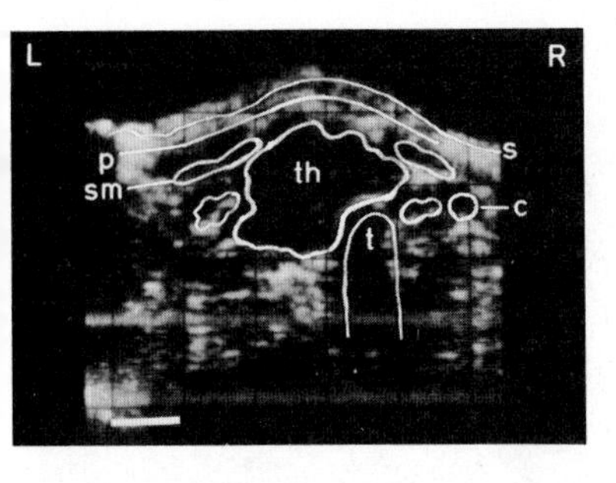

Figure 9.7 Thyroid scan. A transverse scan made with a water-bath showing an adenoma in the thyroid (th) displacing the trachea (t) to the right. The platysma (p) and sterno-mastoid (sm) muscles as well as the carotid bundle (c) are shown.

anatomical disturbances such as elevations of the retina due to choroid melanomas, tumours of the iris and ciliary body may be seen. The extreme lateral portions of the globe are often difficult to image and there is frequently some distortion of the foveal region due to the high speed of sound in the lens. Most of the lesions visualized by ultrasound can, of course, be seen via the ophthalmoscope. The value of ultrasound is in establishing the depth of penetration of the globe by such lesions, and in patients with opaque media (cataract or vitreous haemorrhage).

In the orbit the optic nerve can be imaged in almost all cases. Ocular muscles are sometimes seen, but the orbital fat is always displayed. Small tumours of these structures can be shown, usually regions of reduced reflection, the limit of resolution being around 1 mm (Fig. 9.7).

HEAD AND NECK

The important organs to be considered here are the salivary glands and the thyroid. Salivary gland scanning has been rather neglected to date, essentially because palpation is usually adequate. Contact scanning for parotid tumours has been employed with promising results.

In the thyroid, however, tumours are often impalpable, and the differentiation between benign and malignant nodules may be baffling even with histology. Ultrasound scanning through a water-bath provides good images of the thyroid (Fig. 9.8); tumours are readily identified and very reliably differentiated from cysts, which can be pin-pointed for aspiration biopsy. Several enthusiastic reports give promise of ultrasonic differences between carcinomas and adenomas, the former being poorly echogenic because of the destruction of the parenchymal fibrous stroma. If this can be substantiated then ultrasound would prove a most valuable adjunct to isotope scanning, aiding the sorting out of cold lesions, i.e. those failing to concentrate iodine. However, it seems unlikely that this technique can hope to make a definite diagnosis in those cases where even histology is misleading! (Jellins *et al.*, 1975).

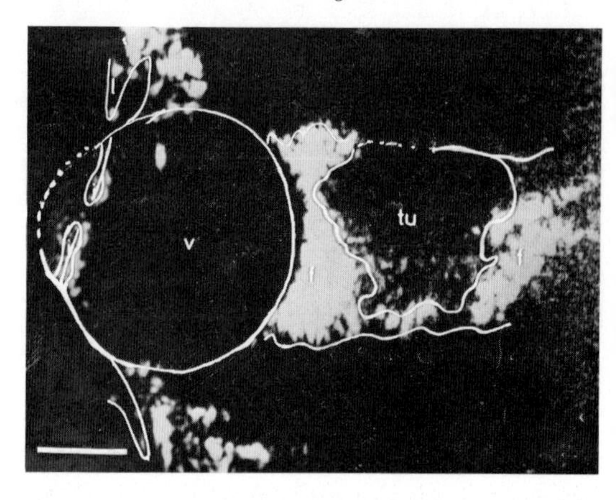

Figure 9.8 Eye scan. A water-bath scan with the lids (l) open of a patient with a retrobulbar lymphoma (tu = tumour) displacing the fat pad (f). The iris (i) is shown anteriorly. (v = vitreous humour). (Courtesy of Dr Marie Restori, Moorfields Eye Hospital, London.)

THORAX

Intrathoracic masses cannot be investigated ultrasonically due to air in the lungs, but superficial masses can be outlined and their depth estimated, even in the presence of pleural fluid, a situation in which conventional X-rays cannot be used because of lack of contrast. Such measurements are useful in planning fields for radiotherapy in the same way as in the abdomen (*vide infra*) and in following the changes of lesions during therapy.

A major application of ultrasound is examination of the breast. A water-bath technique is used, the most convenient being to arrange for the transducer to be moved in the water and pointing upwards. The patient then lies over the water-bath with the breasts immersed. As with the thyroid, breast ultrasonography is a developing rather than an established field, the major problem being the great normal variation in structure that is encountered. However, initial reports are encouraging and since this method is free from radiation hazard, it could be especially valuable in population screening (Kossoff *et al.*, 1976).

ABDOMEN

Abdominal Masses

Because of its capability of visualizing soft tissues, ultrasound has a major role in the management of tumours involving the major abdominal organs. Indeed it is probably as valuable as radiology in this field and in hospitals where ultrasound facilities are available this technique has often become indispensable.

A common problem is a patient presenting with an abdominal mass. Clinical clues as to its origin are often helpful, but an ultrasound

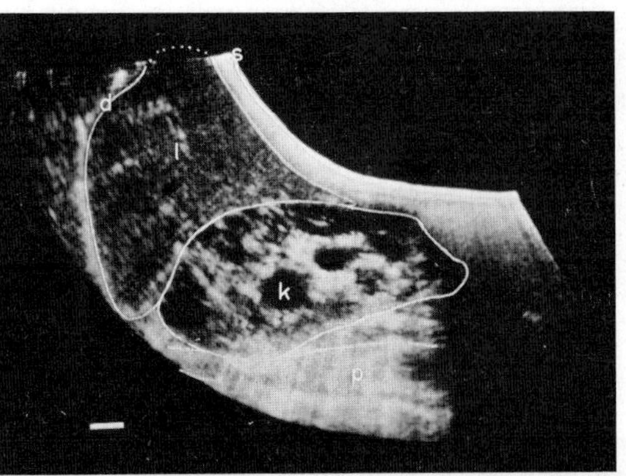

Figure 9.9 A right upper quadrant mass. The longitudinal section 5 cm from the midline shows it to be due to a large polycystic kidney (k) which is distorting the otherwise normal liver (l) (s = skin, d = diaphragm, p = psoas major muscle).

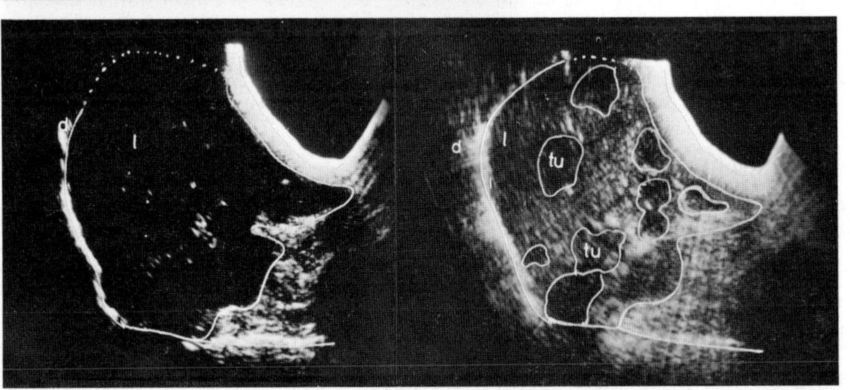

Figure 9.10 Bistable vs. grey scale imaging – liver metastases. The same longitudinal section through the right lobe of the liver (l) shows only the outline in the black and white image (a). On the grey scale display (b) the liver parenchyma is seen and metastases appear (tu) as darker regions which were not visible on the bistable picture (d = diaphragm).

examination will usually provide definitive information not only on its source, but on its size, relationship to nearby organs (compression, infiltration etc.) and will often indicate whether it is benign or malignant (Figs. 9.9, 9.16, 9.19) (Holm, 1971).

Liver

Because of its importance in oncology, the liver has become a prime target for ultrasonic diagnosis especially as it is difficult to detect liver tumours by any other means. Indeed it was this goal in part which prompted the development of the grey scale machines. The problem was beyond the reach of the older bistable machines which would allow only the liver size to be estimated (Fig. 9.10) (Taylor and Carpenter, 1974).

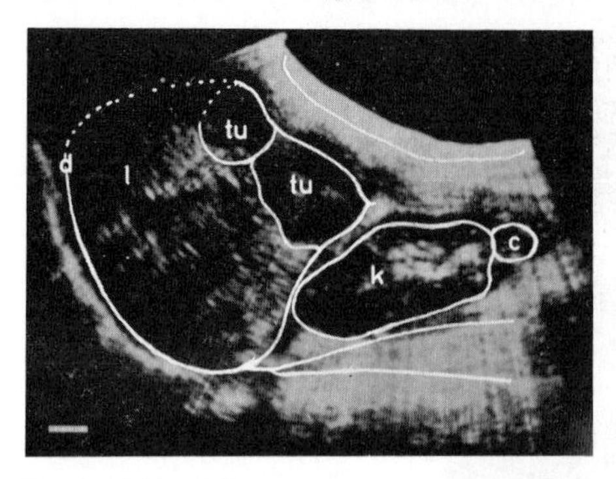

Figure 9.11 Primary hepatoma in the right lobe of the liver. The bilobular tumour (tu) is a poorly reflecting region in the liver (l) but some internal texture is retained (d = diaphragm, k = kidney, c = transverse colon).

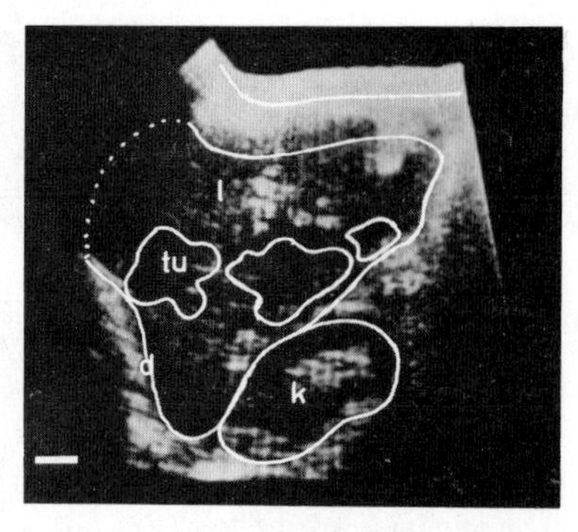

Figure 9.12 Lymphoma deposits in the liver. A longitudinal section through the right lobe of liver (l) and right kidney (k) showing three anechoic circumscribed lymphoma deposits (tu) (d = diaphragm).

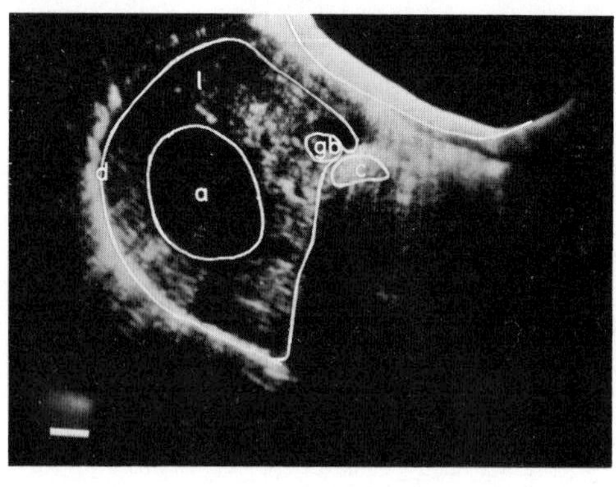

Figure 9.13 Liver abscess. Longitudinal section through the right lobe of liver (l) and gall bladder (gb) showing an amoebic abscess (a) (d = diaphragm, c = transverse colon with acoustic shadow).

Given display of liver parenchyma, then tumours of about 1 cm diameter are readily detected. They usually show as darker regions with stippled echoes that are very similar in pattern to those of surrounding normal liver (Figs. 9.11, 9.12). The difference in echogenicity may be very small (as little as 2 dB), so that the settings of the ultrasound machine and of the recording photographic apparatus can be extremely critical. When the echo intensity is very low as occurs with some lymphoma and sarcoma deposits, the appearance may suggest a cystic or abscess cavity. Simple cysts are transonic and give a strong TGC induced brightup; abscesses commonly return some reflections and are usually not transonic. However, these rules are fallible, and metastases that have undergone necrosis to become part fluid filled may be identical to abscesses (Fig. 9.13). The clinical features are often helpful and the ultrasonographer will usually note that there is liver tenderness over an abscess; this is unusual over a metastasis. In difficult

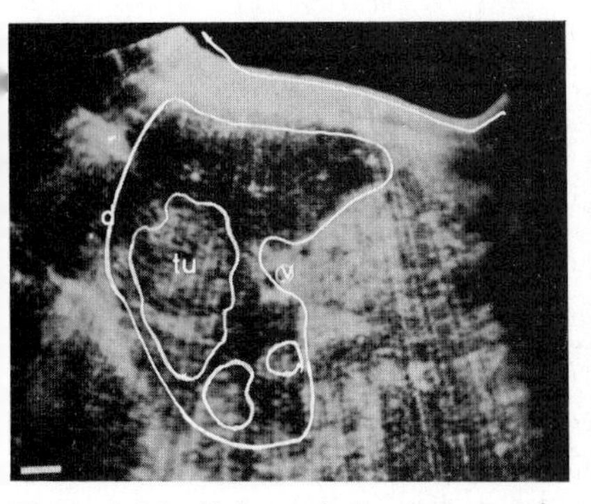

Figure 9.14 Echogenic liver metastasis. Three brightly reflecting tumour deposits (tu) in the liver near the porta hepatis; the primary was in the bladder. An increase in reflectivity is seen in tumours of gut and urogenital tract origin though it is not a constant feature. It also occurs following treatment (d = diaphragm, v = portal vein).

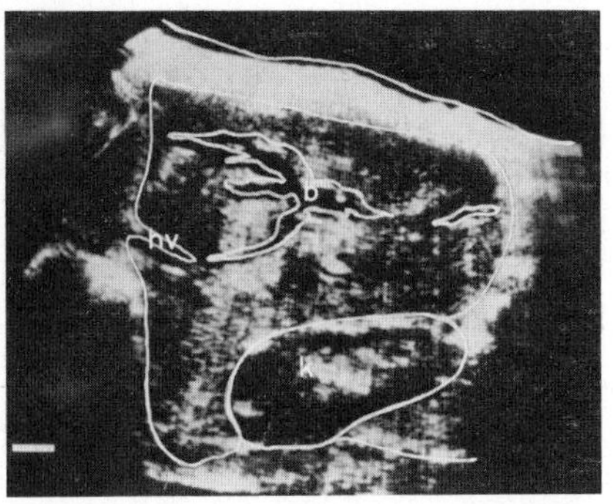

Figure 9.15 Extra hepatic biliary obstruction. In this section through the liver near the porta hepatis the stellate complex of dilated biliary radicles (b) can be seen (k = kidney, hv = hepatic vein).

cases repeated views may be needed when the growth of a tumour will aid the diagnosis.

Nearly all tumours are poorly reflective and this appearance is of no help in suggesting the tissue of origin of a liver metastasis. Under two circumstances, however, liver metastases appear as brightly reflecting regions. One of these represents one mode of response to treatment, when some deposits become more echogenic (it should be noted that many do not behave in this way, but simply shrink and disappear). This may relate to a fibrous reaction to therapy.

The other type of bright deposit occurs in a small proportion of those originating from primaries in the gut (e.g. stomach, pancreas, colon, Fig. 9.14). Some are calcified radiologically and perhaps some of the others have small microscopic calcifications. If a bright metastasis is encountered before treatment, then a gut primary is likely.

A third pattern of liver involvement should be mentioned. It is rare, occurring when there is widespread diffuse liver involvement with small, often confluent tumour deposits. The ultrasonic appearance is of a rather subtle uniform alteration in texture; unfortunately this pattern can be rather similar to that found in cirrhosis and fatty change and this poses a diagnostic problem.

Jaundice is a frequent occurrence in malignant disease in the abdomen, and may be the presenting feature in carcinoma of the pancreas. The problem is to differentiate jaundice due to widespread liver metastases from that due to obstruction of the biliary tree outside

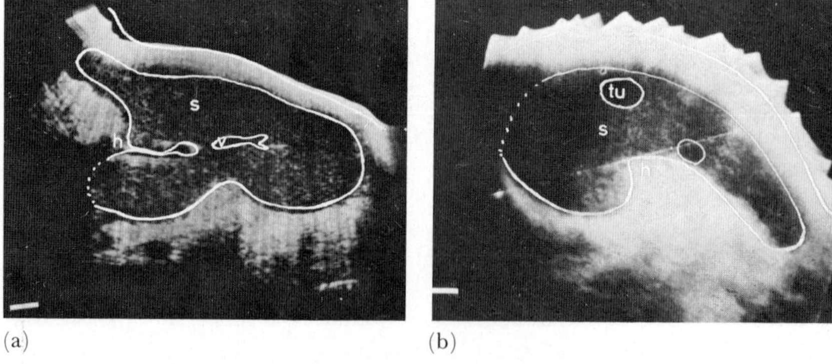

(a) (b)

Figure 9.16 Splenomegaly. (a) Longitudinal sector scan of a spleen (s) involved with chronic granulocytic leukaemia. The tortuous central vein (v) running to the hilum (h) is shown. (b) Compounded scan of an enlarged spleen (s) in Hodgkin's disease. Taken in the tenth intercostal space, it shows two focal deposits (tu) and the overall low level of echoes typical of the lymphomas.

the liver. Ultrasound has proved a reliable method for detecting dilated biliary vessels (Fig. 9.15), and will often localize the site of obstruction as being at the porta or at the head of the pancreas. This will allow the appropriate selection of therapy (surgical, chemo- or radiotherapy), and enable accurate planning of a radiotherapy field to be made.

Spleen

Access to a normal sized spleen is rather difficult since it is subcostal, and there is usually gas in the splenic flexure infero-anterior to it. Oblique intercostal views through the tenth or eleventh space are required and it may be difficult to cover the whole organ in a single sector sweep, so that compound scans are often used. Spleen size is readily determined, and this may be useful in the lymphomas and leukaemias. The normal spleen has an echo texture similar to that of liver, but at a rather lower intensity. Lymphomatous spleens are commonly poorly echogenic, and those involved with leukaemias are often strongly echogenic (Fig. 9.16(a)). Some of these changes may be due to treatment and at present are not well enough understood to be diagnostically useful. Focal splenic lesions are rarely due to tumours, except in Hodgkin's disease (Fig. 9.16(b)). Cystic masses are easily detected with ultrasound.

Kidney

The kidneys are readily examined through the paraspinal muscles with the patient lying prone. In this position the twelfth rib may obscure the

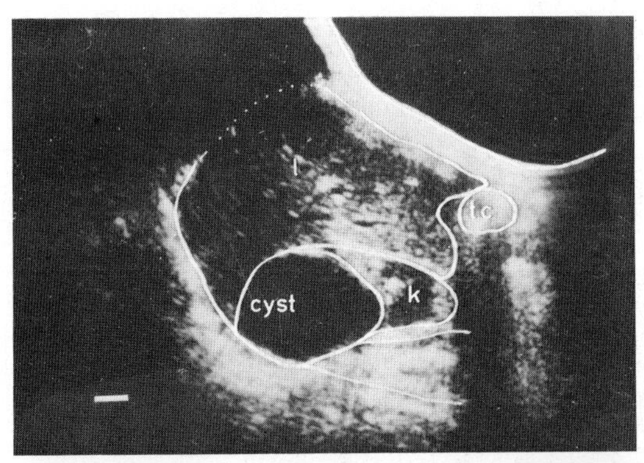

Figure 9.17 Renal cyst. This IVP defect in the right kidney (k) was shown to be a cyst on this longitudinal section through the liver (l) (tc = transverse colon).

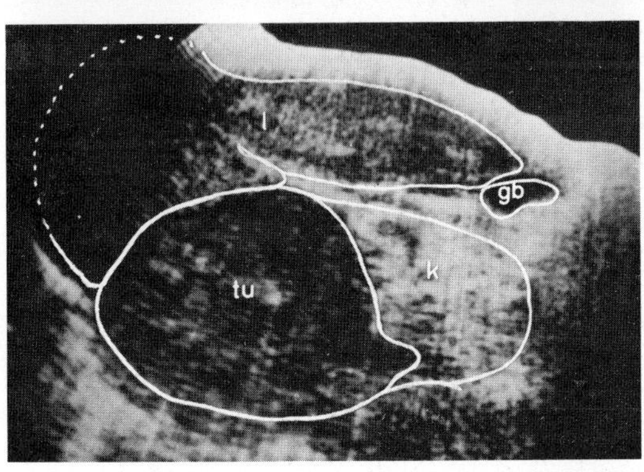

Figure 9.18 Renal tumour. This right renal mass proved to be solid (tu) and was a Wilms's tumour. The liver (l) is distorted by the tumour (gb = gall bladder).

upper pole; deep inspiration is usually helpful and the right kidney can also be reached from the front using the liver as a window.

Renal ultrasound examinations are useful in determining whether a mass seen on the Intravenous Pyelogram (IVP) is solid or cystic (Figs. 9.17, 9.18). Cystic masses are almost all innocent, and may be punctured under ultrasonic guidance, whereas solid masses are usually tumours. The extent of local and lymph node involvement can usually be assessed ultrasonically and transverse tomograms are useful for determining the mass's relationship with the liver and spine for radiotherapy planning.

A minor but sometimes helpful application is in detecting early hydronephrosis, usually visible as a separation of the layers of the pelvis before the IVP becomes abnormal.

Abdominal Lymph Nodes

Although the resolution at present obtainable does not allow normal lymph nodes to be identified, when enlarged they appear as poorly reflecting masses. All groups of nodes can be imaged, provided the abdomen is gas free (an aperient or colon washout may be required),

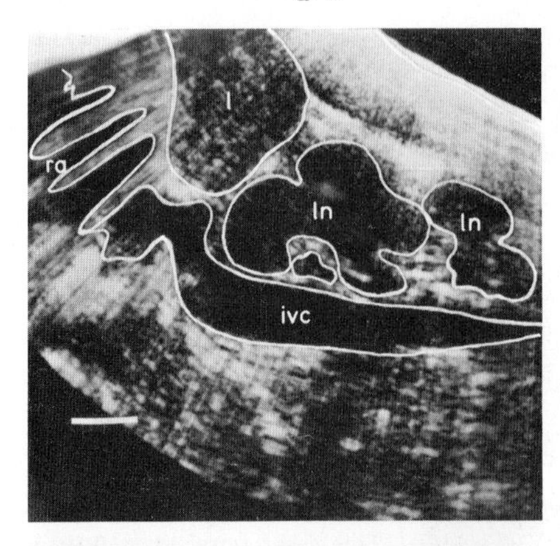

Figure 9.19 Abdominal lymphadenopathy. (a) Longitudinal section 1 cm to the right of midline through the inferior vena cava (ivc) as it enters the right atrium (ra) in which the moving tricuspid valve can be seen. Inferior to the left lobe of the liver (l) is a lobulated mass of precaval nodes (ln) which were involved with metastases from a bronchial carcinoma.

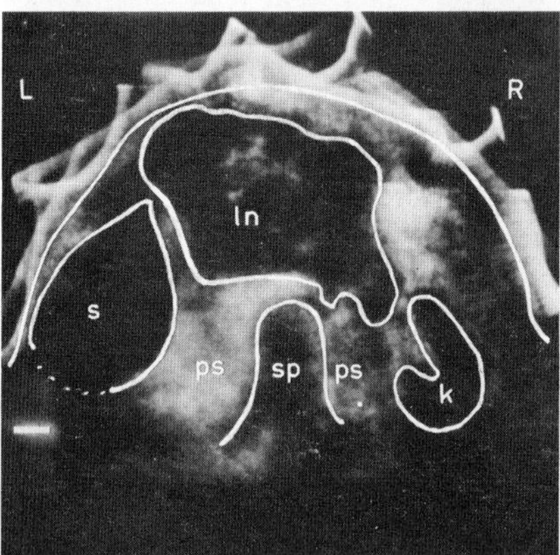

(b) Epigastric transverse section to show a large mass of lymphomatous pre aortic nodes (ln) and an enlarged spleen (s) (sp = lumbar spine, ps = psoas muscles, k = right kidney).

and the relationship between the nodes and other organs can be delineated in three dimensions, and their positions noted relative to skin markers. Thus although the resolution and specificity as to cause of enlargement are inferior to contrast radiography (lipiodol lymphangiography), the anatomical limitations of this technique do not apply. Nodes in the mesentery, porta hepatis and upper para-aortic region can be outlined (Fig. 9.19) and this remains true where there is a great bulk of nodes that is not filled on lymphangiography.

This technique has proved to be of great value in radiotherapy planning, allowing accurate placing of the X-ray field, with frequent repeat examinations to tailor the field to improvement during the course. During response the involved nodes shrink away and may finally disappear at the limit of resolution (about 2 cm in this area). Sometimes one notes persistent and stable residual masses, and it is not possible to distinguish between residual involved nodes and scarring resulting from treatment, except by their long-term behaviour on follow-up examinations (Tyrrell *et al.*, 1976).

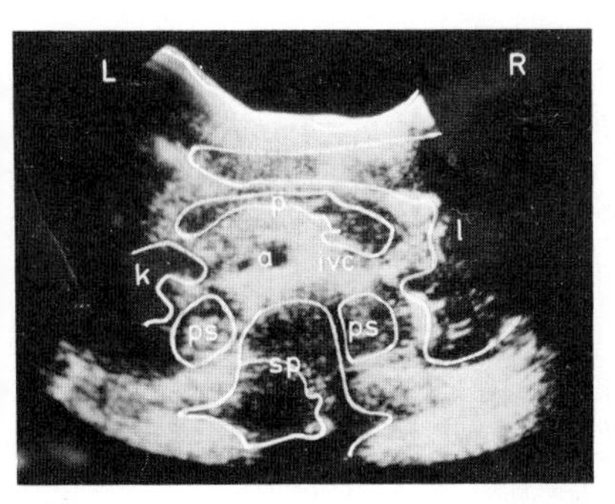

Figure 9.20 Normal pancreas. Transverse section in the epigastrium showing the pancreas (p) lying across the aorta (a) and the ivc, posterior to the left lobe of the liver (l) (sp = lumbar spine, ps = psoas muscle, k = kidney).

Pancreas

The pancreas is difficult to investigate short of rather complex tests such as by endoscopic retrograde canulation (ERCP), which though reliable requires skilled operators, has a rather high failure rate and may precipitate pancreatitis. Ultrasound offers a simple solution to the problem, but unfortunately one that has proved somewhat difficult to realize in practice. The difficulty lies in obtaining acoustic access to the pancreas, since the transverse colon usually overlies the organ (e.g. see figure in King *et al.*, 1973). However, when good views can be obtained (Fig. 9.20) then the method is reliable, lesions over some 2 cm in size can be detected, and the position of the gland defined by its relationship with the superior mesenteric vein as it joins the splenic vein to form the portal vein. Usually the normal gland can be visualized but the echo pattern will not differentiate reliably between pancreatitis and tumour unless a large lesion is present when signs of invasion may be seen with tumours. Biliary obstruction is readily detected, and tumours may be localized for radiography.

Pelvis

A window is required for examining the pelvis and this is provided by a full bladder which also has the effect of elevating adjacent organs such as the uterus out of the pelvis, improving exposure. As with other parts of the abdomen most organs in the pelvis can be examined, saving those that are too deeply placed. Masses of all sorts are amenable, e.g. enlarged nodes, ovarian and uterine tumours, sarcomas etc. (Fig. 9.21). Bladder tumours are especially well seen (Fig. 9.22) and often the extent of bladder wall involvement can be delineated also. Ovarian cysts are readily imaged but it is often impossible to decide whether a cyst is malignant or benign.

The prostate is usually too deeply placed to be imaged suprapubically. Probes especially designed for rectal use promise to be very valuable in diagnosis of prostatic and rectal tumours.

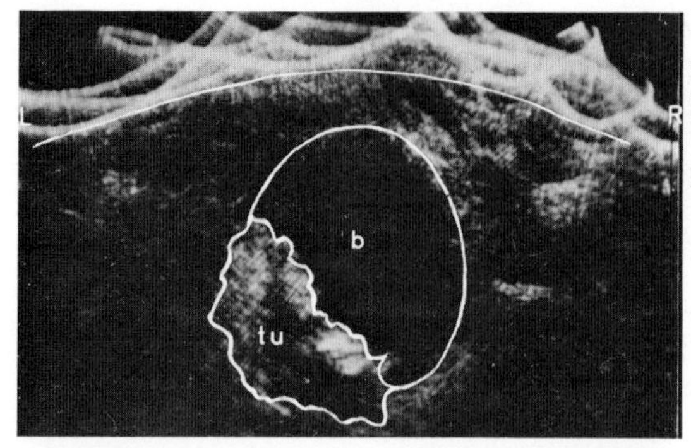

Figure 9.21 Carcinoma of ovary. Transverse section suprapubically through the bladder (b) to show the tumour in the pouch of Douglas (v = vessels in the iliac group).

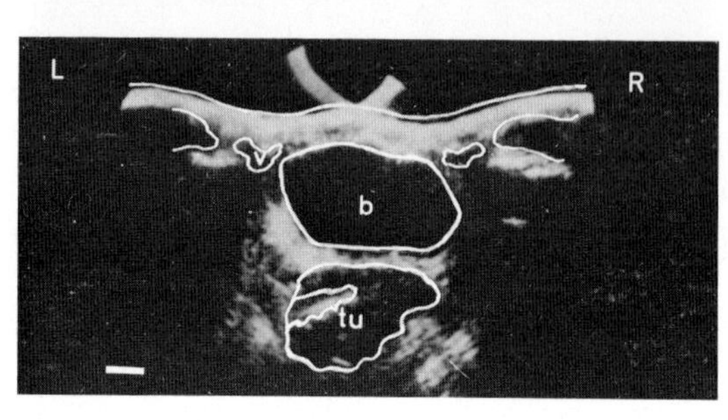

Figure 9.22 Bladder tumour. In this transverse compounded section just over the pubis the bladder (b) wall is distorted posteriorly and to the left by a mass which is an invading carcinoma (tu) of the bladder.

Limbs

Ultrasound examinations are of limited value in the peripheries, simply because clinical examination is usually adequate. However, when this is not so ultrasound will provide the same sort of data on anatomy as in the abdomen, delineating the extent of relationships of masses.

The Uses of Ultrasound in Oncology in Relation to Other Imaging Techniques

Radiology, the longest established imaging technique, has the advantages of high resolution, reproducibility and of being well understood. But plain X-rays will not generally show soft tissue abnormalities, except in the chest where they impinge on the normal lung. Contrast media are required to allow most soft tissues to be outlines (e.g. IVPs, myelograms, lymphangiograms, arteriograms), and these cause discomfort and occasional injury as well as not being readily repeatable.

Isotope techniques depend on functional peculiarities of organs allowing selective uptake of labelled compounds to obtain images. Thus they give both functional and anatomical information, which may be unique (e.g. dynamic brain and renal studies), but they suffer from poor anatomical resolution. They are usually readily repeatable.

Ultrasound scans, like plain X-rays, are solely anatomical. Their value is in imaging soft tissues without the need for contrast injections; they offer, under ideal conditions, high resolution with the facility for easy repetition, and with newer devices, the facility of real time imaging. But they suffer from severe interference by gas and sometimes by adipose and muscle tissue, which limits the areas of application. Computer assisted tomography (CAT or EMI scans) also images soft tissues with high resolution. Its role in the head is well established where it has proved invaluable and there is every reason to hope that the same will be true of the whole body machines. It is, however, expensive and takes rather a long time to make a whole abdominal study. In addition, this method lacks the mobility of ultrasound machines so that views can only be transverse and there is no likelihood of portable versions appearing. The physical means by which the soft tissue images are obtained are quite different from those exploited by ultrasound, and further experience may indicate hitherto unsuspected relative advantages and limitations.

Whereas conventional radiology has reached a high degree of perfection, the other three approaches are new; spectacular improvements are to be expected in all of them making it difficult to assess their relative roles at present. It seems likely that they will prove to be complementary means of aiding patient management.

Acknowledgement

This work was carried out with support from the MRC and from EMI, which is gratefully acknowledged. Much assistance was given by Dr V. R. McCready, Dr K. J. Taylor and Dr C. R. Hill, Mr P. Garbutt and Miss E. Holmes.

References

Hellman, L. M. *et al.*, Duffus, G. M., Donald, I. and Sunden, B. (1970) Safety of diagnostic ultrasound in obstetrics, *Lancet*, **1**, p. 1133.

Hill, C. R. (1976) Review of ultrasonic imaging, *Journal of Physics E*, **9**, pp. 153–62.

Holm, H. H. (1971) Ultrasonic scanning in the diagnosis of space occupying lesions of the upper abdomen, *British J. Radiology*, **44**, pp. 24–36.

Holm, H. H. *et al.* (1976) *Abdominal Ultrasound.* Copenhagen: Munksgaard.

Jellins, J., Kossoff, G., Wiseman, J., Reeve, T. and Hales, I. (1975) Ultrasonic grey scale visualisation of the thyroid gland, *Ultrasound in Medicine and Biology*, **1**, p. 405.

King, D. L. (ed.) (1974) *Diagnostic Ultrasound.* Kimpton.

King, W. W., Wilkiemeyer, R. M., Boyce, W. H. and McKinney, W. M. (1973) Prostatic echography, *Journal of the American Medical Association*, **226**, p. 444.

Kossoff, G., Carpenter, D. A., Robsinson, D. and Garrett, W. (1976) Ultrasound imaging of the breast with the 'Octason', *Proc. 2nd European Congress on Ultrasonics in Medicine.* Amsterdam: Elsevier.

Kossoff, G., Robinson, E. E., Liu, C. N. and Garrett, W. J. (1964) Design criteria for ultrasonic visualisation systems, *Ultrasonics*, **2**, p. 24.

MacIntosh, D. C., Brown, R. C. and Coakley, W. T. (1975) Ultrasound and *in vitro* chromosome abnormalities, *British J. Radiology*, **48**, p. 230.

Prospectives for Ultrasonic Imaging in Medical Diagnosis. National Science Foundation, Washington, 1973.

Saunders, R. C. (ed.) (1975) B-Scan ultrasound, *Symposium in the Radiological Clinics of North America*, **3**, 13.

Taylor, K. J. N. and Carpenter, D. A. (1974) Grey scale ultrasonography in the investigation of obstructive jaundice, *Lancet*, **2**, pp. 586–7.

Taylor, K. J. N., Carpenter, D. A. and McCready, V. R. (1973) Grey scale echography in the diagnosis of intrahepatic disease, *J. Clinical Ultrasound*, **1**, pp. 284–7.

Thurstone, F. L. and Ramm, O. T. von (1974) Electronic beam scanning for ultrasonic imaging, *Ultrasonics in Medicine.* M. de Vlieger, D. N. White and V. R. McCready (eds.) Exerpta Medica, Amsterdam.

Tyrrell, C. J. T., Cosgrove, D. O., McCready, V. R. and Peckham, M. J. (1977) Ultrasound in diagnosis of involved abdominal nodes in teratoma. *Clinical Radiology*, **28**, pp. 475–481.

Wells, P. N. T. (1969) *Physical Principles of Ultrasonic Diagnosis.* Academic Press.

Wells, P. N. T. (1975) Ultrasonic diagnostics: a look into the future, *Biomedical Engineering*, **10**, 247–51.

White, D. N. (1975) The use of ultrasound in Neurology, in G. Baum (ed.), *Fundamentals of Medical Ultrasound.* Putnam.

Chapter 10

Surgical Oncology

HARVEY WHITE,
M.A., D.M., M.Ch., F.R.C.S.
Consultant Surgeon,
Royal Marsden Hospital
London and Surrey

Introduction

Since classical times, surgery has played a leading role in the treatment of cancer. The belief that surgery could be curative is based on the view that malignant change in a tissue remains localized at the primary site for long enough to be diagnosed and excised. We now know that this is an oversimplified view and there are, for example, many documented cases of surgical 'cure' in which malignant cells have been recovered from the blood at the time of excision of the primary lesion. Why these cells do not produce distant metastases and why patients may remain disease-free for many years following excision of a tumour before the development of secondaries, remains a mystery. These paradoxes do, however, indicate a complex relationship between malignant cells and normal tissue involving local defence mechanisms as well as natural host immunity.

It is now accepted that a tumour is often not confined to the primary site by the time it can be diagnosed, so we have to redefine the position of surgery in the management of cancer. The technical feats of radical surgery which are possible, although having a limited place in treatment, are seldom now the rule. Despite this change in emphasis, however, surgery plays no less important a part in treatment, although it is now merely one facet of a multidisciplinary approach. The diagnostic and palliative aspects of therapy may be of greater benefit to the patient than some of the misguided extensive operations of the past in situations which could in no circumstances be 'curative'.

The surgeon's objectives in the treatment of cancer have recently been elegantly expressed by Sir Rodney Smith, past President of the

Royal College of Surgeons of England:

> All of us are going to die and, travelling in the same direction through life, each one of us does 'nightly pitch his moving tent a day's march nearer home'. When a patient has a serious ailment and seeks our help what we are trying to do, surely, is to see that he does not, on this journey, take some short cut he would rather avoid, and also that the terrain over which he travels shall be as smooth and as agreeable as possible.

Diagnosis

Surgeons are often called upon to provide a diagnostic service in oncology. This usually entails obtaining tissue for pathological examination.

EXCISION BIOPSY

Certain tumours – notably skin cancers such as basal cell carcinoma and malignant melanoma are easily visible and can often be completely excised. Other tumours such as breast cancers may be palpable below the skin and can be completely excised. Occasionally lymph nodes are felt to be enlarged; these are sometimes associated with tumours of organs lying within the field drained by the node. Biopsy will often enable a diagnosis to be made more easily than obtaining tissue from an inaccessible primary – as in the case of an enlarged supraclavicular node associated with a carcinoma of the stomach. Nodes may also be enlarged in haematological malignancies and lymphomas and be of great value in establishing a diagnosis.

INCISION BIOPSY

Occasionally it is felt unwise to excise a suspicious lump or skin cancer completely. In these circumstances an incision biopsy is performed so that treatment can be planned following a definite tissue diagnosis.

NEEDLE OR DRILL BIOPSY

This has been practised sporadically for many years and provides a small core of tissue or merely cells for examination. Recently – especially with the development of satisfactory disposable sampling needles, this method is proving useful in many sites including breast, prostate and liver. Liver biopsies can be made 'blind' or under direct vision using a laparoscope introduced into the peritoneal cavity, thus enabling the needle to be inserted under direct vision. The instrument may also have built-in biopsy forceps. The expertise of cytologists is now so advanced that when a hypodermic needle is inserted into a tissue and withdrawn, cells from the needle smeared onto a microscope slide may be enough for diagnosis.

EXFOLIATIVE CYTOLOGY

Cells are sometimes shed by a tumour such as a carcinoma of the bladder, or they may be contained in a discharge such as that from the nipple, or can be removed from a tumour by scraping or brushing. Now that cytologists can recognize the origin of many of these cells, the possibilities of early diagnosis and screening are greatly increased.

ENDOSCOPY

The technique of looking into various sites normally inaccessible to direct vision and so obtaining not only a view but a tissue biopsy under direct vision is now an important and rapidly expanding field of diagnostic medicine which may involve the surgeon. Rigid optical instruments such as the bronchoscope, oesophagoscope, sigmoidoscope, cytoscope and laparoscope are still in use, but in addition many newer instruments using flexible fibre-optic systems are now used. The gastroscope and colonoscope are particularly useful in surgical oncology. The tissue obtained is usually a bite by special cupped forceps but may be brushings or even a larger piece of tissue (e.g. when a polyp is snared).

There are some theoretical dangers in biopsy for it has been alleged that the process may spread a tumour by implantation – especially along the track of a biopsy needle or by seeding in the skin over an excision biopsy. There is little evidence for this but precautions such as wide excision of a suspected malignant lesion are naturally advised. Fresh towels, gowns, gloves and instruments are used when preliminary biopsy confirms a malignant lesion and definitive surgery immediately follows.

The advantages of immediate tissue diagnosis during an operation in order to plan the extent of surgery have led to the development of frozen sections. By this method, tissue can be frozen, cut and examined under a microscope within a few minutes of being obtained rather than undergoing the long process of being fixed in formalin and embedded in paraffin wax which takes several days. The technique of frozen sections allows the surgeon to plan the extent of an operation without the patient being subjected to a second anaesthetic and operation.

STAGING

The diagnostic biopsies discussed so far have been used to establish the nature of the tumour. However, it is of paramount importance to know the extent of a disease process in order to select the most appropriate form of therapy, for neither clinical staging nor X-rays, ultrasound and scanning are as accurate as actual tissue examination. Occasionally the biopsy of a gland from a regional node or a distant site is taken to establish how far a disease process has spread. The extent or stage which the disease process has reached can therefore be determined in the hope of predicting the prognosis or survival or in order to determine what particular form of treatment is most appropriate. Occasionally staging requires tissue biopsies from several sites, e.g. liver and bone marrow, and a laparotomy may even be required. Recently, the necessity of biopsy of the liver and abdominal lymph nodes and resection of the spleen in order to stage Hodgkin's disease has become almost routine practice.

Treatment

The objectives of surgical treatment of cancer have already been mentioned in general terms. The surgeon must keep these principles in the forefront of his mind in order that he can plan the most appropriate treatment which may be an attempt at cure, palliation, or even on rare occasions prevention. The information determining the treatment will, in addition to the special diagnostic procedures mentioned, include all the other vital aspects of patient care (e.g. family and social history) which should contribute to the overall management of any surgical case but come together in an especially important way in oncology.

CURE

Theoretically, cure can be taken to imply the absence of residual viable tumour after treatment, which of course should not itself significantly reduce the life expectancy of the patient when compared with the normal population. In practice, precise knowledge of whether or not any residual tumour remains sometimes cannot be established until death. It may require studies on a large group of patients for twenty years or more before statisticians can determine whether the survival of treated patients approaches that of the normal population or not. A compromise is adopted and the success of treatment is often expressed in terms either of the disease-free interval following treatment or the survival of patients in years.

These results bear some relation to the histological grade (or differentiation) of the tumour and the stage of spread at which it is diagnosed. Neither of these criteria, however, has a universally predictable association with survival or even disease-free survival. There are many reasons for this, including the fact that a tumour may spread either via the blood or lymphatic system while the primary is small (even too small for clinical detection), and also the variable host resistance.

Although our knowledge of the natural history of tumours suggests that most primary tumours have the capacity to spread, and may well have disseminated cells in the vascular or lymphatic system before diagnosis, cures are reported even if this is known to have occurred. Therefore, not all cells which have disseminated would appear to have the capacity to implant. This, and the hope that removal of the primary tumour bulk will allow such disseminated cells to be prevented from developing by the host's natural immunity, forms the basis of our attempts at cure. If there is no clinical evidence of spread, therefore, it is theoretically reasonable to attempt surgical cure. Even today, however, our methods of determining spread and staging are relatively crude and undoubtedly many patients who are manifestly beyond cure are regrettably subjected to 'curative' operations.

The principles of curative surgery are simply to remove the primary by a process which will not itself lead to dissemination. The primary is handled as little as possible during surgery and spread via the vascular system and lymphatics is reduced by early ligation and division of the vessels draining the area. Rupture of an encapsulated tumour and spillage of cells must also be avoided. If an organ such as a breast is known on occasion to be subject to multiple primary tumours, the whole organ is often removed. In this way, the possibility of another tumour developing in residual tissue of an organ which has experienced the same genetic, familial and environmental factors which provoked the original neoplasm is avoided. It is, of course, not the practice to remove both breasts if cancer is discovered in only one. Careful follow-up of the remaining breast is therefore required.

When removing a primary tumour, it is reasonable to perform a wide excision in case there has been some minimal local spread. The disappointing results of such operative treatment in apparently 'curable' lesions has led to more extensive radical operations, taking not only the tissue in the immediate neighbourhood of the tumour but also the regional lymph nodes. Frequently this turns out to be ill-conceived for survival prospects may not be improved. However, surgeons can often justify such treatment for the distressing problems of local recurrence, as in the breast, or mechanical obstruction, as in the bowel, are reduced. In addition, such operations are performed in good faith, without proof of spread, and may occasionally be dramatically successful. With more sophisticated methods of diagnosing spread, the selection of cases will be improved.

PALLIATION

The possibilities of surgery playing an important role in the palliation of malignant disease are numerous. The distress of local ulceration can be overcome by mastectomy in patients with cancer of the breast, even if spread is known to have occurred. Obstruction of the gastrointestinal tract at almost any level causes pain and systemic disturbances from which great relief may be afforded by resection, bypass or colostomy. The effects of peritoneal ascites or pleural effusion associated with secondary deposits may cause distressing symptoms which can be relieved by abdominal paracentesis or pleural aspiration.

The result of pressure on a nerve or the spinal cord from metastases or following collapse of a vertebral body destroyed by tumour may lead to pain or loss of sphincter control and surgery (laminectomy) may relieve some of the symptoms.

Pain from and growth of certain tumours can sometimes be limited by chemical means which may involve operative expertise such as arterial or venous canulation to allow antitumour agents to be infused or perfused. Occasionally the ligation of the hepatic artery is undertaken to reduce the blood supply to hepatic secondary deposits.

Ablation of endocrine glands such as the pituitary, adrenals, ovaries or testes is often able to alter the hormonal environment of some apparently hormone 'dependent' tumours.

With all these therapeutic tools for manipulating the course of malignant disease, it is important that the objectives of treatment should be examined by the surgical oncologist at each stage. An improved quality of life for the patient must be the overriding aim. There is, perhaps, no branch of cancer medicine which depends so much on the multidisciplinary approach to total management than the field of palliation.

PREVENTION

Premalignant conditions can now be identified in certain circumstances. These may be congenital as in familial polyposis coli or acquired as in leucoplakia of the tongue following chronic irritation and infection. Metaplasia in the epithelium may be recognized as premalignant and treated surgically, for example the diathermy of such areas in the bladder or excision of areas of solar keratosis in the skin and epitheliosis of the cervix uteri. It also seems likely that the new techniques of fibroscopy will enable certain changes such as atrophic gastritis to be correlated with the subsequent development of cancer. Gastrectomy may then be performed at a stage before the actual development of cancer or when the malignant change only involves a few cells and is said to be '*in situ*'. It is known that a patient who has suffered from colitis for more than ten years and whose colitis has involved the whole colon at some stage and has been severe or 'fulminating' runs an increased risk of developing cancer. In this case colectomy may be the right course of action. A more common condition which predisposes to the development of malignant change is that of gall stones. Carcinoma of the biliary tree is more common in those who have had stones for many years and this fact encourages surgeons to recommend cholecystectomy in cases of asymptomatic cholelithiasis.

Special Surgical Considerations

Preoperatively the patients are often somewhat debilitated and anaemic with low plasma proteins. It may be impossible to correct this without a period of intravenous feeding and blood transfusion. Some malignant conditions (e.g. leukaemia), and some forms of treatment such as chemotherapy, affect blood clotting and may lead to haemorrhage if surgery is undertaken unless preoperative platelet infusions are given. Occasionally, the patients will have fistulae making both electrolyte and fluid balance difficult.

During surgery special care is taken to avoid touching a malignant lesion either during excision or mobilization. The vascular pedicles supplying the tumour are ligated as early as possible to minimize the chance of spread via the blood-stream. This technique is especially important during the resection of a kidney tumour when the renal pedicle can be ligated; during resection of a testicular tumour when the cord can be ligated; during resection of a colorectal carcinoma when the inferior mesenteric pedicle is ligated early in the operation.

A wide excision of malignant lesions is undertaken to reduce the risk of local recurrence. This means that the tension on skin edges may be greater and sutures are therefore sometimes left in longer on account of this as well as the delayed healing in these debilitated patients. If the skin cannot be closed after a wide excision, skin grafting may be necessary.

Following laparotomy in some malignant cases – especially if ascites is present or after radiotherapy – deep tension sutures are often thought to be a wise precaution. Previous radiotherapy may also delay healing and demands special caution in suturing. Drains should be brought out wherever possible within the field of any subsequent radiation because of the danger of seeding along the tract.

During the postoperative period the wound should be observed for signs of haemorrhage, dehiscence and infection in view of the special circumstances which increase the dangers of these various complications. Skin care is particularly important if subsequent radiation is likely and therefore zinc oxide dressings are best avoided because of possible reactions.

Patients with cancer are frequently committed, by the nature of their disease, to several operations and often uncertainty about further treatment. Sympathetic concern and supportive nursing is, therefore, essential during all stages. Easy access to the other supporting services – such as the medical social department – can help to alleviate many of the tensions and worries in the postoperative period.

Surgical Examples

COLON AND RECTUM

An example of a malignant lesion which may often be treated successfully by surgery alone is cancer of the colon and rectum.

The distribution of carcinoma of the colon is shown in Fig. 10.1. The lesions may be papillary, ulcerative or annular (Fig. 10.2). The annular lesions, especially if they occur in the descending colon where the faeces are less fluid, may cause early obstruction. Sigmoidoscopy, barium enema and colonoscopy are the most common methods of diagnosis. Rectal bleeding and haemorrhoids may be associated with

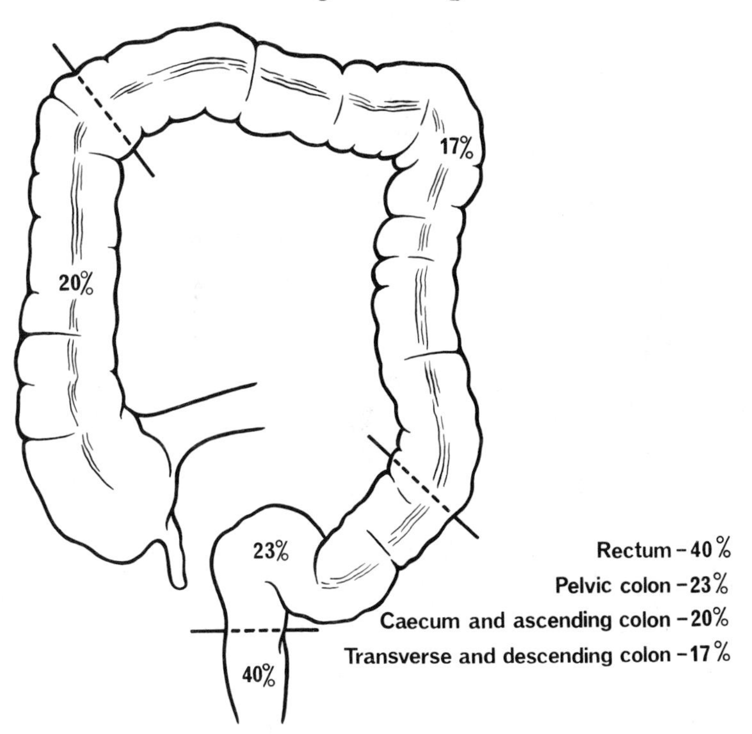

Figure 10.1 Distribution of cancer of the colon.

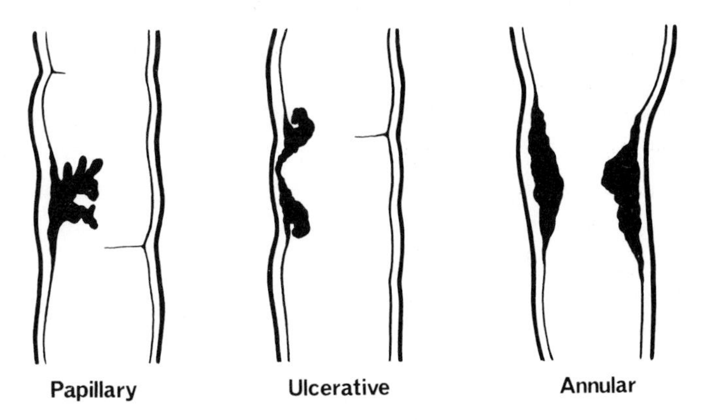

Figure 10.2 Pathological types of cancer of the colon.

colonic tumours which should be excluded by investigating patients with these symptoms.

Following preparation of the bowel by enemas, salts and sulphonamides, resection is usually attempted. Ideally, the tumour, associated mesentery, adjacent colon and the region of immediate

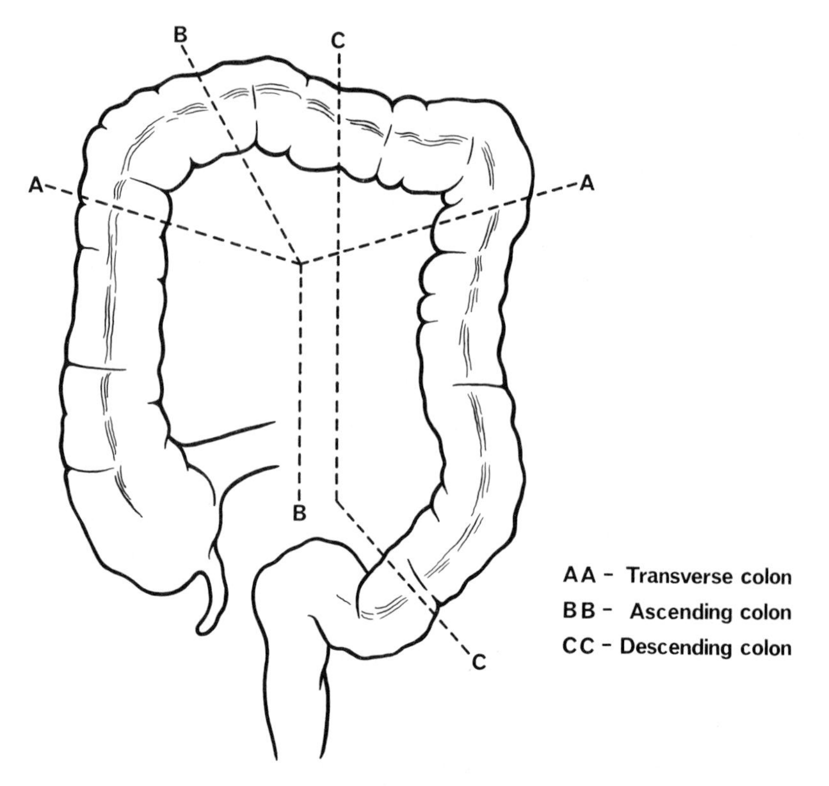

Figure 10.3 Areas requiring resection in cancer of the colon.

lymph drainage are resected (Fig. 10.3) by right (or left) hemicolectomy (Fig. 10.4) or transverse colectomy (Fig. 10.5) and continuity restored. Occasionally a temporary colostomy (Fig. 10.6) or caecostomy (Fig. 10.7) is performed to protect the anastomosis until healing is complete. The colostomy has to be closed formally at a second operation but the caecostomy will close spontaneously once the tube is withdrawn. For lesions of the sigmoid colon, an anterior approach and resection which restores the continuity of the bowel can be performed (Fig. 10.8). If the tumour is very low (below the peritoneal floor) the rectum has to be completely excised and following this 'abdomino-perineal resection' the patient is left with a permanent left iliac fossa colostomy (Fig. 10.9).

A tumour of the colon may be found unexpectedly when a patient with obstruction is explored as an emergency. A 'staged' resection may then be performed, a temporary colostomy being fashioned so that the patient can be prepared for subsequent elective resection when the obstruction has been relieved.

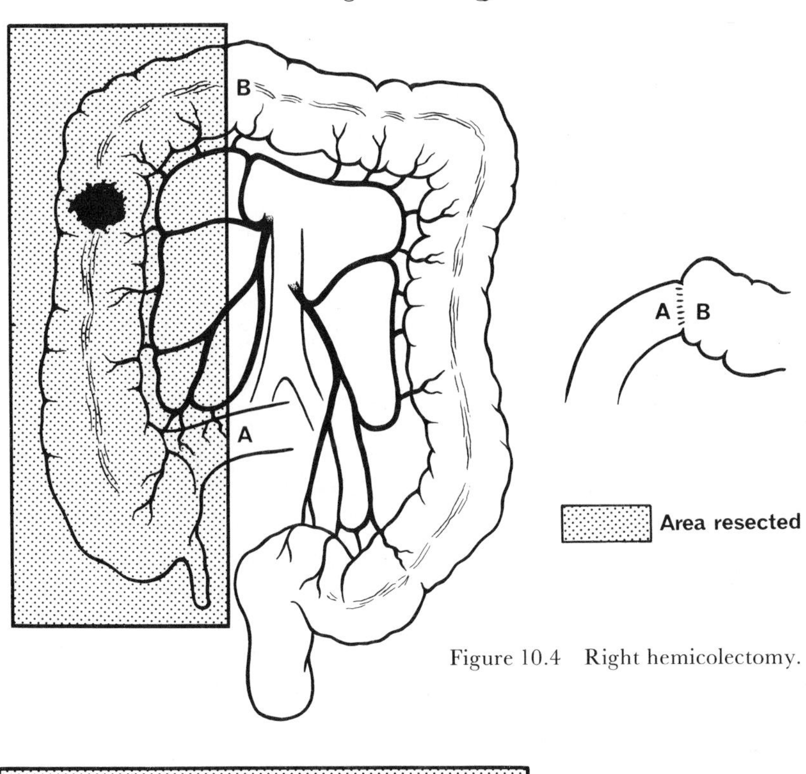

Figure 10.4 Right hemicolectomy.

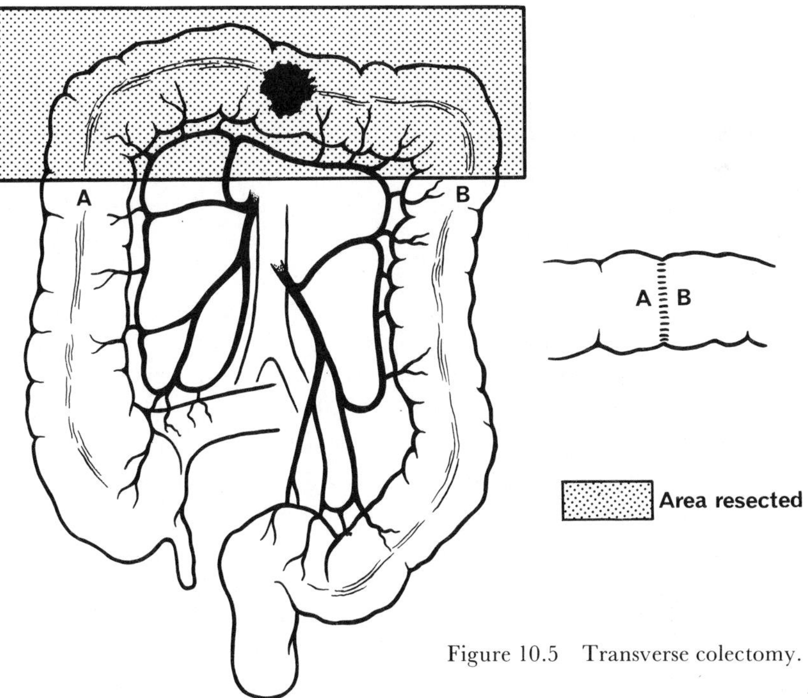

Figure 10.5 Transverse colectomy.

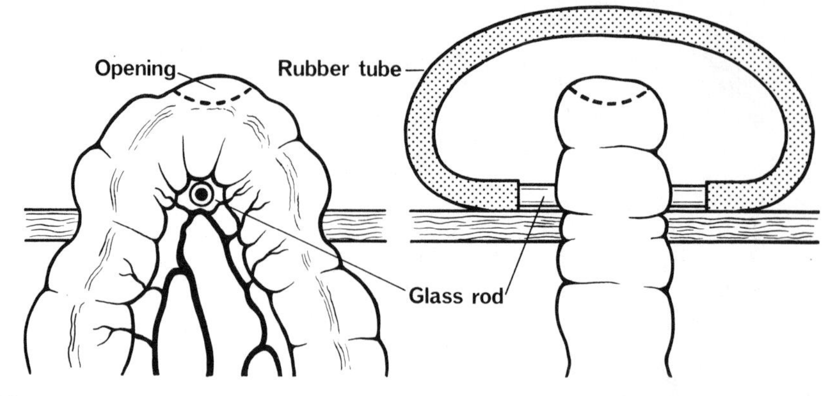

Figure 10.6 Temporary colostomy.

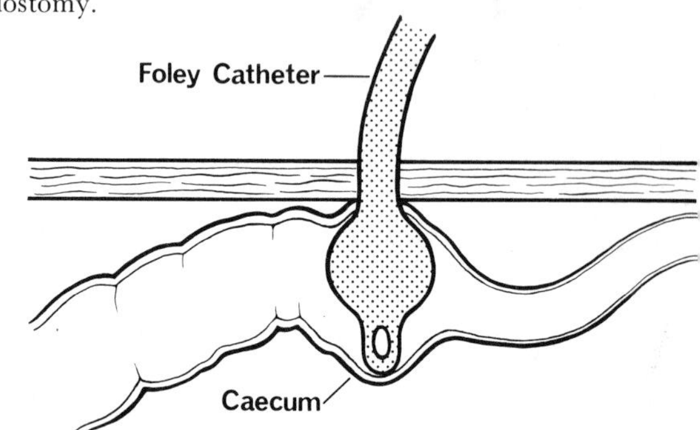

Figure 10.7 Caecostomy.

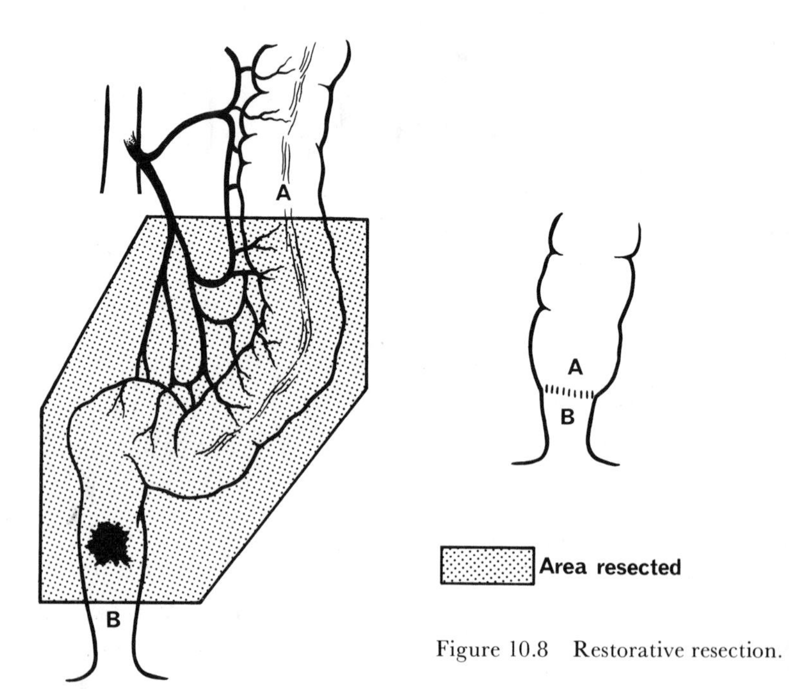

Figure 10.8 Restorative resection.

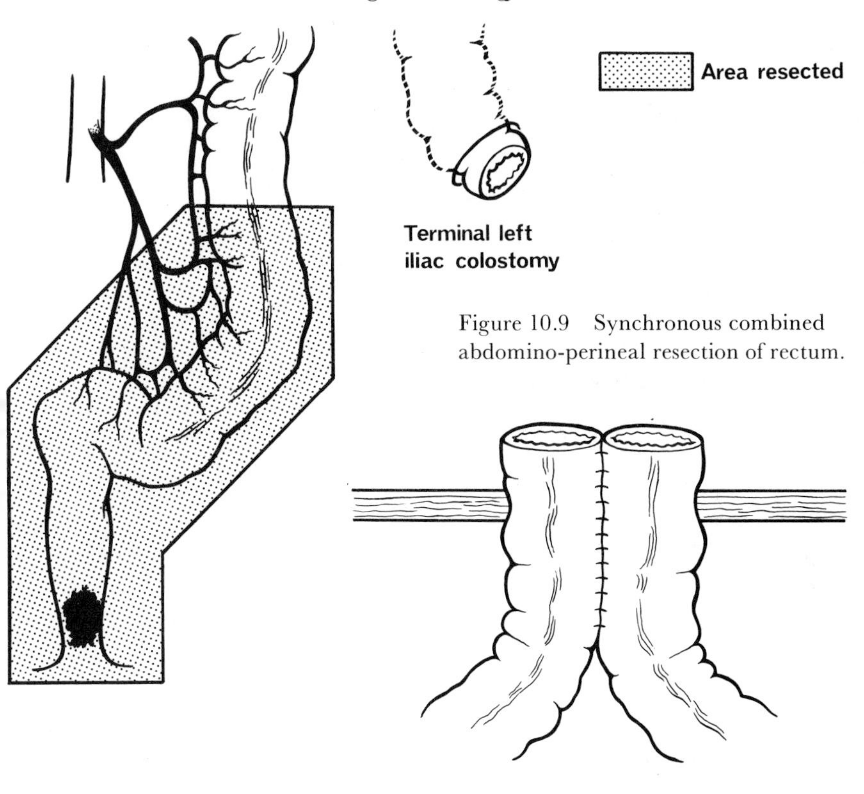

Figure 10.9 Synchronous combined abdomino-perineal resection of rectum.

Figure 10.10 Spur colostomy.

Palliative Paul-Mikulicz resection resulting in a spur colostomy (Fig. 10.10) or Hartmann's resection (Fig. 10.11) is sometimes performed in elderly or infirm patients. It is now accepted that 'second look' operations may be justified to resect recurrences in certain cases of colorectal cancer. It must also be borne in mind that a second primary tumour may occur in the remaining colon.

BREAST

An example of a malignant lesion which may often be treated successfully by surgery and radiotherapy is cancer of the breast. Nearly 30 per cent of all female malignancies arise in the breast, affecting about 5 per cent of women. Those who have not had children appear most susceptible, as do mothers who have not breast fed.

Histologically the tumours may be classified as being intraduct (growing within the ducts of the breast) or infiltrating. If the malignant cells are arranged in a glandular pattern resembling normal breast

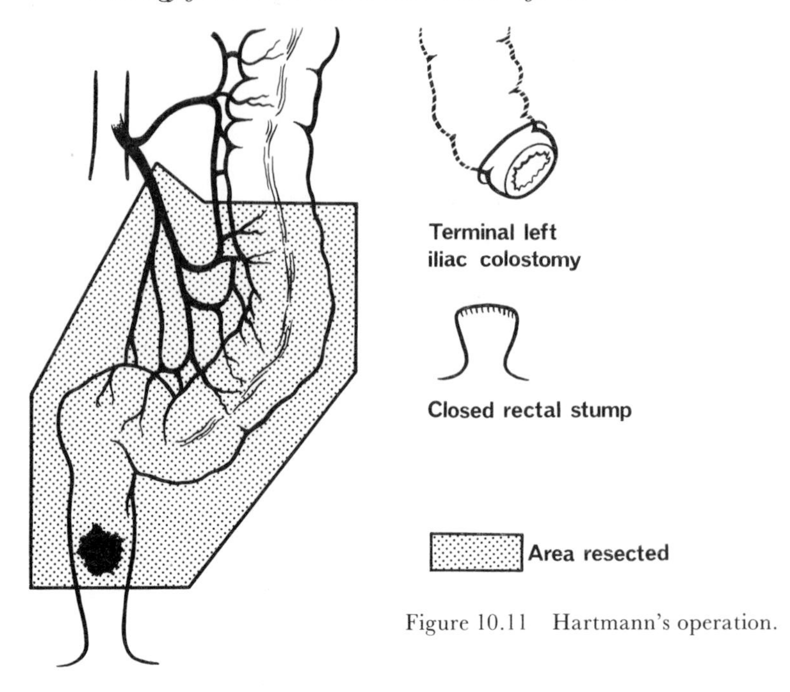

Figure 10.11 Hartmann's operation.

tissue (alveolar), the tumour is less aggressive. The proportion of glandular tissue and fibrous stroma varies and there is thus a variety of tumours ranging from soft (medullary) cancers to fibrous (scirrhous) lesions. Spread is by local infiltration and via the lymphatic and vascular channels (Fig. 10.12). Secondary deposits in the lungs, liver and bones are most common. In an attempt to rationalize operative treatment, the extent of spread of the tumour is assessed before surgery is undertaken.

The aim of surgical treatment is to excise the tumour before it has spread – remembering that primary malignant change may occasionally be multifocal. This has usually led surgeons to remove the entire breast if it contains a cancer (simple or total mastectomy). However, a limited *wedge resection* can very reasonably be defended on theoretical grounds and will undoubtedly be performed more often in the future. If there has been some clinically detectable spread, an attempt to block further spread by removing the lymph nodes in the axilla can be made (*simple (or total) mastectomy and anxillary clearance*). Even without clinical spread, we know that microscopic spread may often have taken place and this leads some surgeons to perform a mastectomy and *en bloc* dissection taking the pectoral muscles – *radical mastectomy* (Fig. 10.14). If more distant nodes such as those above the clavicle

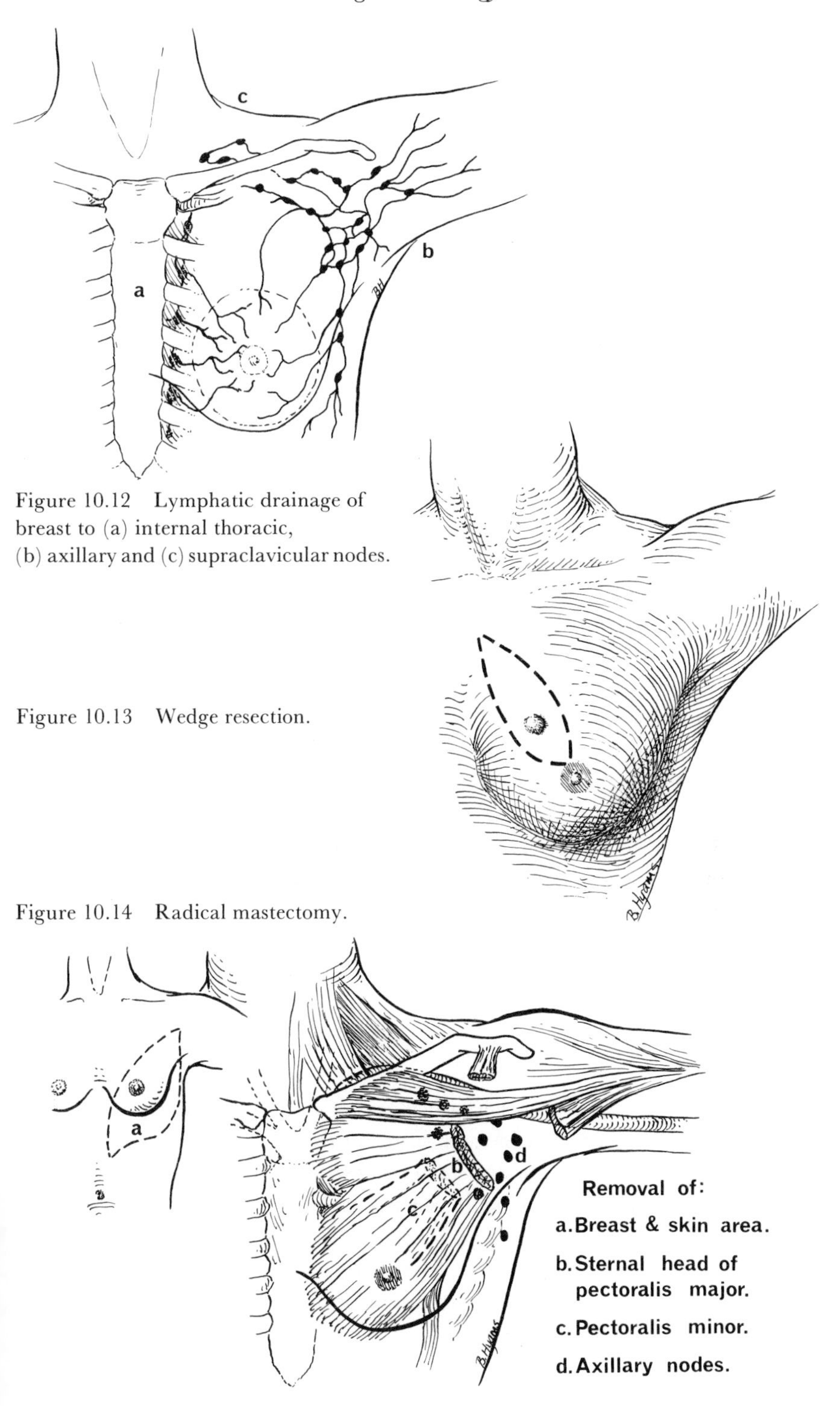

Figure 10.12 Lymphatic drainage of breast to (a) internal thoracic, (b) axillary and (c) supraclavicular nodes.

Figure 10.13 Wedge resection.

Figure 10.14 Radical mastectomy.

or in the internal mammary chain are removed, the operation is called a *super-radical mastectomy*.

Usually skin closure following mastectomy is possible but occasionally a skin graft is required. Suction drainage to prevent fluid collecting under the skin flap is now generally employed.

Surgery is sometimes indicated, even if cure is clearly impossible, in order to reduce the risk of offensive local ulceration. Occasionally this is undertaken after initial radiotherapy and is called '*toilet mastectomy*'.

After mastectomy, if the axillary glands are found to contain deposits of cancer cells, postoperative radiotherapy is usually given in order to destroy any malignant cells which remain in the axilla. Radiotherapy is also given to the chest wall if the lesion has become fixed to the muscles or fascia lying beneath the breast. When the cancer is in the medial half of the breast, radiotherapy is given on the assumption that the internal thoracic glands (which cannot be felt) may have small deposits even though they may not have been biopsied.

Chemotherapy is now being used in addition to surgery and radiotherapy in breast cancer either as 'adjuvant' therapy in an attempt to reduce recurrence or in advanced cases where metastases have not been controlled by other measures.

The knowledge that breast cancer is to some extent hormone dependent has led to medical and surgical attempts to alter the hormone environment of the tumour. Surgical removal of the ovaries in premenopausal patients may cause dramatic regression. Occasionally, removal of the adrenal glands (which are a major source of sex hormones in postmenopausal patients) or hypophysectomy (pituitary ablation) is undertaken. Following both these procedures, substitution hormone therapy is required and it is now more common to suppress adrenal function with corticosteroid therapy.

KIDNEY

An example of a malignant lesion which may often be treated successfully by surgery, chemotherapy and radiotherapy is kidney tumour (e.g. Wilms's tumour in children). Tumours of the kidney usually present with haematuria, pain which may be due to clots of blood causing obstructive colic, and a palpable mass. All three of these features only occur together in about 15 per cent of cases. The most common adult tumour is an adenocarcinoma (hypernephroma) and that found in infants and children most commonly is the nephroblastoma (Wilms's tumour).

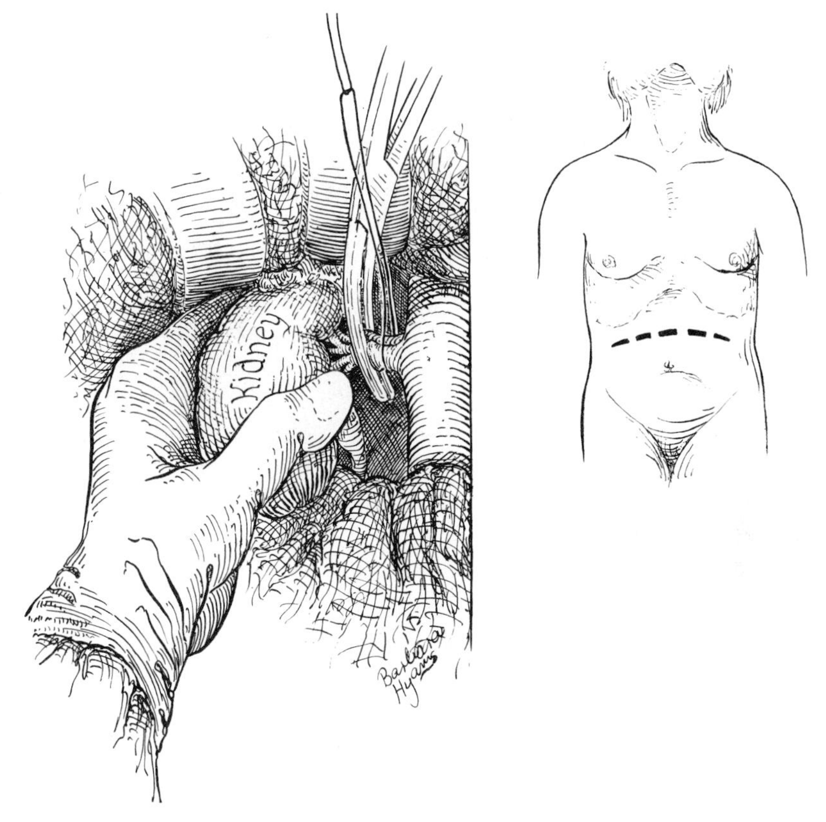

Figure 10.15 Nephrectomy – transperitoneal approach.

Although not usually necessary in children, the surgeon may have to undertake cystoscopy as a diagnostic procedure and even insert a fine tube into the ureter via a cystoscope in order to perform retrograde pyelography. Removal of the kidney together with the perinephric fat (nephrectomy) is performed in both adults and children if the lesion is curable. In children an anterior, transperitoneal, approach is commonly used (Fig. 10.15). This has some technical advantages and also allows the other kidney to be examined. In adults the classical loin incision is often used (Fig. 10.16). The renal pedicle is ligated as early as possible during mobilization and great care undertaken to avoid rupturing the capsule of the kidney and spilling cells.

Chemotherapy starts at the time of diagnosis before surgery according to a prescribed schedule. That used in the children's solid tumour protocol at St Bartholomew's Hospital in Stage 1 disease is as follows: Vincristine 1·5 mg/m² is given weekly starting before surgery

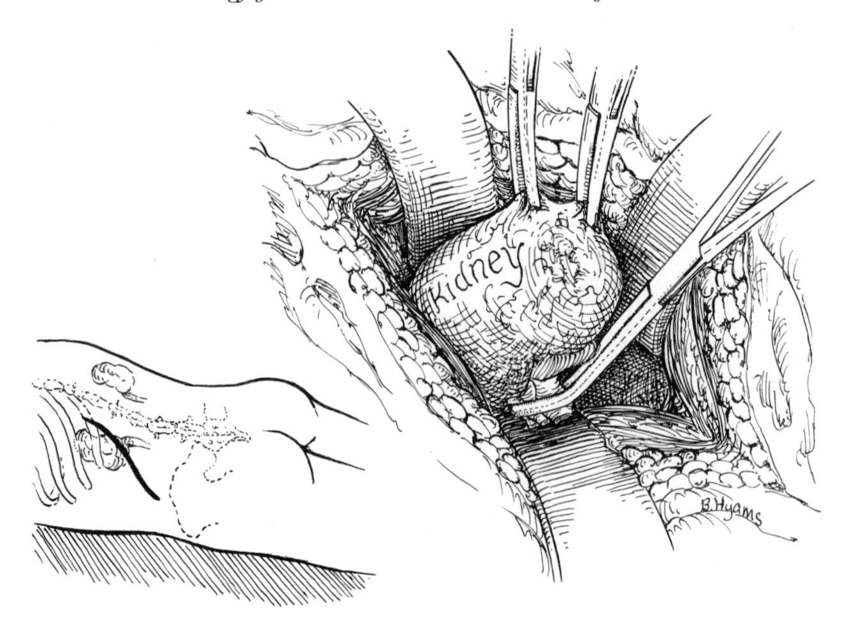

Figure 10.16 Nephrectomy – loin approach.

and extending through the period when the child is having post-operative radiotherapy to the renal bed and para-aortic glands. After a four-week rest period this weekly injection cycle is repeated regularly, giving a three-week course with a four-week rest period between. Actinomycin-D (1·4 mg/m² IV) is given in addition at the start of each cycle. This treatment may be continued for a year. The complications of synchronizing surgery, radiotherapy and these drug regimes require the closest co-operation between all groups working in the hospital and underline the special multidisciplinary approach now required in cancer treatment.

Chapter 11

The Nature of Radiotherapy

M. RUTH SANDLAND
M.B., B.S., F.R.C.S., F.R.C.R.
Consultant Radiotherapist
St Bartholomew's Hospital, London
Hospital for Sick Children, Gt Ormond Street

Introduction

One does not have to be involved for many months in the care of patients having radiotherapy before one realizes that to ask a person to undergo a course of such treatment very frequently evokes a response of extreme fear.

It is not altogether surprising that patients react in this way, however. Most adults know of relatives or friends who have been treated with irradiation (often called 'radium treatment' or 'cobalt bomb treatment' by lay people). They know that these people have often been diagnosed as having cancer. Many of them will have died, often soon after their treatment. Some of them, especially in years gone by, will have had severe skin reactions (radiation 'burns') and some will have been quite ill during treatment. A general air of hopelessness probably surrounded them.

Once treatment has commenced and other patients – some apparently very fit and others obviously very ill – have been met in the radiotherapy department, familiarity with the routine and the helpfulness which we like to think exists among the staff involved, should dispel this fear to some extent. However, there is one important aspect which probably contributes to the continuance of depression and dislike of the treatment, quite apart from the particular disease or any disturbance resulting from the treatment.

Many radiotherapy departments are housed in basements, without natural lighting. The entrance to many of the treatment rooms is not direct; one has to traverse a 'maze' corridor, turning corners before reaching the part of the room containing the unit. The 'setting-up' of the treatment position by the radiographers is accompanied by much adjustment of the couch on which the patient lies; and lights will frequently be turned on and off. When everyone is satisfied with the position, the patient will be left alone, with the light on, while the machine is turned on by remote control and the staff watch through a small, distant pane of lead glass for any movement or signal of discomfort. At the actual time of its administration the patient will not feel anything that can be identified as coming from the irradiation. This makes such treatment a little mysterious, unlike the taking of tablets, or subjecting oneself to the surgeon's scalpel.

In the following paragraphs, some of these points are considered in an endeavour to see how the unseen irradiation works and why the conditions under which it is given have to operate, as well as discussing some of its short-term and long-term side effects. The techniques and equipment have been improved, so the side effects may not be so prominent as previously.

Radiotherapy is not used just as a palliative treatment for someone who has a limited life expectancy, but it is commonly used as part of a planned treatment programme for malignancies in which surgery and chemotherapy may also be involved with a curative intent.

What are X-rays?

A large spectrum of electromagnetic radiations operates in the universe. By these radiations, electromagnetic energy moves from one place to another. Energy is usually spoken of as moving in space as 'bundles' or 'quanta' in a wave-pattern. The distance between one point on a wave and a corresponding point on the next wave is known as the wavelength. The shorter the wavelength of the quanta, the greater the wave frequency, and hence the greater the energy. The 'intensity' of the radiation gives a measure of the flow of energy, that is the amount passing through a particular area in a particular time. The unit in which this intensity is measured is the electronvolt. The electromagnetic irradiations most familiar to us are those of visible light. Light itself is composed of a spectrum of radiations of different wavelengths, separately giving the colours of the rainbow. Of greater wavelength (and lesser energy) are infrared rays and radio-waves. Of lesser wavelength (and greater energy) are the ultraviolet radiations, while of even smaller wavelength are the X-rays and gamma-rays which we must now consider.

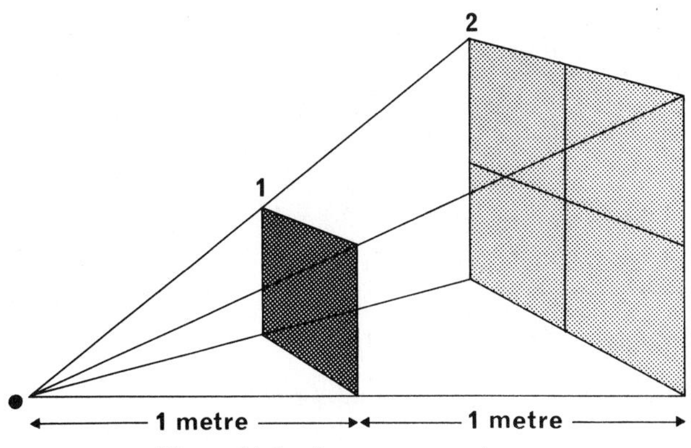

Figure 11.1 Inverse square law.

X-rays have energies ranging from a few thousand electronvolts (or kilovolts, kV) to several million electronvolts (or megavolts, MeV). The particular name given to a quantum of X-radiation is a photon. The greater the energy of the photon, the greater its penetration in matter. Also of practical importance, as we shall see, is a basic law of physics – the Inverse Square law. This can be roughly stated thus – the radiation intensity at a point varies inversely as the square of the distance from that source.

For example, if there is a radiation intensity of 1,000 units at 1 metre from a source, there will be an intensity of $\frac{1}{4}$ of 1,000 (250 units) at 2 metres, and one-ninth of 1,000 (111.1 units) at 3 metres from the source. Figure 11.1 shows this diagrammatically.

The term gamma-ray is used interchangeably with X-ray and this is a broadly valid transfer of terms. However, the radiation known strictly as gamma-radiation is differently produced from X-radiation as we shall see later.

HOW ARE X-RAYS PRODUCED?

X-rays were first detected by Röntgen in 1895 when he was experimenting with passing a high voltage current through a vacuum tube. Present-day production makes use of the same principle – that X-rays will be produced when high-speed electrons are arrested by a target of high atomic number. Not all the kinetic energy of the electrons is converted to X-radiation; much of it is converted to heat. The electrons are usually produced by thermionic emission, from an electrically heated tungsten filament which is the cathode, and are brought to rest on a target or anode which is made of a heavy metal such as tungsten, and which if placed at a suitable angle to the path of the

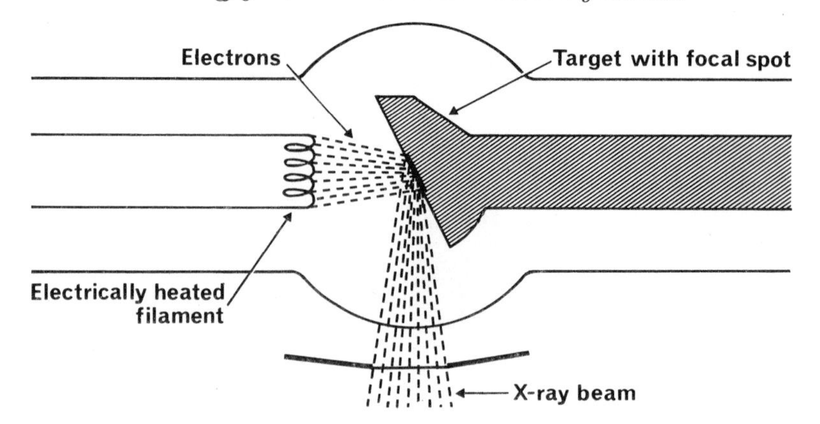

Figure 11.2 Diagram of a tube for the production of X-rays by an electric current.

bombarding electrons can reflect the resultant X-radiation away in a suitable direction for use. The equipment has to incorporate a cooling system for dispersing the heat generated at the target, and a collimator to direct the beam (see Fig. 11.2).

The spectrum of energies of the X-radiation varies with the voltage of the electric current applied. Therefore, at a particular applied voltage, the quality or penetrating power of the X-radiation will be the same, though its quantity or intensity will vary with the material used in the target anode.

GAMMA-RAYS AND RADIOACTIVITY

Gamma-rays are identical with X-rays in their behaviour, though not in their mode of production. For an understanding of their formation we have to discuss the concept of radioactivity.

All matter is made up of atoms which, in turn, are combinations of neutrons and positively charged protons characteristic of the particular element and making up its nucleus. Electrons (negatively charged) are arranged around this nuclear structure in shells or orbits and are bound to the nucleus at a characteristic binding energy for the particular element. Some of these neutron–proton combinations are not stable, and when this is the case, a spontaneous disintegration of them may take place to form a more stable combination. This process is called decay and the unstable combination is described as being radioactive, because of the by-products of the decay. In the process of disintegration, energy is released, frequently in the form of high-speed electrons or other particles. In addition, non-particulate and uncharged electromagnetic radiations called gamma-rays may be released and these have

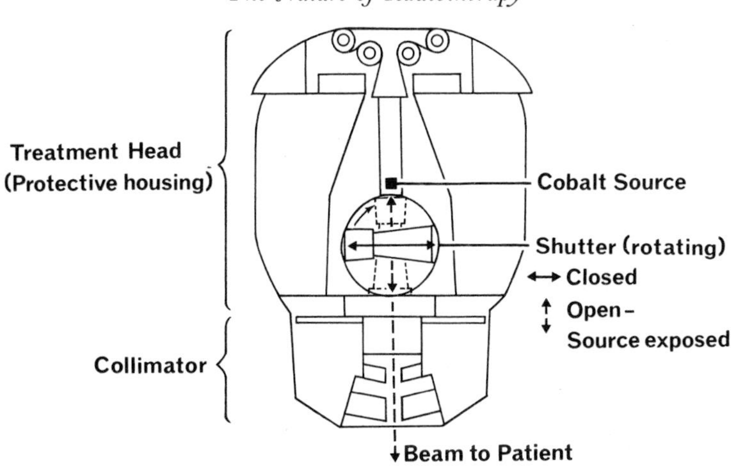

Figure 11.3 Diagram of cobalt unit with protective housing and shutter mechanism.

energies in the same range as X-rays. Thus, for practical purposes, the terms X-rays and gamma-rays are interchangeable.

An example of such decay is that of radioactive cobalt which is written thus:

$$^{60}\text{Co} \rightarrow {}^{60}\text{Ni} + \text{electron} + \text{gamma-ray}$$

The radioactivity of several elements is made use of in radiotherapy. While some radioactive elements, such as uranium, occur naturally, most clinically useful radioactive elements are produced artificially. In the case of radioactive phosphorus or cobalt this may be by neutron bombardment or nuclear fission in a cyclotron or nuclear reactor. Radium is not used very much in therapeutic situations today, though formerly it was the most frequently used radioactive element. ^{60}Co and ^{137}Cs are two of the most commonly used radioactive materials today.

Figure 11.3 shows the basic structure of a cobalt unit for external beam therapy. The radioactive cobalt is constantly undergoing decay as described above, and is therefore built into a protective housing. To release the gamma-rays for treating a patient, the radiographer operates switches which allow the protective lead to move aside so that the gamma-rays pass down the collimator instead of being absorbed within the housing.

Radioactive elements give off less radiation as time passes. This fact is expressed in the concept of 'half-life' which is defined as the time taken for half of the radioactive material to decay or for the rate of emissions to fall to half. Thus, if an element has a half-life of ten days, its radioactivity will be half as much on day ten as it was on day one,

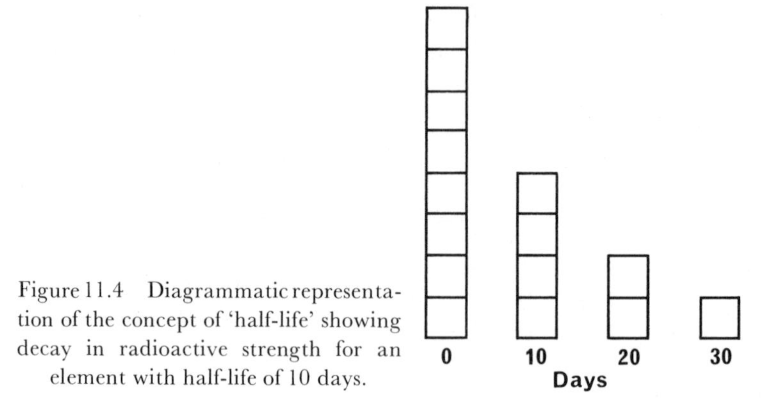

Figure 11.4 Diagrammatic representation of the concept of 'half-life' showing decay in radioactive strength for an element with half-life of 10 days.

it will fall to one-quarter strength at twenty days, and to one-eighth strength at thirty days as shown in Fig. 11.4. Table 11.1 lists the half-life of some of the radioactive elements which have been used in radiotherapy. It will be clear that these facts have important corollaries so far as their storage, handling and disposal in clinical use are concerned, and these will be discussed later in the chapter.

Table 11.1 *Half-life of elements used in radiotherapy*

Element	*Symbol of Radio-active form*	*Half-life*
Radium	Ra 226	1620 years
Caesium	Cs 137	30 years
Cobalt	Co 60	5·3 years
Tantalum	Ta 182	115 days
Iridium	Ir 92	74 days
Phosphorus	P 32	14 days
Iodine	I 131	8 days
Gold	Au 198	2·7 days
Yttrium	Y 90	2·5 days

IONIZING RADIATIONS IN TISSUES

It is beyond the scope of this book to explain with any completeness the complexity of the interactions which occur when X-rays pass through tissues. But it is important to mention the basic factors affecting the passage of an X-ray beam in order that we can understand better a patient's treatment.

It is obvious to state that the intensity of a radiation beam decreases as it penetrates the tissues. But how does this happen? In general, this process, known as attenuation, has two main components, absorption and scatter. There are several other processes of photon attenuation, but these are relatively unimportant as the energies of practical concern to us.

ABSORPTION

To express it simply, there is more absorption of radiation from the beam the greater the thickness and also the greater the density of tissue placed in its path. For each centimetre of tissue in the path of the beam, the fractional decrease in energy will be the same, the exact fraction depending on the energy of the particular beam.

In human tissues, this process is not an important constituent of the attenuation process as the elements making up the tissues hold their electrons in their atomic shells at a very low binding energy relative to the range of photon energies in use. Thus, very little beam energy is required to eject electrons. However, if the beam is passed through lead or other material of high atomic number, much more energy is absorbed in overcoming the binding power of the inner orbits of electrons.

SCATTER

Photon scatter is a common phenomenon when the X-ray photon collides with the peripheral electrons of the atom. Some of its energy may be given to the electron which, freed from its linkage to the more central atomic particles, moves away at an angle to the path of the beam. The photon also will be scattered, with diminished energy, at an angle which may be as great as 180°, i.e. continuing its journey back along its original path.

Photons of low energy may be scattered in any direction, but the higher the photon energy, the more likely is scatter to occur in a forward direction. Thus the scattered photons of a high energy beam continue to make a large contribution to its intensity as it travels onwards in the tissues. This fact is utilized much in modern radiotherapy.

Another corollary of this predominance of forward scatter with high energy beams is the phenomenon known as 'skin-sparing'. With low energy irradiation, backward scatter from collisions occurring just under the skin surface contributes to the dose received at the surface

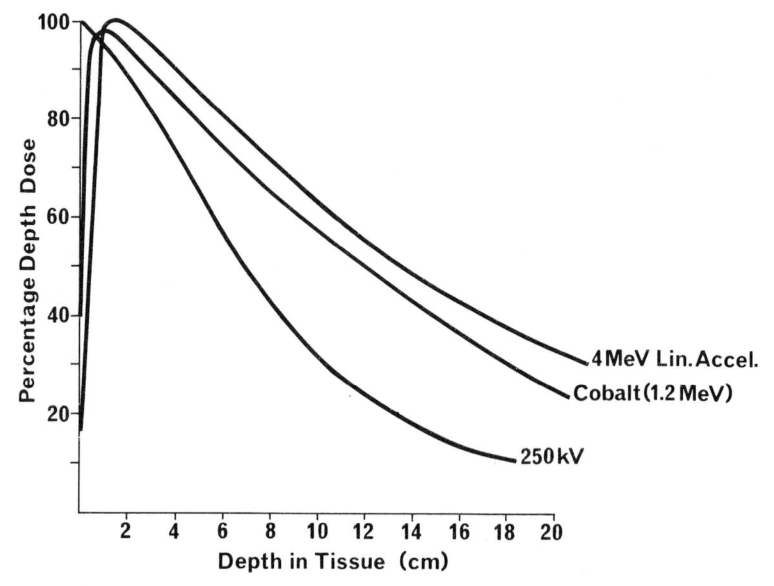

Figure 11.5 Depth–dose curves for beams of different energies.

in such a way that the maximum dose occurs at the surface. With virtually no back-scatter at higher energies, the maximum dose is not reached until several millimetres of tissue have been penetrated, thus sparing the skin. This principle is illustrated in Fig. 11.5.

In the days when only low energy irradiation was available, it had to be used for all tumours, whether superficially or deeply situated. High doses had to be administered to achieve a satisfactory dose in a deeply seated lesion. The skin therefore received a much higher dose and this could result in a very uncomfortable skin reaction. This need not happen nowadays with megavoltage equipment due to the skin-sparing effect, and the administration of a lower dose will be adequate for a deep tumour because of the higher penetration.

There are times when one wishes to overcome the usual advantage of the skin-sparing effect, i.e. to give a tumour-killing dose to the whole thickness of a scar or when the tumour involves the skin as well as much deeper tissues. In such a case, 'build-up' material, equivalent to a few millimetres of normal tissue, may be placed over the skin, thus ensuring that the skin surface receives full dosage.

Similarly, in some tumour sites where great precision in positioning of the patient is required, as in the head and neck area, a cast or shell several millimetres thick may be made to immobilize the patient so that each day's treatment is in precisely the same position. When this is the case, we may again see a skin reaction at energies and doses at which it would not normally be expected.

EXIT BEAM

With the use of penetrating megavoltage therapy, another factor has to be allowed for in planning the patient's treatment. Figure 11.5 shows the relative intensity of beams of various energies at different depths from the skin surface. If we look at the intensity of each beam at 15 cm it will be very low for the 250 kV beam. When using the 4 MeV beam, the intensity at 15 cm will not be inconsiderable, and at such a depth may even have penetrated the full thickness of the patient's tissues in that site. In such situations we say that we have to allow for the 'exit beam' and this becomes especially important if we are giving additional treatment from the opposite side of the patient, as is often the case.

PENUMBRA

We have already seen that with low energy irradiation scattered photons may move in any direction, whereas at high energies scatter is predominantly forwards. This has important consequences at the edge of the X-ray beam so, if there is much sideways scatter, there will be a zone of tissue which, though not receiving as much radiation as that in the centre of the beam, will still receive a significant dose. This zone is termed the penumbra.

A megavoltage beam has a very narrow penumbra or, put in another way, it is said to have a sharp 'cut-off'. This fact is of value in planning treatment as we can therefore ensure that the irradiation given to surrounding normal tissues is minimized.

Particle Beams Used in Radiation Therapy

Much less commonly, a beam of particles, charged or uncharged, is used clinically to produce ionization. Electron beams of high energy have now found a place of great usefulness in practice, and the use of neutron beams is being explored in order to find their best role. We will mention other particles which are of much less established value.

ELECTRONS

These are negatively charged particles, and light in mass relative to the neutrons and protons of the atomic nucleus. They are often called beta-particles in contrast to the positively charged alpha-particles, and both are emitted quite commonly in the disintegration of radioactive nuclei.

Electrons behave in tissue as ionizing radiations, but their range is very dependent on their energy. Radioactive phosphorus (^{32}P) pro-

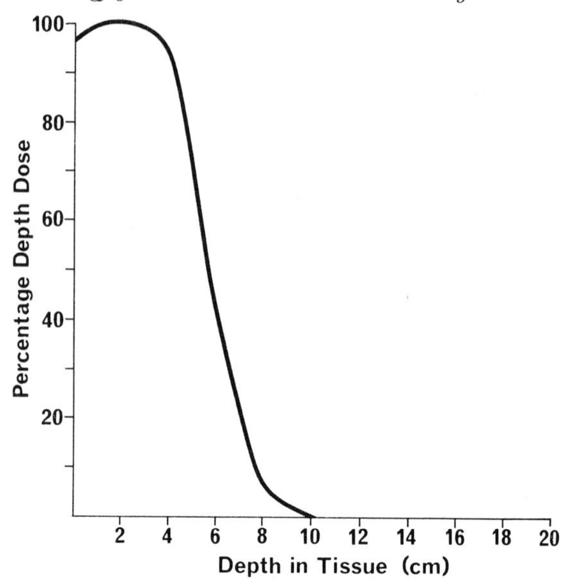

Figure 11.6 Depth–dose curve for 15 MeV electrons.

duces electrons in its decay and their range is only a very few millimetres. But there are clinical situations where use can be made of this property. Electrons of much higher energy are produced by an electric current and are accelerated down the wave-guide of a linear accelerator. It is possible on some machines to make use of these accelerated electrons rather than the X-ray beam which would be produced by their bombardment of the target. In such a case, their energy is in the range 2–15 MeV.

The Betatron is a unit specially designed to produce electrons at an energy of 20 MeV or greater, using a unit which is much more compact than would be required for the production of a beam of this energy in a linear accelerator.

Figure 11.6 is the depth–dose curve for a 15 MeV electron beam. If we compare the shape of this curve with those of Fig. 11.5, it will be seen that though the range is about 8 cm in tissue, there is a rapid fall-off in intensity at a greater depth, unlike the gradual fall-off of the X-ray beam. This characteristic is particularly obvious in a lower energy range, e.g. 2–5 MeV. In treating a superficial tumour, if the appropriate electron energy is used, normal tissues beneath the tumour will receive a rapidly decreasing dose.

Electrons are very readily scattered. In order to minimize this, the collimator of the generator has to be brought down close to the skin. Even so, there is considerable scatter deep in the tissues at the beam edges, resulting in a wide penumbra.

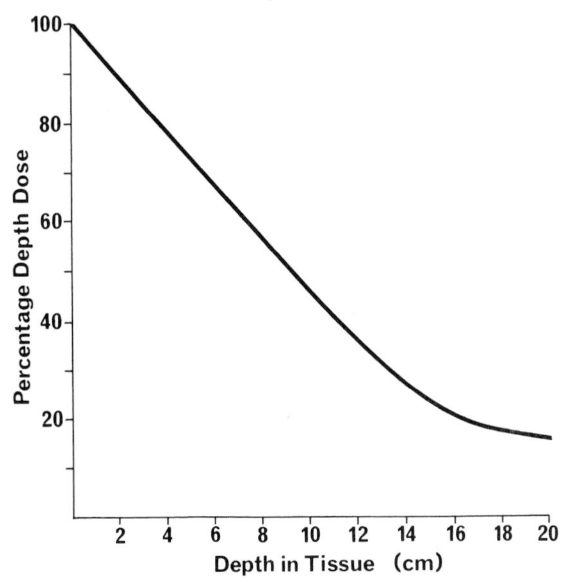

Figure 11.7 Depth–dose curve for 14 MeV neutrons.

NEUTRONS

These particles are present in the atomic nucleus in association with protons. They are liberated in the radioactive decay of some elements and produced artificially in cyclotrons in a wide range of energies. Between 6 MeV and 15 MeV is a clinically useful range, in that they have sufficient penetrating power (Fig. 11.7), and can be produced on a relatively small and less expensive generator.

It is their effectiveness in killing cells in the absence of oxygen, shown experimentally, which has made them attractive, though these theoretical advantages have not found wide application as yet.

PROTONS

These positively charged particles travel in straight lines through matter and, at an energy of 100 MeV, have a range of about 10 cm. Most of their ionization in tissues occurs at the end of their track, resulting in a very limited depth at which they can be useful (Fig. 11.8). This high dose area can be brought nearer the surface by the insertion of wax blocks in the path of the beam. The use of protons has been confined to the treatment of very small lesions such as pituitary tumours, with the purpose of minimizing radiation to the normal brain tissue through which the beam passes. Production, however, calls for a very costly and large cyclotron.

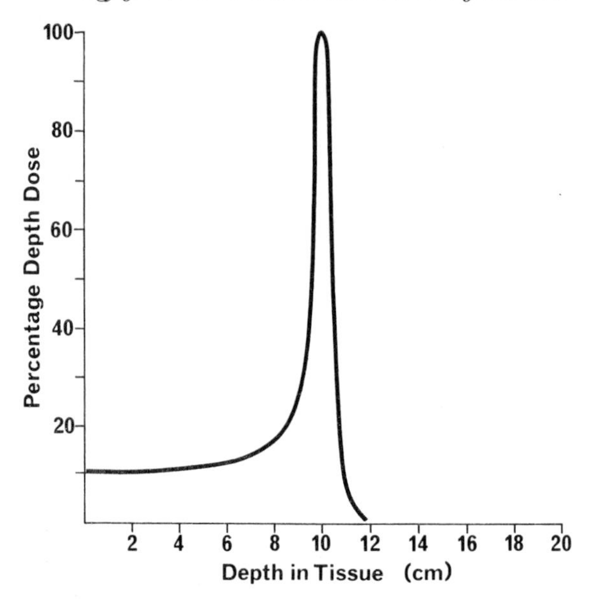

Figure 11.8 Depth–dose curve for 100 MeV protons.

ALPHA PARTICLES

These have a double positive charge and are of considerable mass. They travel slowly and lose their energy quickly and are of no clinical usefulness.

NEGATIVE PI-MESONS

These heavy, negatively charged particles are produced in large cyclotrons and have a depth–dose pattern at 50 MeV, very similar to that of the proton beam illustrated above (Fig. 11.8). Their theoretical attraction is the same as that of neutrons in that they are not dependent on the presence of oxygen for their effectiveness. Wide use is never likely to be achieved because of the expense of production.

Biological Effects of Ionizing Radiations

One of the chief effects of the passage of photons through matter is the ejection of electrons from the shells of the atoms which make up matter. The ejected electron interacts with the surrounding atoms, being deflected by the negative charge of their outer shell electrons in many cases, resulting in a tortuous course and a rapid loss of energy. Or, if this interaction occurs at greater energy, other electrons may be ejected by it from the shells of their parent atoms, leaving them ionized and capable of entering into chemical reactions or open to receive another electron and return to their normal state.

Where the 'matter' through which the ionizing radiations are passing is living tissue, these subatomic and chemical effects result in biochemical changes which, in turn, cause cell damage. The exact mechanisms by which these occur are imperfectly understood, and to introduce even a preliminary discussion of this large field of enquiry would be unhelpful at this stage.

However, some of the observed effects of radiation damage at a cellular level include rapid death of some cells and the impairment of DNA synthesis in others. If the latter is the case, the process whereby the nuclear material replicates itself prior to cell division is delayed, and when the cell division (mitosis) eventually occurs it may be abnormal, and the abnormality, if severe enough, may lead to cell death.

One of the questions naturally arising in this context is that of the variable response of the tissues of the body to irradiation and why it is that irradiation can be used to destroy tumour cells without destroying in the same way the normal cells in its path.

While in a full discussion of this subject it would be seen that many other facets would require amplification, it is fairly accurate to say that a greater proportion of tumour cells are undergoing cell division than in most normal tissues and that, in general, radiation destroys a greater proportion of cells where mitoses are frequent. This does not, of course, explain this phenomenon, but it is consistent with the observed differences in radiosensitivity of normal and tumour cells. It also correlates with the differences in radiosensitivity between various normal tissues. For example, the rapidly dividing cells of normal bone marrow or of the bowel epithelium are much more susceptible to irradiation than muscle cells where the mitotic rate is slow.

OXYGEN EFFECT

Other factors have been shown to play their part in the susceptibility of a living tissue to damage by irradiation; important in this respect is the presence of oxygen in the cells at the time of irradiation. It has been shown experimentally that two or three times the dose of irradiation may be needed to inflict the same damage on a tissue in the absence of oxygen. One assumes that normal tissues, in communication with their oxygen-carrying blood supply are well oxygenated. But this is not always so in a tumour, where the central cells may be poorly oxygenated and thus protected from the effect of radiation.

Various methods to overcome this 'oxygen effect' have been tried experimentally and some have been applied in the clinical field, especially the use of the hyperbaric oxygen tank (Fig. 11.9). In this apparatus the patient is placed in the treatment position while breathing oxygen under three atmospheres of pressure. Over several minutes the oxygen tension of the tissues is thus increased including the hypoxic portions of tumour masses. Once the oxygen tension is believed to be uniformly raised, the radiation is given. Encouraging results from such methods have been reported in tumours of the head and neck, as well as bladder and gynaecological malignancies, but they have not been sufficiently convincing to result in their widespread use, quite apart from the considerable practical difficulties of using these time-consuming methods.

As already mentioned above, neutrons and pi-mesons are not so dependent for their efficacy as the most commonly used X-rays and gamma-rays on a good oxygen tension in the tissues. As yet, these theoretical advantages have not been widely applied therapeutically.

FRACTIONATION: DOSE–TIME RELATIONSHIPS

Much of the theoretical basis of therapeutic radiation has been established in the animal laboratory. Large single doses of irradiation may be given to the whole or portion of the animal and its effects studied. This is not possible in humans, but we know from these experiments and from experience of atomic explosions and radiation accidents, that exposure of the whole body to a high dose may be fatal or severely damaging, while a smaller dose has lesser effects. In addition, a total exposure over many days may not have anything like such a severe effect as a single exposure to the same total dose.

This will, perhaps, be more readily understood if one likens exposure to ionizing radiation to sunbathing. If one lies with a large portion of the skin exposed to a hot sun for five hours on the first day of one's summer holiday, one is not surprised to have a rather uncomfortable erythema of the exposed skin the next day. However, if instead, the same skin area had been exposed for one hour each day for five days, there may be some erythema, increasing over this period, but it would not be so severe. And it would be even less severe if the five hours of exposure were achieved in ten doses of half-an-hour on each of ten consecutive days.

This is the principle on which 'fractionation' (the dividing up of the total dose of radiation into smaller 'fractions') is based. If all one had to consider was the tumour, it could, perhaps, be eradicated in one

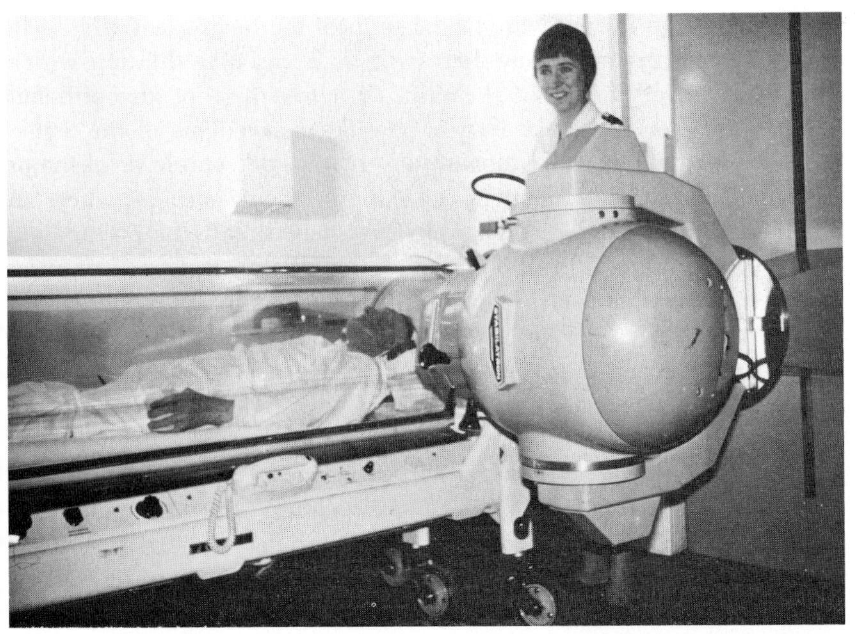

Figure 11.9 Patient ready for treatment in the tank breathing hyperbaric oxygen.

large dose. But the normal tissues would not tolerate this and so the treatment is extended to allow for some recovery of the normal tissues to occur between doses. One could imagine that this would allow time for the tumour activity to recover as well, or for it to continue its growth between fractions. Some allowance is made for this in that the final total dose is somewhat larger than if all the treatment had been given in a single dose.

EFFECTS OF RADIATION ON NORMAL TISSUES

The most obvious radiation effect known to an earlier generation of radiotherapists was the erythema of the skin, the severity of which was related to the factors of time and dose discussed above. While megavoltage equipment presently in use has, by its skin-sparing quality, removed this helpful evidence from us in many cases, the fact remains that there is a response to radiation damage similar to that inflicted by any injurious agent. Whether it be a chemical burn on the skin, or an operation wound, or a bacterial infection in the bladder, the body's response is basically the same once the harmful agent has been removed. The difference in the response evoked by irradiation is that the blood vessels and connective tissue components normally activated in response to tissue damage may themselves have been damaged by the radiation if they were in the path of the beam. Initially, as in any inflammatory reaction, there will be a vascular dilation which may result in erythema of the skin, or a mucositis of an epithelial surface (as when the oral cavity is irradiated). Oedema of the tissues may also occur, but this is not usually readily detectable or of major significance in the management of a patient except, perhaps, where an advanced tumour of the laryngopharynx may already be prejudicing the airway and any additional swelling may be critical.

When a course of treatment is finished and the total dose given has not been excessive, nor the time in which it has been given too rapid, return of the tissues to normality may occur, at least to all superficial appearances. However, this is not always the case, especially if a large volume of tissue has required inclusion in the treatment fields. It can be readily appreciated that if a small volume of tissue is irradiated, none of it is very far from unexposed tissue which is able to respond with the normal healing processes. But, if a large volume has been irradiated, as for example in a large carcinoma of the bronchus or an advanced bladder carcinoma, the more central parts of the volume will have a blood supply which has, itself, been damaged to some extent. Thus, it is likely that healing will only occur in association with some fibrosis and contracture, and the diameter of the damaged blood vessels may be reduced by sclerosis. Having said this, there is wide individual variation in the severity of damage done with apparently identical treatments.

In summary, three main factors are of importance in the amount of radiation damage inflicted on normal tissues:

1. Total dose given.
2. The number of doses given and the time over which they are spread.
3. The volume of tissue treated.

RADIOSENSITIZERS

It has been an attractive idea to radiotherapists for many years that chemical substances might be found, which, if given to a patient before or at the time of radiation, would potentiate its action. This would mean a lower total dose requirement. An ideal radiosensitizer, as such a substance is called, would be one which preferentially protects the normal tissue cells from radiation damage without protecting tumour cells.

Many agents have been tried and thought to confer some advantage in experimental animals, but in the clinical situation they are often unsafe because of severe toxic effects if given in adequate dose to achieve their purpose. Such agents are not in general use, but one called misonidazole is showing promise.

CYTOTOXIC DRUGS AND RADIATION

Irradiation is often used in combination with cytotoxic drugs which, when first produced, were often called 'radiomimetic' because of their similarity to irradiation in their action against tumour cells. It is clear that some at least of those agents potentiate the action of irradiation in normal tissues both at the time of its administration and acute reaction, and also in its long-term effects. An example of the former is the increased severity of the skin reaction in a treated area sometimes seen when methotrexate is used. Another is the known increased incidence of radiation hepatitis when actinomycin-D is used and the liver is being irradiated. An example of more long-term potentiation is the increased severity of pulmonary fibrosis when actinomycin-D and irradiation of the lungs are both employed.

These effects, as with all the acute and long term results of radiation, are dependent on the relationship of total dose of radiation given, the number of fractions and the volume of tissue treated.

Practical Considerations in Treating a Patient with Radiation

Having considered some of the underlying principles of the production and use of ionizing radiation, some of the factors in the choice of treatment for a particular patient can now be discussed. External beam therapy is only one, albeit the commonest, of three main ways of delivering radiation to a patient.

A. External Beam Therapy (Teletherapy)
B. Moulds, Implants, Applicators (Plesiotherapy)
C. Radioactive Isotopes used systemically

A. EXTERNAL BEAM THERAPY

Four questions must be in the therapist's mind when planning a patient's treatment.

1. What is the tumour?
The histology report given by the pathologist about a tumour provides important information about its likely radiosensitivity and its anticipated pattern of spread.

2. Where is the tumour?
This is not such a foolish question as might at first appear. Sometimes we may be able to locate a tumour on the patient ourselves,

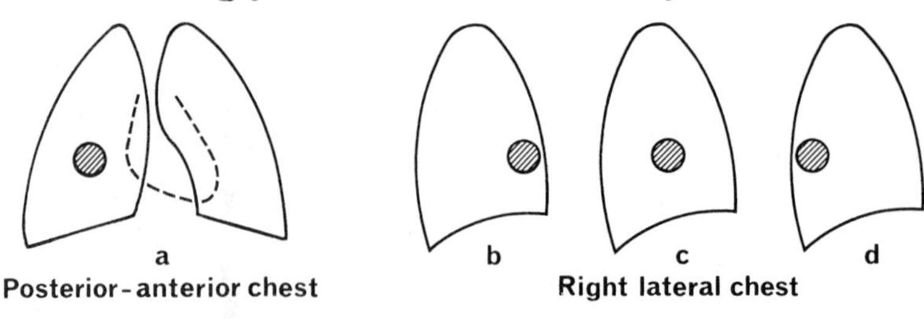

Figure 11.10 Diagram of lung tumour showing that its position must be defined in three planes before planning irradiation.

using our eyes and our hands. More often, information about its position may have to be obtained from X-rays, scans, ultrasonic examinations or the surgeon's findings at operation. Whatever the sources of our information, we have to answer this question in three dimensions. Just looking at a routine posterior–anterior chest X-ray may reveal a tumour in the midzone of the right lung as in Fig. 11.10(a). But, unless we look at the lateral chest films as represented diagrammatically in Fig. 11.10(b), (c), and (d), we may not realize that the tumour could be at any one of the three depths illustrated or, indeed, extend through the complete thickness of the chest from front to back.

3. What volume must be treated?
This question reminds us that very commonly a malignant tumour, by its very nature, will have spread microscopically beyond the limits which we have palpated with our hands or seen on X-ray or scan. It is usually wise to include a margin of apparently normal tissue around the tumour to allow for this, as well as including the lymphatic drainage areas if this is appropriate in the light of the answer to question one.

4. What normal structures are nearby?
This question must not be dominant in one's thinking, unless possible damage to normal structures by including them is likely to be disabling. One must always try to minimize normal tissue damage but this must not be done at the expense of inadequately treating the tumour. For example, great care is always taken to spare the dose to the spinal cord as radiation myelitis is a recognized and severe complication in a proportion of patients if well-documented limits of dose and speed of administration of radiation to it are exceeded. Occasionally, however, one must take risks in relation to normal tissues, keeping in balance the risks of undertreating against those of damage to normal structures.

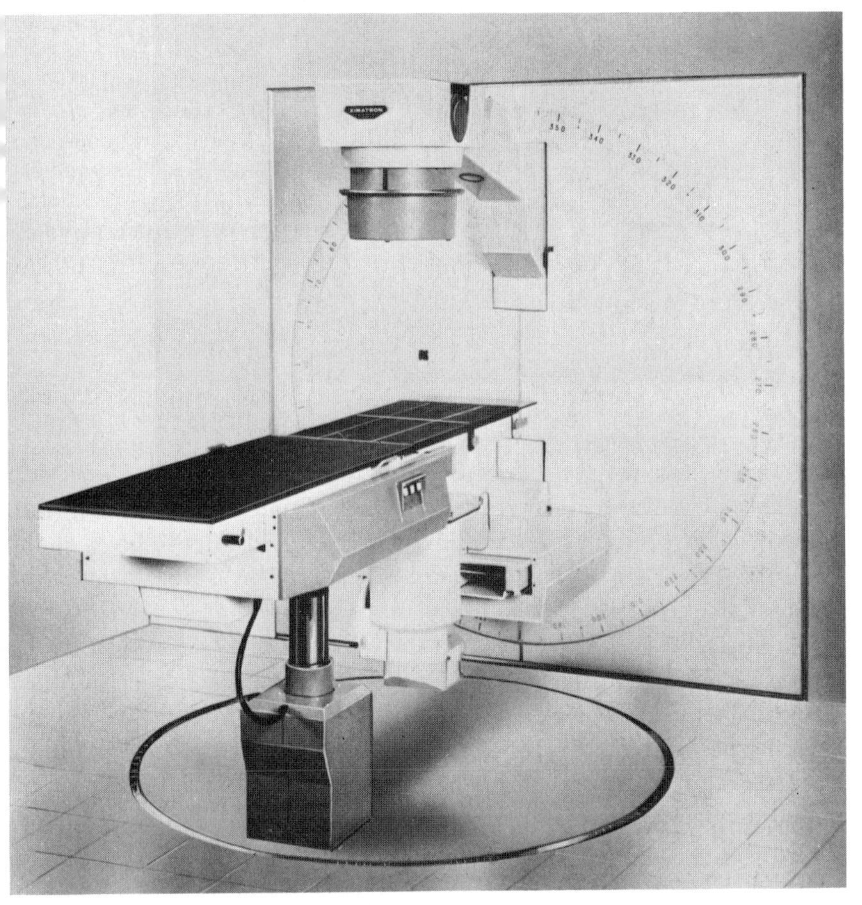

Figure 11.11 Ximatron simulator with X-ray tube and image intensifier.

Preparing the Plan of Treatment

Having answered these preliminary questions it is possible then to proceed with the formal planning.

Most modern radiotherapy departments have a simulator. This is an X-ray unit with image intensifier which, with the aid of a television screen, is used to locate quickly X-ray and skin landmarks which the radiotherapist has already defined as the boundaries of the treatment volume. The patient is positioned on the simulator couch in the same posture and at the same distance from the X-ray machine source as is planned for use in treatment (Fig. 11.11). X-ray pictures are taken with markers indicating the boundaries of the tumour, this being done in more than one plane if feasible. The central level of the planned volume has been marked both on the X-rays and the patient (Fig. 11.12).

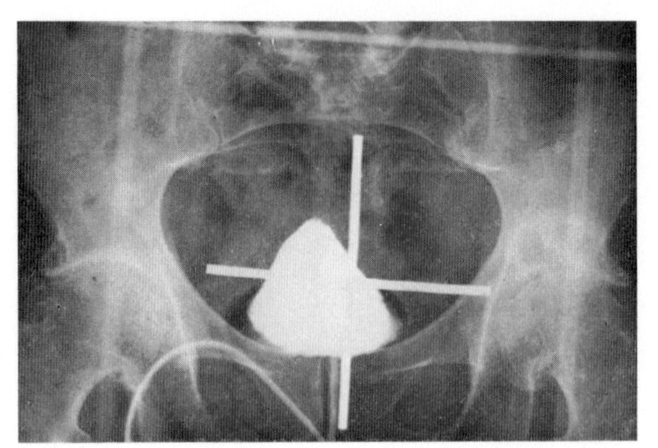

Figure 11.12 Simulator X-ray of a patient being planned for pelvic irradiation for carcinoma of bladder. Dye, instilled by urethral catheter, outlines the bladder. The metal cross, on the patient's skin, is reference point for measurements.

The physicist takes an outline of the patient's contour while lying in that position and through that central plane. (For example, if an intrathoracic tumour to be irradiated extends from the level of the upper border of the second thoracic vertebra to the lower border of the sixth thoracic vertebra, it is likely that the patient's contour will be taken at the level of the middle of the fourth thoracic vertebra.)

The physicist transfers the patient's contour on to a piece of paper and this 'outline' is passed to the radiotherapist for him to transpose the 'volume' requiring a tumour-killing dose of radiation from the planning X-rays on to paper. He also draws on (by measuring their position accurately from the X-rays) the position of any normal structures such as the spinal cord or rectum, the dose to which must be considered. (See Fig. 11.13).

The physicist then sets about producing a 'plan' of treatment which as nearly as possible gives a uniform dose across the whole of the volume outlined by the therapist, with as rapid as possible fall-off in dosage to the surrounding normal tissues and vulnerable structures. (See Fig. 11.14).

In some departments, this task has to be done manually, with the use of charts of the depth dose produced by the particular unit chosen. In other departments, this phase of the planning is made easier by the use of a digital computer which has in its store of information these depth–dose charts. To obtain a satisfactory plan, at least two, and sometimes three, four or more fields facing the patient from different directions may be required. The production of such a plan is sometimes far from straightforward, and several factors may contribute to difficulty.

First, the chosen tumour-bearing volume may be an irregular shape, or biased to one side of the body, making it asymmetric, or close to a

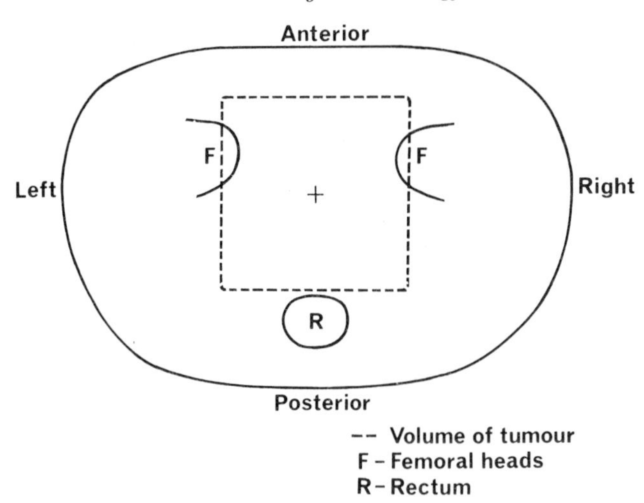

Figure 11.13 Outline of patient's contour taken through centre of planned treatment volume, taken from planning X-ray.

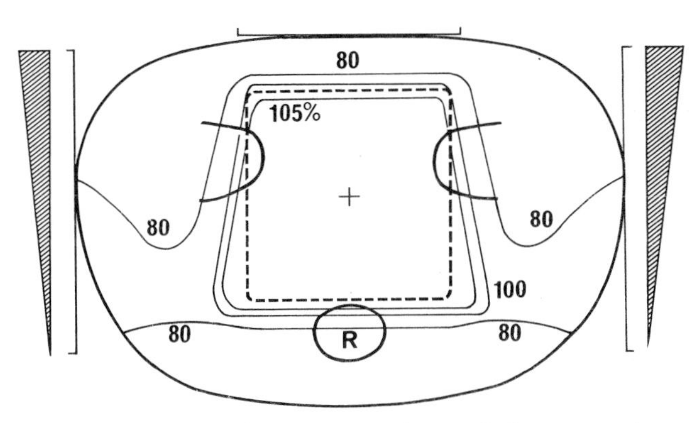

Figure 11.14 Physicists' plan of treatment to give marked tumour volume as uniform dose as possible. In this case, one anterior beam and two lateral beams are used.

vital structure. In these cases it is often necessary to apply the X-ray beam at oblique angles or to use a combination of 'wedged' fields. A 'wedge' is a piece of lead which can be mounted on the head of the X-ray machine and which is of a size to cover the dimensions of the field required. The thickness of the lead increases across its width and, as the X-ray beam passes through it, the thick end absorbs more irradiation than the thin end which thus allows more irradiation to reach the patient on that side of the field and is therefore called the 'hot' edge of the wedge. In this way, the contribution of a particular treatment field can be varied across its width, catering for a particular tumour volume. (See Fig. 11.15).

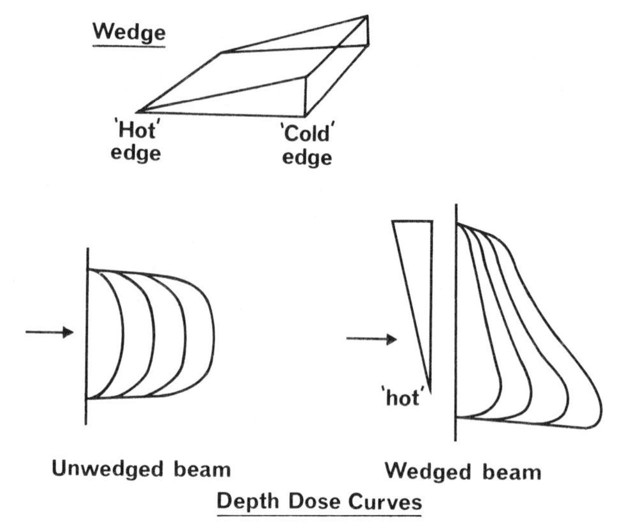

Figure 11.15 Wedge – a device for modification of the X-ray beam.

Second, the surface on which the X-ray beam falls may not be flat, or even regularly curved. A wedge, as described above, may be sufficient to compensate for the difference in intensity of the proportion of the beam which has to traverse more air before reaching the tissue surface than does another portion. But, if there is marked irregularity of shape, or irregularity in more than one plane, other methods are called for.

Compensators, (Fig. 11.16), which are individually fashioned blocks of lead for each patient, are also able to be mounted on the head of the X-ray machine and make use of the same principle of variable X-ray absorption of the X-ray beam as do the wedges. The difference is that they allow for variations in the patient's contour in both the vertical and horizontal plane.

A less sophisticated method of compensation for the irregularities of a patient is often used, especially when a uniform dose to the skin surface as well as in deeper tissues is required. By the use of bolus bags, which contain material of density comparable to that of human tissue and which are flexible enough to fit into irregular contours, the X-ray beam then strikes a uniform block of tissue or its equivalent. Similarly, a wax mould or plastic shell may be used to make a rectangular block onto which that X-ray beam falls, as in the treatment of a skin cancer of the bridge of the nose. (See Fig. 11.17).

Third, the tissues through which the irradiation passes may not be homogeneous. In particular, the density of normal lung tissue is less

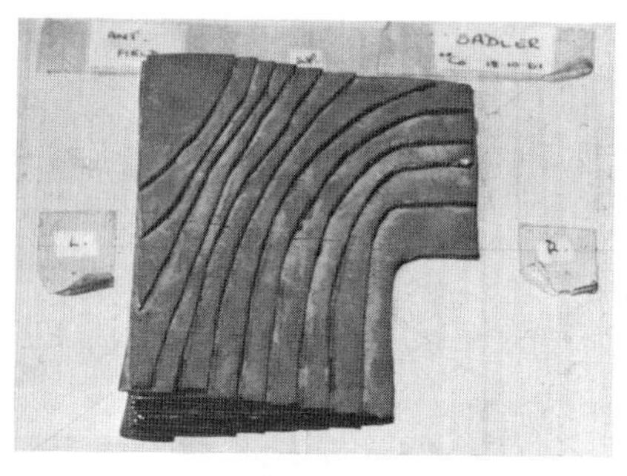

Figure 11.16 Compensators – layered lead adjusts for variations in a patient's contour.

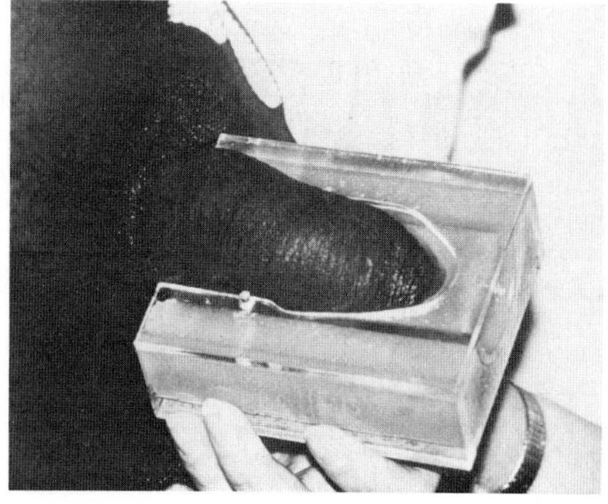

Figure 11.17 Half of wax mould used for lesion of penis. With both halves in position, the organ is part of a rectangular block, ensuring uniform dosage.

than that of body tissue generally, and this results in less radiation absorption. This factor does not apply, of course, if the area of lung in question is infiltrated by a solid tumour, but it should be allowed for in calculating the dose which a deeply-seated intrathoracic lesion such as a carcinoma of the oesophagus will receive.

The presence of bone in the path of a low-energy (kilovoltage range) X-ray beam results in increased absorption of radiation. In the megavoltage range most commonly used today, bone absorption, however, is not significantly different from that in other tissues.

Fourth, the shape of the beam emerging from the treatment unit is rectangular. The diaphragms on the collimator can be adjusted to alter the length and width of the field, but lead blocks must be placed in the path of the beam if protection of tissues in a portion of that field is required. In Fig. 11.18(a), the field for treating a child's pelvis is shown. It is possible to shield the growing ends of the upper femora by triangular blocks of lead of appropriate thickness without shielding the pelvic tumour.

Similarly, when treating the nasopharynx by lateral fields (Fig. 11.18(b)), it is possible to protect the eyes with a lead block which absorbs scattered rays in the 'penumbra' and also insert a lead block into the upper posterior corner of the field to protect the brain.

After all these factors have been considered, it is sometimes necessary for the physicist and radiotherapist, in consultation, to allow a small degree of compromise in the finally accepted plan, but with experience on all sides the occasions on which this is necessary will be few.

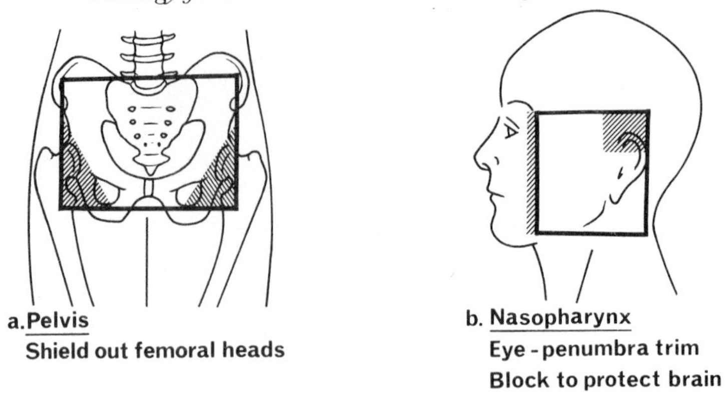

Figure 11.18 Diagrams showing use of lead blocks in protection of normal tissues not involved by tumour.

Treating a Patient

The patient is positioned on the treatment couch in the same way as on the simulator, and with the treatment head at the same distance from him as when the planning X-rays were taken. The machine's light beam, marking the central axis of the X-ray beam is focused on the centre mark made on the patient at the time of simulation. (In some situations, this central point may have been made more permanent by the carrying out of a pin-prick tattoo, or there may be several marks on the patient's skin to enable greater checks on accuracy.) The jaws of the collimator of the treatment machine are set at the dimensions previously determined and any wedges or compensators needed are inserted by the radiographers and their position checked. (See Fig. 11.19). The patient is then left alone in the room during the time of exposure to the treatment. While the field is being set up by the radiographers, the overhead lights in the room will probably have been turned off, but when the patient is ready for treatment they will be turned on again.

The dose of radiotherapy to be administered over the course of treatment will have been decided by the radiotherapist and calculated for each treatment by the physicist. The radiographer sets the appropriate time on the machine controls so as to give the required dose. With megavoltage equipment, such as the linear accelerator, the dose rate is often of the order of 100 rads per minute. Thus, if 250 rads is the prescribed dose, it will take about two and a half minutes to give. With a cobalt unit, one has to allow for the radioactive decay of the source which has a half-life of 5·3 years. In practical terms, if it takes five minutes today to administer 400 rads, it will take ten minutes to administer the same dose in 5·3 years time. Adjustments are therefore

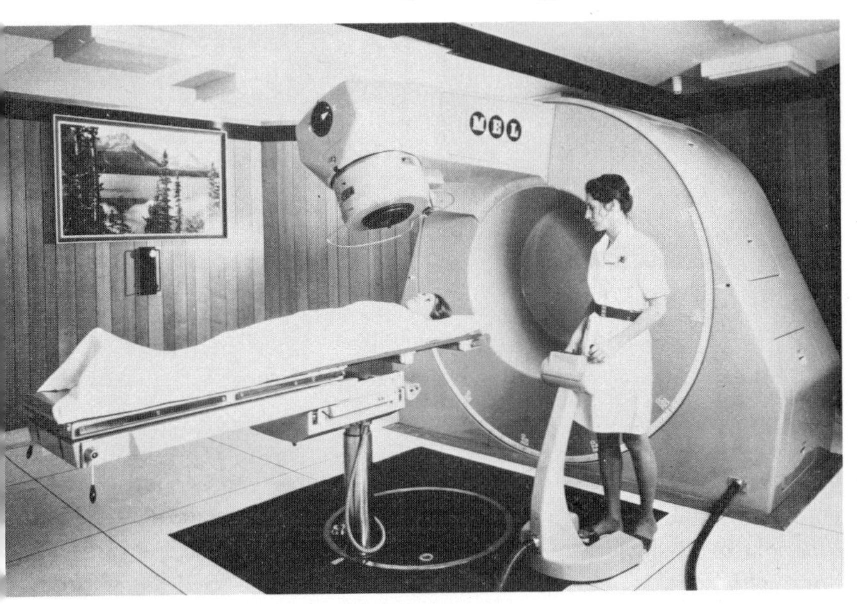

Figure 11.19 Patient positioned for treatment on Linear Accelerator (SL75-10 by courtesy, Churchill Hospital, Oxford).

made to the output figures each month so that the correct dose is given according to the time for which the patient is exposed. The cobalt source itself is replaced every three years or so, in order that treatment times do not become too protracted and the department become unable to treat as many patients in a working day as the source gets 'weaker'.

B. PLESIOTHERAPY: MOULDS, IMPLANTS AND APPLICATORS

Plesiotherapy (by derivation, short-distance or near-therapy) is much less commonly used than previously, though there seems to be a recent revival of interest in its use at selected sites.

In principle, with the use of radioactive sources immediately adjacent to, or within, the tumour-bearing tissue one is able to administer continuously or, by certain techniques, intermittently, a high dose of radiation. The sources used for each therapy are usually of low intensity compared to the strength of the source contained permanently in a unit designed for external beam therapy. The intensity of the source when measured at a distance from it obeys the Inverse Square law as discussed earlier. This means that there is a rapid fall-off in intensity at a short distance from the source, ensuring that nearby normal tissues are not heavily irradiated.

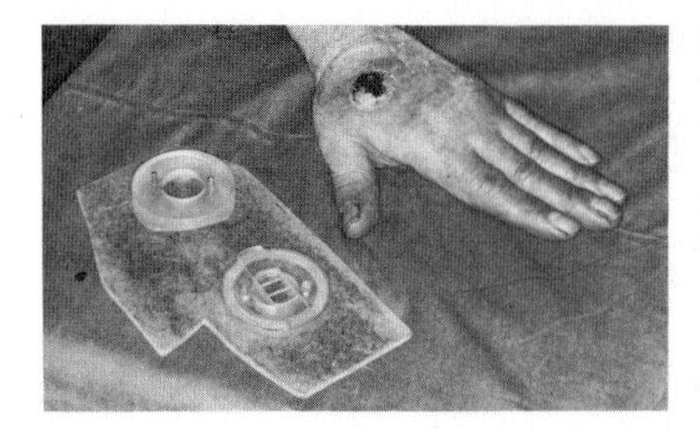

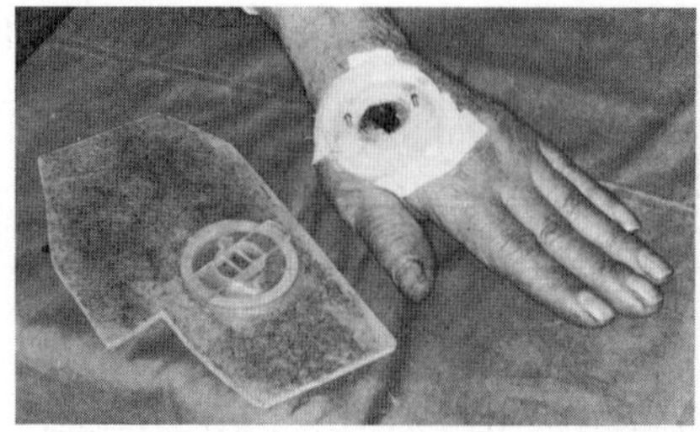

Figure 11.20 (a) Lesion on dorsum of hand. (b) Base of mould positioned over lesion ready to receive sources embedded in mould at left.

Moulds

Not commonly used today, this is a method whereby a mount or cast of some plastic or other material is made to apply precisely to the tissue containing the tumour. In it are mounted the required radioactive sources. Sites where moulds have been used include the dorsum of the hand, the lip, the penis, and for large scalp lesions. (See Fig. 11.20).

When the radiotherapist has decided on the area and the depth of tissue which should receive a tumour-killing dose, the physicist uses specially calculated tables to determine the number, the strength and the spacing of the sources needed to give the required dose in a particular time. He also determines the distance from the skin at which the sources have to be stabilized within the mould to give this dose.

In practice, it may necessitate the patient wearing the mould for six or seven hours a day for several consecutive days. For the patient, this may be no more than tedious and inconvenient, and perhaps uncomfortable. But for the department arranging it, problems of protection from radiation exposure to staff and other patients arise and this has been one reason for its decline in popularity as a treatment method.

Implants

In this method, the radioactive material is inserted into the tumour itself. In recent years, with the advent of a greater variety of sources of increased flexibility of use, there has been more widespread application of this technique.

The principle of treatment is again that of deciding the amount of radioactive material and its distribution on the basis of the volume of tissue requiring the tumour dose. The physicist can then advise the strength and length of sources to employ.

We may use this technique with caesium needles for a large tumour

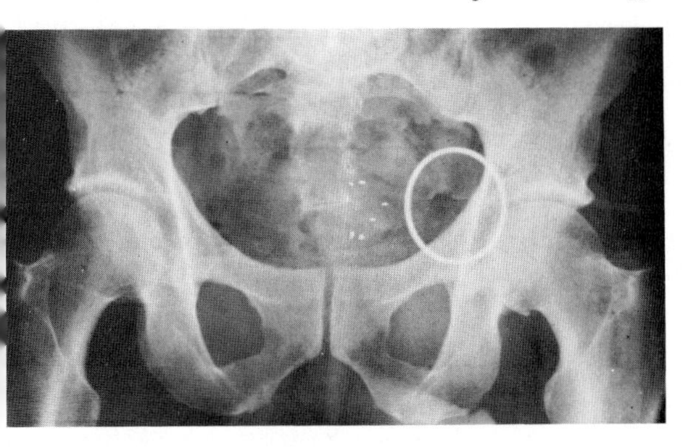

Figure 11.21 Gold grains shown on X-ray after insertion into bladder tumour at operation.

involving the tongue and floor of the mouth, or with gold grains for the base of a superficial tumour of the bladder the rest of which has been diathermied by the surgeon. (See Fig. 11.21). Also, iridium wires, mounted in flexible nylon tubing, may be inserted into residual lymph node masses in the neck or into a breast lump where there has been previous external beam therapy.

Again, the advantage is that one can limit the dose to surrounding normal tissues, and this may be a critical factor in satisfactory treatment if these tissues have had prior heavy irradiation.

Intracavitary Applicators

This method has been in continuous use for many years as part of the treatment for many cases of carcinoma of the uterine cervix and body. Anatomically, the uterus is situated approximately centrally in the pelvis, with the rectum close to it posteriorly and the bladder nearby anteriorly. Both these organs could be damaged severely and irreversibly if the doses which are known to be required to deal with these tumours are given entirely by external beam therapy. Instead, part of the treatment is given by applying the sources close to the cervix and within the uterine cavity. Radium was the material used previously but it is now largely replaced by caesium. (See Fig. 11.22).

The accurate positioning of these sources and the packing of them so that they do not slip or give unnecessarily high doses to the bladder or rectum can be difficult in inexperienced hands. Even with experience, the procedure may take some time, and as it is carried out under general anaesthetic in an operating theatre it involves many staff in some exposure to irradiation. In a later section of this chapter some of the ways in which this risk can be minimized are discussed.

Techniques have been developed whereby the sources are not loaded

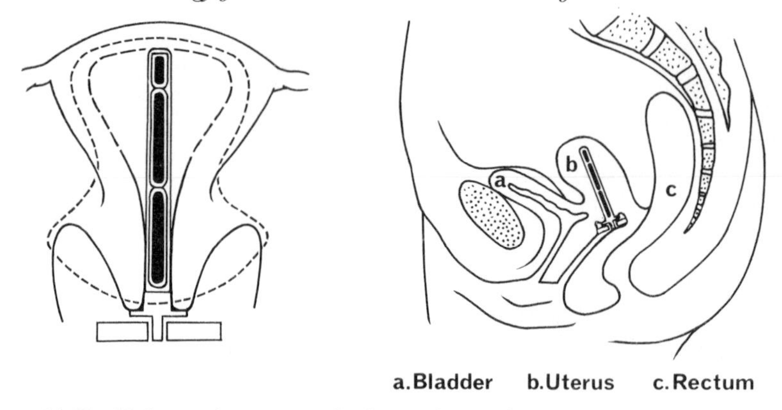

Figure 11.22 Tube caesium sources in the uterine cavity and against the cervix at the vaginal vault shown in diagrams of the anterior and lateral views (as used for carcinoma of cervix).

into the applicators until the position of them has been shown by X-ray to be satisfactory. Such techniques are known as 'after-loading' and in these cases, the sources are not usually put into the patient until she is back in the ward. Sophisticated equipment such as the curietron or cathetron is in use in some hospitals, and by this means the sources can be loaded mechanically, by remote control, thus minimizing the exposure of staff. The length of time for which the applicators are in position varies with the strength, number, and position of the sources and with the dose required.

C. SYSTEMIC USE OF RADIOACTIVE ISOTOPES

Elements which normally participate in the body metabolism and which are selectively taken up by certain tissues may, in their radioactive form, be of clinical usefulness. Two such elements are radioactive phosphorus (^{32}P) and radioactive iodine (^{131}I).

In the case of ^{32}P the range of the emitted alpha particles is only a few millimetres. But when incorporated into bone in the course of its metabolism, its ionizing power may be of use in at least two clinical situations – in polycythaemia rubra vera, a condition in which the blood-forming bone marrow is hyperactive, and second, the diffuse bone metastases of prostatic cancer, though its value in this latter condition is small.

^{131}I is used in relatively small doses in non-malignant overactivity of the thyroid gland. The thyroid takes it up from the circulation as if it were normal dietary iodine and it can then destroy a proportion of the cells secreting excess thyroid hormone. In some cases of thyroid cancer, especially those where the cells are well differentiated, it can be shown by the use of small tracer doses that they are metabolizing iodine. This may even be true of some thyroid cancer metastases in bone. Where this is demonstrated, it is sometimes appropriate to administer large doses of radioactive iodine to destroy the activity of these tumour deposits.

Radiation Protection

We introduced this chapter by mentioning some of the factors which may contribute to a patient's fear when subjected to a course of irradiation. What we did not discuss was the publicity given to the risks of exposure to radiation from nuclear fall-out or from accidents in industries using radioactive chemicals which has brought an additional element of fear because of the uncertainties about the consequences of radiation in the long term, quite distinct from the disease for which it is being given.

Some of the risks in irradiation treatment are known and well documented and, in most cases, avoidable in the running of a radiotherapy department. Some of the risks are only being recognized as fragments of evidence are pieced together.

Protection of the Patient

The treatment of a life-threatening disease is of the first priority, but, where irradiation is being given with the expectation of recovery, one must be mindful of possible harmful consequences in the long term. Particularly is this so in children and young adults. In the next chapter the long term effects of radiotherapy at various sites in the body are discussed, while some effects which tend to cause particular concern to the patient are described below.

Irradiation of the gonads. We know that a dose of 500 rads to 1,000 rads to the ovaries will make most women sterile; the younger the patient, the higher the dose required. When a woman needs extensive pelvic irradiation for a tumour, it is inevitable that the ovaries will receive a sterilizing dose, unless it is therapeutically safe to shield them by the positioning of a lead block in the appropriate part of the beam. In young female patients having pelvic lymph nodes irradiated in Hodgkin's disease, it is sometimes feasible to transpose surgically one or both ovaries into a midline position where lead shielding would be placed to protect bladder and rectum. Many successfully treated patients who have had this operation performed have conceived and delivered normal children.

In males, the shielding of the testes by specially made gonadal shields is a means devised to absorb scattered irradiation and is used when abdominal or pelvic irradiation is being administered, but only if by so doing one is not protecting potentially tumour-bearing tissues which are at risk.

It is important that efforts are made to do this in men having irradiation for lymphomas and testicular tumours of the seminoma type as the likelihood of survival is high. Even with gonadal shields in position during treatment, careful monitoring of the dose received by the testes should be arranged and the patient should have the risks of sterility, as well as the measures being taken to avoid these, explained to him.

The dose of irradiation which will produce permanent sterility in men is difficult to document, but a single dose of 500 rads or 600 rads may do this, whereas arrest of spermatogenesis and temporary sterility commonly occur at lower doses.

What is extremely difficult to determine is the precise risk of genetic damage (with the subsequent birth of abnormal children in future generations) when the gonads receive a lower than sterilizing dose from scattered radiation. Experimental evidence from animals suggests a strong possibility of mutations occurring, but it will take many generations before such a trend could be clearly demonstrated in humans. Meanwhile, it behoves us to keep very careful follow-up information on the children born to parents who have been exposed to radiation.

Carcinogenesis. It is one of the ironies of cancer therapy that irradiation of a tumour may, in a very small proportion of cases, result in a new tumour in the irradiated area. This occurrence has been observed at relatively low dosage where the X-rays were not used for malignant disease. For example, in years gone by, it was not uncommon for children with thymic enlargement to have the upper mediastinum irradiated. A proportion of these children developed thyroid carcinoma.

Many cases of second tumours, such as fibrosarcomas and osteogenic sarcomas have been reported in the medical literature. These have developed in the soft tissues and bones years after courses of radical radiotherapy, especially when it has been given in childhood. It would seem likely that, with the increase in numbers of children who have had malignancies successfully treated, we will be confronted with this problem more frequently. And it may be that the use of adjuvant chemotherapy will aggravate this trend.

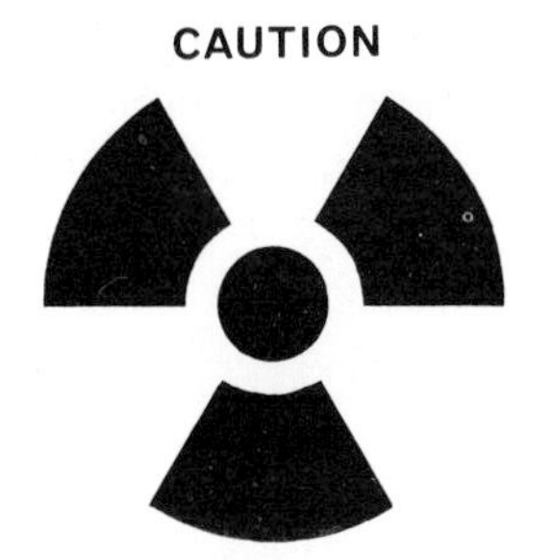

Figure 11.23 Radiation warning sign.

The increased risk of developing leukaemia after exposure to radiation has been well publicized, especially in relation to the victims of the Japanese atomic bomb explosions. The latent period between exposure and the appearance of leukaemia is usually about 5–10 years.

For these reasons, it is obvious that one should limit the use of X-ray therapy to necessary procedures, but in the treatment of malignant conditions, the risk of the primary disorder usually far outweighs the slight risk of developing a second tumour or leukaemia.

Protection of Relative and Visitors

Patients having irradiation are often concerned that they will contaminate members of their family and any others in close contact, and may even ask, 'Am I radioactive?'

The simple answer is that most radiotherapy patients are not 'radioactive' as they are undergoing external beam therapy. However, if radioactive sources in the form of moulds, implants or applicators are in position or if the patient has had a recent therapeutic dose of an isotope such as ^{131}I or ^{32}P, he must be considered as a potential radiation risk to others.

In these circumstances, a patient is, if possible, nursed in a single room or, at least, in a corner bed, with a warning notice on the door or the bed indicating that radioactive materials are in use. (See Fig. 11.23).

Precise limits of time which visitors' stay must not exceed each day are calculated by the physicist according to the intensity of the sources in use on that day (or the amount of decay and excretion which has occurred in the case of a systemically administered isotope). Pregnant women and children are not permitted to visit these patients as the risk of damage to a developing foetus or a child is greater than in the mature tissues of adults.

A patient is allowed to go home and to travel on public transport only after the sources have been removed, or, in the case of the short half-life gold grains, when sufficient decay has occurred. Similarly, with systemic isotopes, daily monitoring of the patient and his excreta will enable a decision to be taken as to when the patient may safely leave hospital.

Protection of Staff

Staff in the Wards. When a ward patient has radioactive material *in situ*, the radiation warning notice has a similar significance for nurses and other ward staff as for the patient's visitors. For each patient, guidelines are laid down as to how long any one staff member should spend at the patient's bedside in one day.

In some hospitals, specially made low lead screens (on castors for mobility) are placed along the sides of the bed to protect the bodies of the staff attending the patient. Whether or not this facility is available, staff should work in such a position as to minimize their exposure. By the Inverse Square law, the further one stands from the sources, the less will be the radiation dose received.

It is mandatory for all patients who have radioactive sources in position to have a lead pot at the bedside so that, should a source become dislodged inadvertently, it can immediately be placed in a container which will absorb the radiation being given off and can then be removed promptly to the radiation safe in the radiotherapy department. Careful routines are followed in the ward, so that the number of sources is checked regularly and linen is checked before being sent to the laundry.

Special precautions are taken in the care of patients having systemic isotopes, as in these cases the excreta are likely to be contaminated. The patient should have the exclusive use of a toilet, and all bed-linen, excreta, etc. are monitored for radioactivity with special arrangements being made for their disposal, as advised by the physicist who has been designated radiation protection officer for the hospital.

All ward staff caring for a radioactive patient will be issued with a 'film-badge' (see Fig. 11.24), and this detects the amount of radiation received by its wearer. It should be worn at all times while on duty, as the film within it is later 'developed' and the dose received calculated from the exposure detected by the film. There are well-defined limits laid down in the United Kingdom for any staff exposed.

Radiotherapy department staff. In many ways, there are less risks to the staff working with radiation at all times than to the ward staff mentioned above. The department's design should minimize the hazards, most

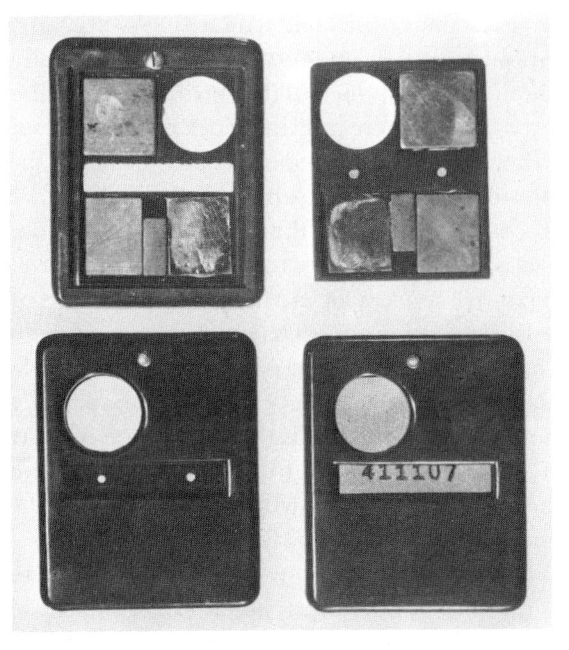

Figure 11.24 'Film Badge' worn by staff in contact with radiation.

people involved will have been trained to an understanding of the principles governing radiation protection, and it is laid down that regular checks are performed under the direction of the radiation protection officer.

Where an external beam is being produced by exposing the patient to a radioactive source as in a cobalt unit, the machine head embodies a very bulky shielding device which absorbs all the radiation which is being given off constantly, except when the switch is turned on. It is possible for 'leaks' to occur through this shielding and, if so, the radiographers and other staff involved in the setting-up of a patient could be repeatedly exposed to small doses. The physics staff are required to make regular inspections to ensure that this is not happening.

If the X-rays are being produced by an electric current, as with the kilovoltage units or the linear accelerator, a risk of radiation only exists when the machine is turned on. Various precautions are taken both with these units and with cobalt units to ensure that staff, visitors, or other patients waiting for treatment are not inadvertently irradiated while the patient is having treatment.

The design of the room is such that as a person enters, the thickness of a radio-absorbent wall is between him and the unit. The walls and ceiling are constructed to absorb X-radiation, and the treatment head is positioned so that it can never be turned in the direction of a patient waiting area or towards the console desk from which the radiographers operate the controls. The glass panel through which they watch the patient to check his comfort and position under treatment is of specially absorbent lead glass, but again it is positioned so that no direct radiation can reach it, only scattered rays. There are interlock switches, too, on these machines so that they cannot be turned on while the door of the room is open. This is a reminder to the staff to check that all people are out of the room during exposure and ensures that the machine cuts out automatically if the door is opened during treatment.

Limited supplies of radioactive sources for use in moulds, implants or applicators are stored in the radiotherapy department. If their half-life is long, such as with caesium, they will be part of a regular stock, the storage of which has to be carefully supervised in a specially designed and locked safe in the storage room. If the sources are of short half-life, as with iridium wires, they will be obtained to order for a particular patient from the manufacturer and will only be stored for the short time immediately prior to insertion into the patient.

The physicist who prepares these sources for use and who cleans them afterwards should work with long-handled instruments over the top of a thick lead shelf which protects his body from unnecessary irradiation. Similar precautions must be taken by staff working in a radioisotope (Nuclear Medicine) department. Because many of the preparations which they handle will be in liquid form, they are issued with gloves, boots and other protective clothing as required to prevent skin contamination.

As with all ward staff nursing patients who are radioactive, all staff in a radiotherapy department should wear their 'film-badge' at all times while on duty. The film is replaced each month, the film developed and the dose for that month calculated. The 'Code of Practice' lays down the 'Maximum Permissible Dose' (MPD) for workers in the United Kingdom (see Table 11.2). These values have been agreed after advice from the International Commission on Radiological Protection in consultation with the Medical Research Council's Committee on Protection against Ionizing Radiations.

The rem is the unit in which personal exposure is stated. For X-rays and gamma-rays this figure can be taken as the equivalent of rads (the unit in which the absorbed dose of radiation is expressed). If it is considered that a person's annual exposure may exceed three tenths of the annual MPD, a staff member is titled a 'designated person' and is subjected to special medical supervision, including a medical examination and a full blood count at the beginning of employment and annually thereafter. Those under the age of sixteen years are not permitted to engage in work which should require them to be designated persons.

Table 11.2 *Maximum permissible dose for designated persons*

Part of body	*Annual dose*	*Quarterly dose*
Gonads, red bone-marrow and whole body	5 rems	3 rems (1.3 rems to the abdomens of women of reproductive capacity)
Bone, thyroid and skin of whole body	30 rems	15 rems
Hands, forearms, feet and ankles	75 rems	40 rems
Any single organ (excluding gonads, red bone-marrow, bone, thyroid and skin of whole body)	15 rems	8 rems

So far as can be determined, these dose limits give more than reasonable safety margins for the staff at risk. In the past, when the risks were not recognized and when mould and implant techniques were more frequently used, and without present day precautions, it was common for staff to develop problems associated with long exposure. Today, this should be a rare occurrence if the guidelines for safety are observed.

Chapter 12

The Role of Radiotherapy

M. RUTH SANDLAND
M.B., B.S., F.R.C.S., F.R.C.R.
Consultant Radiotherapist
St Bartholomew's Hospital, London
Hospital for Sick Children, Gt Ormond Street

Until recent years, the role of radiotherapy in the management of malignant disease could be discussed under two main headings, curative and palliative, with the possible addition of its adjuvant role where surgical removal of a tumour had been complete.

In current discussion of this subject, the use of irradiation as an adjuvant to both surgery and chemotherapy must be rated as of equal importance with its curative and palliative roles. The reasons for this change in emphasis are several, but the advent of effective systemic chemotherapy for the control of metastases and for the elimination of microscopic residues has been a major one. The technical advantages of the radiotherapy machines developed in the last thirty years permit adequate doses to be given to tumours with less heavy dosage of normal tissues. Similarly, understanding of the natural history of many tumours has improved as well as knowledge concerning the radiation doses required to eradicate them.

Taking an overall view, radiotherapy is used more rationally and, consequently, more effectively than in the past, and we must now examine that role in more detail.

Curative Radiotherapy

If irradiation alone is to be curative, it must destroy all the tumour cells. For this to be achieved, the tumour's boundaries need to be definable with reasonable certainty; metastases outside the irradiation field should not have occurred, and it must be possible to give a high enough dose without undue risk to normal tissues. With these limitations, various circumstances dictate the curative use of irradiation.

ALTERNATIVE TO SURGERY

Many skin cancers, whether basal cell carcinoma or squamous cell carcinoma, can be treated by surgery or irradiation equally effectively and the chosen method may be related to availability of facilities, the preference of the medical adviser or the domestic circumstances of the patient (Fig. 12.1(a)).

Certain sites on the skin are probably best treated by irradiation. One such is the inner canthus of the eye. These skin cancers can be satisfactorily removed surgically and the defect of skin may be covered by the rotation of a skin flap in many cases. However, these lesions are often more deeply infiltrating than suspected and, if one is covered by a skin flap, further damaging growth inwards may occur before it is recognized superficially. Once this has occurred, it is difficult to control the tumour without extensive and, maybe, mutilating surgery.

INACCESSIBLE TO SURGERY

Surgical resection of tumours is not feasible in such sites as the nasopharynx and posterior third of the tongue. Unfortunately, tumours at these two sites tend to present late with extensive lymph node deposits in the neck at the time of diagnosis. This makes them less likely to be cured but, at present, irradiation remains the mainstay of treatment.

INAPPROPRIATE TO SURGERY

It is possible to cure an early carcinoma of the larynx by surgery alone, but this usually involves laryngectomy with all the consequent difficulties for the patient in learning oesophageal speech. Six to seven weeks of treatment with irradiation effects a cure in over 90 per cent of cases of early laryngeal cancer and there are only minor side effects at the time of treatment and few problems in the long term, apart from diminution in the strength of the voice.

Some skin cancers, especially if they are of the more aggressive squamous cell type, or if they are already large at the time of commencement of therapy, may not be suitable for surgical excision because of the subsequent deformity which may be difficult to avert even with skilful plastic surgery (Fig. 12.1(b)). This is not to say that afterwards the site of irradiation will necessarily be invisible but, as we have seen in Chapter 11, the use of carefully fractionated doses can minimize the amount of scarring and deformity. Where the matter of cosmetics is of concern, the alternatives should be explained and discussed with the patient. Hodgkin's disease confined to lymph nodes is a special example

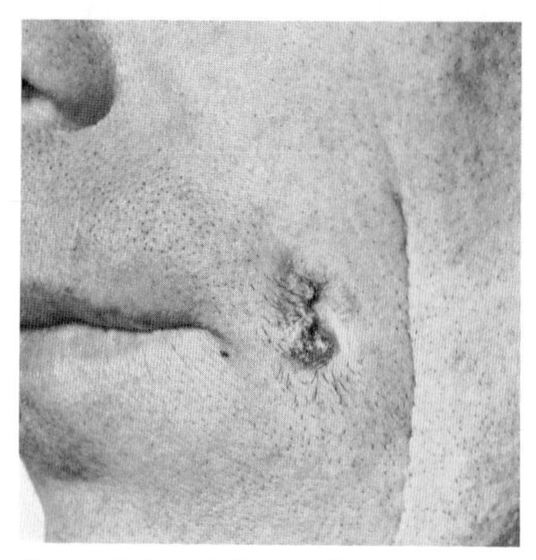

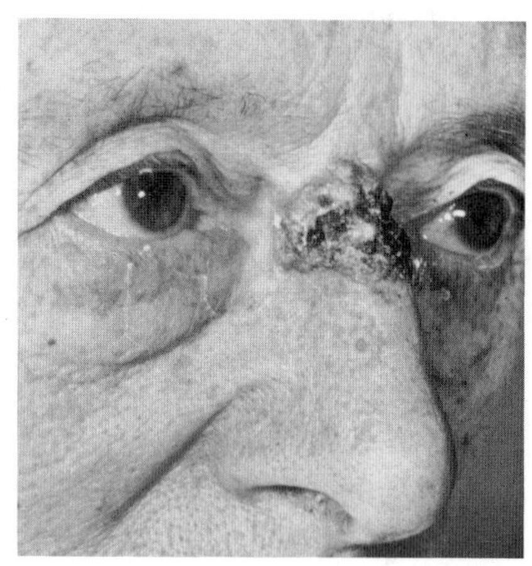

Figure 12.1 (a) Basal cell carcinoma in the nasolabial fold. Treatment by surgery or irradiation should be curative, and leave minimal scar. (b) Basal cell carcinoma of bridge of nose. Careful radiation technique cured this patient with barely perceptible skin changes six months later.

of a disseminated malignancy which may in certain circumstances be curable by irradiation alone.

Another factor in the choice of irradiation for some patients is their unsuitability for surgery due to medical conditions which make them undesirable candidates for general anaesthesia. This may apply in some skin cancers and also in 'internal' cancers such as those involving the bladder where it is uncommon for a patient over seventy years of age to be considered fit for a radical cystectomy.

Adjuvant Radiotherapy

The indications for irradiation as an adjuvant form of therapy are much better defined, because they are better understood, and it is probably helpful to consider this use of irradiation under several headings.

PREOPERATIVE IRRADIATION

Here the purpose may be varied.

(*a*) To reduce the bulk of the tumour to make it possible for the surgeon to perform a curative operation. That is, it is the intention to enable the surgeon to remove the tumour without having to cut into it, and without rupturing it.

(*b*) To reduce the number of viable cells in the tumour. This is an attempt to lower both the chance of microscopic deposits of tumour being left at the site of operation and later giving rise to recurrence, and the risk of dissemination of viable cells during the manipulations of the operation.

Using such a rationale some improvements in survival of patients having irradiation before surgery for carcinoma of the middle third of the oesophagus have been seen. Similarly, this is also the basis of several current studies aimed to improve survival in carcinoma of the rectum.

In these circumstances, it is common to give a short course at a higher than usual dose-rate and to operate within days of its completion before there has been time for development of the late vascular changes and fibrosis due to irradiation in the tissues where the surgeon is operating.

(*c*) To destroy microscopic tumour deposits in tissues peripheral to the primary mass, especially in regional lymph nodes.

Preoperative irradiation in cancer of the bladder may have this effect. Certainly the incidence of tumour involvement in the iliac lymph nodes is noted to be much lower in cases who have had irradiation before surgery than in those who have not.

IRRADIATION BEFORE CHEMOTHERAPY

Here the aim is the control of tumour at the primary site, with chemotherapy added to deal both with any local residue and with metastases whether or not they are detectable.

It is becoming less common to give irradiation before chemotherapy, but the choice of which comes first rests on the knowledge of the behaviour and radioresponsiveness of a tumour, of its histology, as well as the clinical problem in the particular case.

POSTOPERATIVE IRRADIATION

The main rationale for this approach to therapy is either the knowledge in the particular case that some tumour has been, or is likely to have been, left behind, or the experience of the past suggesting that local recurrence is likely to occur in a moderate proportion of cases unless such treatment is given.

In the former case, a radiotherapist is not infrequently asked by a surgeon to give postoperative irradiation after a resection of a carcinoma of the rectum when, in the absence of disseminated disease in the abdominal lymph nodes or liver, it is thought that there is a residue in the pelvis. A surgeon will sometimes define this by inserting at the appropriate place metal clips which can be located on an X-ray of the area, guiding the radiotherapist in siting the treatment beam.

The commonest use of irradiation where a high risk of local recurrence is recognized is after mastectomy for carcinoma of the breast. There is still much controversy about the long term value of giving irradiation to the area of the mastectomy skin flaps and regional lymph nodes, but all recognize the incidence of local recurrence on the chest wall to be lower if postoperative irradiation is given to the skin flaps and operation scar.

Seminoma of the testis is an example of a tumour where irradiation has been found to be part of the curative treatment when given in appropriate sites after orchidectomy. Aided by lymphographic assessment of the extent of such a tumour at the time of surgery, patients found to have no lymph node involvement but who have radiotherapy to the pelvic nodes on the side of the tumour as well as to the para-aortic nodes, should be cured. Similarly, with those who have demonstrable node involvement in the pelvis or para-aortic nodes, the extension of irradiation to the mediastinal and supraclavicular nodes (one step ahead of the apparent disease!) should cure the majority of patients.

IRRADIATION CONCURRENTLY WITH, AND AFTER, CHEMOTHERAPY

This is nowadays the most frequent approach to combined irradiation and chemotherapy.

It is believed to be valuable to shrink the tumour mass with chemotherapy first so that high dose radiation is only given to the area of residual tumour, while a lower dose suffices for the originally involved area. It is also possible that irradiation may render the central parts of the tumour mass less accessible to chemotherapy in the long term due to vascular damage and sclerosis of tissues. This, too, would suggest that the primary tumour should be exposed to chemotherapy first, followed by radiotherapy, with chemotherapy following to deal with residual disease or metastases in unirradiated areas.

This is the usual programme in several paediatric tumours, such as Ewing's sarcoma of bone, in which there have been such encouraging improvements in treatment recently.

With the discovery of chemotherapeutic agents effective in the control of childhood acute lymphoblastic leukaemia in the blood and bone marrow, it became apparent that these drugs were not reaching the meninges in sufficient quantity to destroy all leukaemic cells. Many

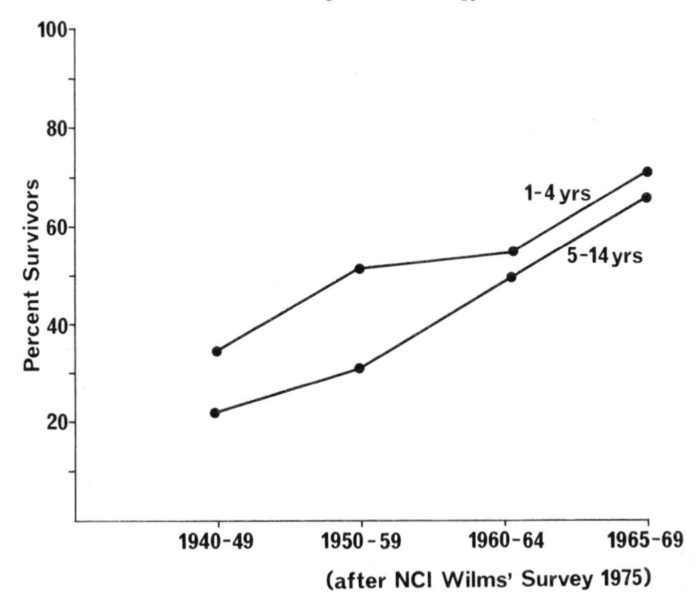

Figure 12.2 Nephroblastoma (Wilms's tumour). Graph to show improvement in survival over recent years with the use of combined treatment methods.

apparently successfully treated children later developed leukaemic meningitis. The addition of preventive irradiation to the meninges, a so-called 'sanctuary site' to chemotherapy, before this problem developed and after induction chemotherapy had brought the bone marrow and blood under control, has improved the survival of these children. Testicular relapse may also occur in boys with leukaemia and it is believed that the testis is another sanctuary site which may be irradiated if a relapse occurs there.

SURGERY, RADIOTHERAPY, CHEMOTHERAPY

All three treatment modalities may have their part to play in the treatment of a particular malignancy. Nephroblastoma, the kidney tumour of childhood, is a very good example showing how the use of all three methods, in that order, has dramatically improved survival over the last twenty years. (Fig. 12.2).

Similarly, rhabdomyosarcoma which arises in various sites in children, frequently involves all three methods of treatment. Nowadays, chemotherapy and radiotherapy are usually given first, with surgery being performed later to resect any residual disease if necessary. Thus it is often possible to perform less extensive and less mutilating surgery without affecting survival.

Palliative Radiotherapy

This term is usually used in relation to radiotherapy in two particular senses. It may be applied to the treatment with irradiation of a primary or recurrent tumour which is considered to be inoperable and incurable but which is causing distressing symptoms. Or, the term may be applied to the irradiation of metastases which are causing discomfort.

In neither case is there any serious intention to cure the patient's malignant condition. Rather, the purpose is to make the patient comfortable for as long as possible. Not that every patient who is given radiotherapy with palliative intent is necessarily terminal. Indeed, many primary tumours may grow very slowly or may cause distressing local problems long before they metastasize or threaten life.

Advanced carcinoma of the cervix presents this problem occasionally. If at the time of diagnosis it is fixed within the pelvis the chances of long term survival are small. The patient may live for a long time, perhaps years, with symptoms related to local disease only, such as vaginal discharge or haemorrhage and the possibility of the development of a faecal or urinary fistula should the rectum or bladder or urethra become involved. Where no fistula has developed radiotherapy can be usefully given to the pelvis resulting in cessation of cervical haemorrhage and decreased vaginal discharge.

Likewise, patients with carcinoma of the breast may not present for treatment until the tumour is inoperable and there is fungation and haemorrhage. Palliative irradiation can cause healing of the ulcerated areas with arrest of bleeding prior to treatment with hormones or chemotherapy. Presentation with such advanced disease is quite commonly, though not always, consistent with several more years of life.

Other tumours can cause distressing symptoms and benefit from irradiation given palliatively. Some examples are listed below:

Carcinoma of the bronchus with chest pain or recurrent haemoptysis;
Carcinoma of the oesophagus with dysphagia due to obstruction;
Carcinoma of the bladder with haematuria;
Carcinoma of the rectum with bleeding and mucus discharge;
Malignant melanoma of the skin with ulceration and haemorrhage.

In this category one particular symptom is worthy of special mention – namely, superior vena caval obstruction. This arises most commonly from a carcinoma of the bronchus and may develop very rapidly over a few days or more slowly over a period of weeks. The symptoms of congestion in the head and arms and the associated sensation of suffocation in the chest are very distressing and irradiation, given promptly, may achieve a measure of control of symptoms while more complete diagnosis and treatment are planned.

One of the commonest uses of irradiation for palliative purposes is the relief of bone pain from metastases or multiple myeloma deposits. Again this does not necessarily mean the patient is terminal, though he may be.

Occasionally the metastasis is solitary. This may be the case in carcinoma of the breast or bronchus, but is relatively much more common in adenocarcinoma of the kidney (hypernephroma). The appearance of a solitary metastasis in such a case is not necessarily the forerunner of a rapid spread of disease. If satisfactorily irradiated, the pain may be relieved, the bone may regenerate, and a long interval ensue before further manifestation of the renal tumour appears.

In breast cancer, prostatic cancer, multiple myeloma, and in other tumours less commonly, skeletal deposits are often extensive and may require palliative irradiation for relief of pain while attempts continue to control the generalized disease process with hormones and chemotherapy. Multiple sites may need to be irradiated concurrently or sequentially when disease is spreading rapidly, and if a long bone such as the femur or humerus shows a deposit which is compromising the cortex of the bone, it is often necessary to have a stabilizing nail inserted along the shaft surgically before commencing irradiation. (See Fig. 12.3(a) and (b)).

Collapsing vertebrae present a particular problem in metastatic malignancy. In the cervical spine, the risks of quadriplegia or lesser neurological deficits are usually managed by the use of a supporting collar to the patient's neck, some restriction of movement, and the administration of irradiation to relieve pain and to destroy tumour, allowing bone reformation to occur.

In the dorsal or lumbar spine, pain may have been present in varying degrees for some time before severe collapse occurs. When it does, the patient may present with signs of spinal cord compression which may include total or partial paralysis of the lower limbs, with or without disturbance of sensation of the legs, buttocks and perineum, as well as loss of tone of the anal sphincter with faecal incontinence and urinary retention.

It depends on how rapidly these symptoms have appeared and how gross the neurological deficit is when diagnosed, as well as the site of collapse and the general condition and prognosis of the patient, as to whether a surgical decompression as an emergency or prompt irradia-

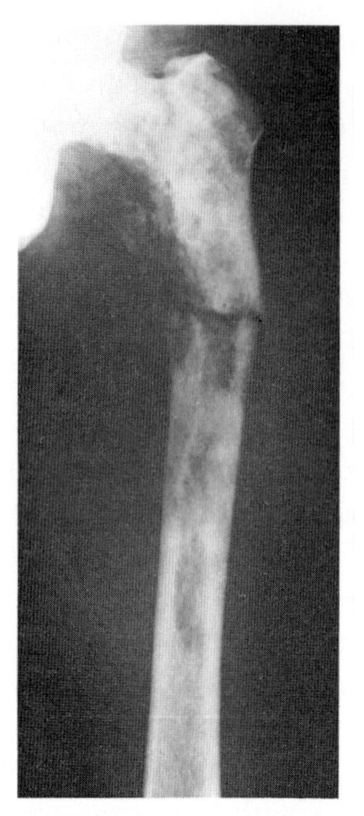

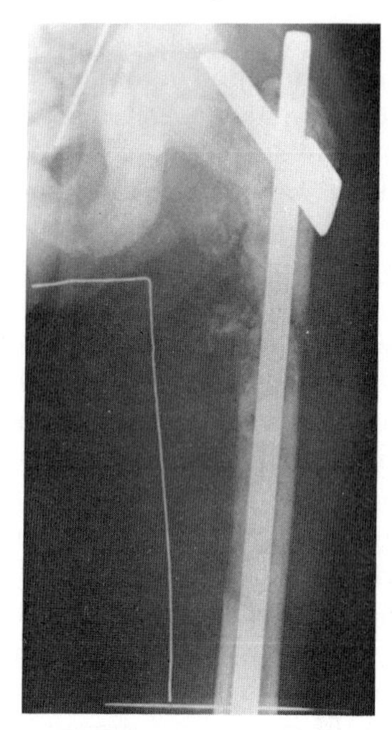

Figure 12.3 (a) Pathological fracture of shaft of femur which is extensively involved with metastatic tumour from carcinoma of prostate. (b) Stabilizing nail has been inserted. Strips of wire (on the patient's skin) outline the area which is to be treated with irradiation.

tion to the affected section of the spine is the appropriate treatment. The aim in each case is to stop the tumour pressing on the cord, so that, whatever the patient's prognosis, he will not end his life paraplegic.

Dosage and Fractionation in Radiotherapy

In Chapter 11, the properties of X-rays and the machines used in a radiotherapy department were discussed, and the ways in which these help in the planning of a particular patient's treatment. Some of the factors which affect the prescribed dose in each patient's case are discussed below.

THE NATURE OF THE TUMOUR

Some tumours are more radioresponsive than others. For example, a lymphoma of the nasopharynx does not need for its eradication as high a dose as a squamous cell carcinoma at the same site. Similarly, a basal cell carcinoma of the skin (rodent ulcer) will be cured by a lower dose

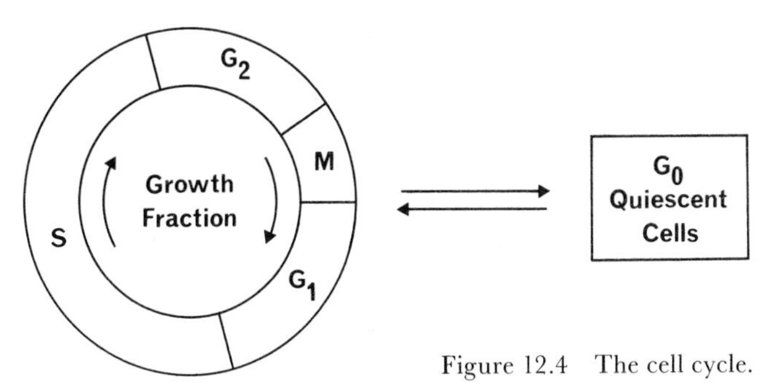

Figure 12.4 The cell cycle.

than will a squamous cell carcinoma. An 'oat cell' carcinoma of the bronchus is responsive at a lower dose than is an adenocarcinoma in the same site, and likewise a seminoma of the testis than a teratoma. The reasons for these differences are complex and incompletely understood. However, it is clear that they are related to biological characteristics of the tumour.

Radiotherapy is known to be most effective when it reaches cells which are actively undergoing mitosis, and even more particularly when they are in the stage of systhesis (S) or of mitosis (M) rather than in the resting phases (G_1, G_2). (See Fig. 12.4).

The number of cells in the 'growth fraction' actively undergoing mitosis varies in different tumours and may even vary at different stages in the life of a tumour or in different areas in the one tumour. In a similar way, the speed of the cell cycle may be variable. In a rapidly growing 'oat cell' carcinoma of the bronchus, for example, the cells would seem to be mostly in the growth fraction and the cell cycle time is short. This presumably contributes to its relatively good response to irradiation.

In the case of a squamous cell carcinoma of the bronchus, the growth rate is usually much slower, the assumption then being that a smaller proportion of cells is in the growth fraction, likely to be damaged by irradiation.

Good cell oxygenation is essential if radiotherapy is to be effective, and it is undoubtedly true that in some tumours the central portions are hypoxic, making their eradication less likely.

AIM OF THE TREATMENT

In practice, tumour dosage is modified not only according to its type but in relation to the purpose for which it is being given, i.e. whether irradiation is being used curatively as the sole treatment, as an adjuvant with surgery or chemotherapy, or palliatively.

If the intention is to cure, the full tumoricidal dose should be given with allowance being made for normal tissue tolerance. If irradiation is being given as part of a combined therapy plan, it may be possible to give less irradiation than a full curative dose, especially if the residue is of small, even microscopic, dimensions. However, if one is irradiating a tumour mass one should go to full dosage for the particular tumour, as the number of cells killed is proportional to the dose given. When irradiation is being given palliatively, there is much more flexibility with dosage. The total dose given tends to be lower than if one is delivering it with curative intent. Side effects are less and it may be possible to give the dosage more quickly without undue upset, thereby reducing the number of visits necessary for a patient whose strength and life expectancy are limited.

NORMAL TISSUE TOLERANCE

The dose-limiting factor in all radiotherapy is the tolerance of normal tissues. They, too, are damaged at a cellular and structural level by irradiation and the reason for dividing up into fractions the total dose to be given, as described in Chapter 11, is to allow for a measure of normal tissue repair.

In the acute irradiation reaction, the most obvious change is arteriolar dilatation, with oedema and erythema. In the long term, there may be sclerosis of small blood vessels with scarring and fibrosis. The extent of this change depends on the degree of damage inflicted by the radiation and this is determined, as we have seen, by the volume of tissue irradiated as well as the number of treatments and the total dose given.

Because of structural variations in different tissues and the different biological characteristics of normal cells, there is a wide range of reactivity of normal tissues to irradiation. The skin is the tissue most obviously evaluable from this viewpoint and most studied in the experimental animal.

In treating a skin cancer, there is much less chance of a noticeable scar or pallor of the treated area the greater the number of fractions used. And, of course, the total dose is greater if a multiple number of small fractions is given rather than a few larger ones.

The spinal cord is a structure well recognized to be vulnerable to irradiation. Its blood supply is segmental with little overlap from adjacent segments. Thus if a long length of cord is heavily irradiated, the consequences can be quite serious, resulting in a radiation myelitis some months later. This may mean patchy sensory and motor disturbances in the limbs but it can be more severe. If, for example, the cervical cord is damaged it can even result in a quadriplegia. There are well-defined limits of both dose and number of fractions below which these changes should rarely occur. But, in the irradiation of many tumours, especially if they are close to the midline of the body, it is inevitable that the spinal cord will receive some irradiation, and it is important that appropriate averting action is taken to minimize the risk of damage.

Other tissues and their sensitivity to irradiation will be mentioned in the following paragraphs when some examples of tumour dosage are given. But, once again, it must be stressed that there is nothing precise or invariable about the dose to kill a particular tumour, or to protect the patient's normal tissues. In both these spheres, as in most biological systems, there is a widespread individual variation which defies the making of absolute rules.

Specific Tumours and Their Treatment

It is obviously not practical to describe the use of radiotherapy for every kind of tumour as well as the techniques at many different sites. Instead, a selection of representative tumours, sites, and techniques has been made for more detailed description, to serve as a guide to the scope of the radiotherapy department's work.

SKIN CANCER

Patients with skin cancer usually present when the lesion is small and curable. Such lesions are commonly on the face and scalp or other parts of the exposed skin. The simplest and commonest method of irradiation is to use superficial X-ray equipment at voltage varying from 60 kV to 140 kV, depending on the thickness of the lesion. Including a margin around the tumour where microscopic spread may have occurred, an applicator of the appropriate size is attached to the machine and approximated to the skin. Where the lesion is of an irregular size, an applicator of larger diameter than necessary is used and lead shielding is taped to the patient's skin to absorb irradiation in areas not involved with tumour.

Particular care must be exercised in the treatment of lesions close to the eye. Especially is this so in the case of a lesion of the inner canthus of the eye, where the tumour may be more extensive than immediately apparent and where it is difficult to position the machine applicator satisfactorily without irregular dosage of the lesion (Fig. 12.5).

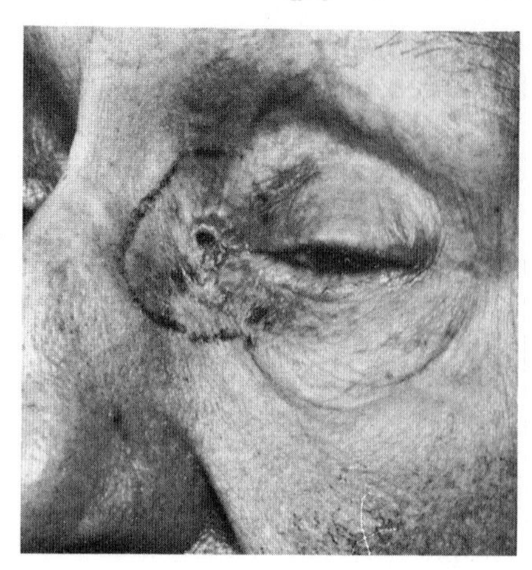

Figure 12.5 Basal cell carcinoma of the inner canthus. The extent of the area to be treated is marked on the skin.

Nowhere is the importance of the factors of dose and fractionation more apparent than in these sites. In an elderly frail patient, three doses of 1,000 rads to a small cancer at weekly intervals should cure it. But the cosmetic result of this regime in a younger person with a lesion in a conspicuous site would not be satisfactory. In such a case, smaller daily fractions are commonly given. 500 rads given ten times for a basal cell carcinoma and given eleven or twelve times for a squamous cell carcinoma is common practice. For more extensive skin lesions, electron therapy may be more appropriate.

BREAST CANCER

It is standard practice to aim to include in the treatment of breast cancer the area of the chest wall over which the skin flaps of the mastectomy were raised as well as the lymph drainage areas of the breast including the ipsilateral axillary, supraclavicular and internal mammary nodes.

The techniques of administration are almost as numerous as radiotherapy departments. A fairly common pattern of treatment is illustrated in Fig. 12.6.

The area of the scar and chest wall is treated by a pair of tangential fields applied from lateral and medial sides from such an angle that the potential area of residual tumour is included without undue irradiation of the underlying lung tissue. The internal mammary lymph nodes are sometimes included in this, depending on the position of the operation scar and the original breast lump, or a separate direct field may be

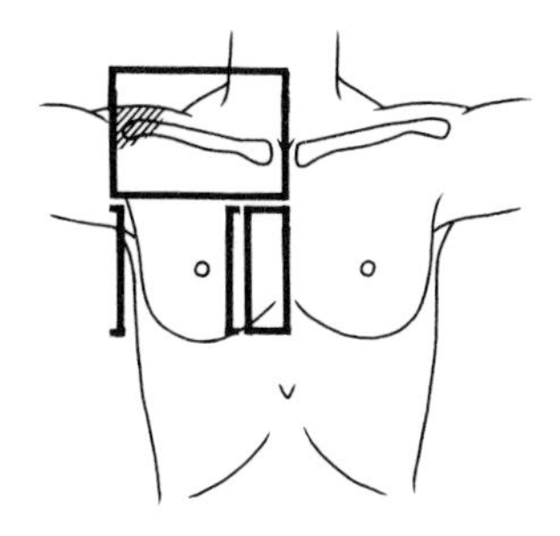

Figure 12.6 Irradiation fields after right mastectomy for carcinoma of the breast (see text).

applied as in the figure. Similarly, a direct field is given to the cervico-axillary chain of lymph nodes and a small additional field may be given from the posterior aspect to ensure that the deepest members of this group are adequately dosed.

When microscopically complete tumour removal is thought to have been achieved, it is common to give doses of the order of 4,500 rads in four to five weeks, depending on the skin tolerance with the different energy of beam used. An additional 1,500 rads may be given to tumour residues such as axillary lymph nodes.

With such a regime it is common for a marked skin erythema to develop by the end of the course of treatment. In moist areas such as the axilla, this may go on to loss of skin epithelium (moist desquamation) and this is more likely to occur in women with fair skins. Some patients develop dysphagia towards the end of treatment. This is secondary to the oesophagitis caused by the medial part of the cervico-axillary field, and perhaps also by the internal mammary field.

A small proportion of patients may, a few weeks later, develop irradiation pneumonitis in the upper lobe of the lung which has received direct exposure to the rays in the cervico-axillary field, and these may go on to develop pulmonary fibrosis in this area. This will be apparent on chest X-ray but does not always cause symptoms.

HODGKIN'S DISEASE

This neoplasm of lymphatic tissue is very responsive to irradiation in the majority of cases. Before lymphography helped us in our understanding of its dissemination, it was common to excise surgically or irradiate only the immediate area where the first mass of glands appeared. Subsequent relapse rates were high and it is now recognized that its original extent may be much wider than at first expected.

In certain cases it has been shown that greater than 80 per cent cure rates can be obtained if wide field irradiation is given. If it is the upper half of the body which is affected, the 'mantle' technique is commonly

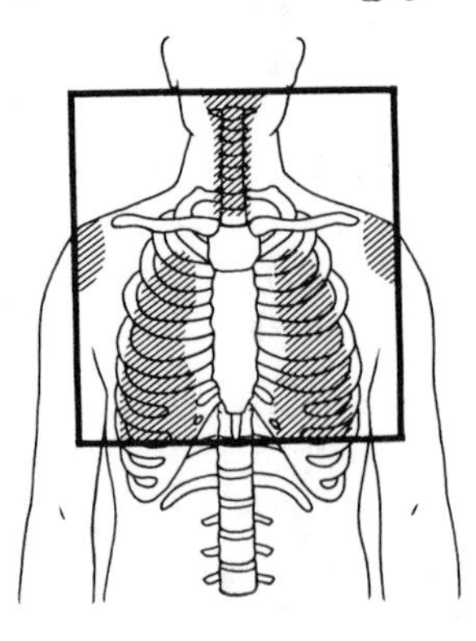

Figure 12.7 Diagram of 'mantle' technique which aims to include all lymph node areas above the diaphragm. Lead blocks protect normal tissues where possible, especially the lungs.

employed (Fig. 12.7) and this should include cervical (extending high enough to encompass postauricular, submandibular and occipital nodes), axillary and mediastinal lymph nodes.

Doses between 3,500 and 4,000 rads daily over a four-week period are commonly given by alternate anterior and posterior fields. Heads of the humeri and all of the lung tissue at some distance from lymph node areas are shielded by lead blocks in the path of the beam as indicated in the diagram. Half-way through treatment the spinal cord is protected by a narrow lead block when treatment is being given from the back. This plan of treatment may result in some nausea and oesophagitis as well as erythema in the axillae and cervical skin folds, but side effects are not usually severe.

Where the Hodgkin's disease is confined to the lymph node areas below the diaphragm (a less common occurrence than involvement above), it is sometimes appropriate to use the 'inverted Y' technique (Fig. 12.8).

Here it is planned to include the para-aortic, pelvic and inguinal lymph nodes. Lead shielding is again used to protect tissues which can safely be

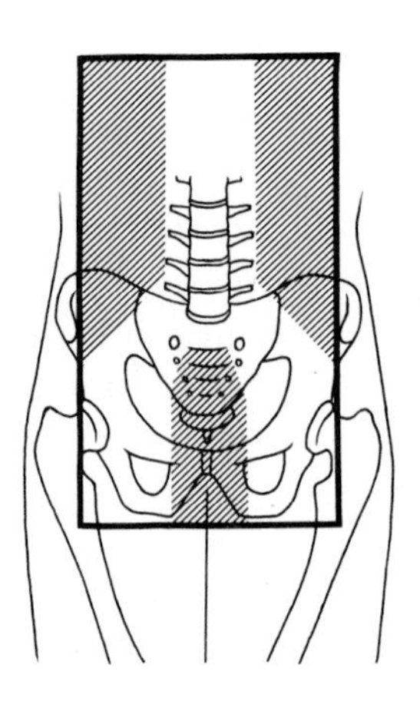

Figure 12.8 Diagram of 'inverted Y' technique which aims to include all lymph node areas below the diaphragm. Lead blocks shield normal tissues where possible, including kidneys, rectum, bladder.

avoided, such as the kidneys, bladder and rectum. Gonadal shields must be used to protect the testes in the male, and in a woman of reproductive age the ovaries can be transposed into a midline position in the pelvis behind the uterus where the exposure dose will be small. There are now many reported cases of women treated for Hodgkin's disease in this way, giving birth to normal children at a later date.

The dose rate is similar to that used in the mantle technique, but side effects may be more marked, especially nausea, vomiting and diarrhoea. A large portion of the bone marrow is being irradiated in the vertebral bodies and the pelvic bones, and this may lead to depression of white blood cells and platelet formation.

BRAIN TUMOURS

The possibility of necrosis if brain irradiation is given too fast or at too high a total dose is always a concern of the radiotherapist. But there is a wide range of brain tumours in which irradiation has an important part to play and there are also wide variations in the amount of brain tissue which must be irradiated for it to be effective.

Pituitary tumours usually present when relatively small and the radiation beams may need only be focused on a volume 5 × 5 × 5 cm or even smaller. In this case the fields, carefully angled so as to avoid scattered irradiation to the eyes, may be of 'postage stamp' size. The commonest such tumour is a chromophobe adenoma of the pituitary and the usual dose is 4,500 rads in six weeks.

The reason for avoiding unnecessary exposure of the eyes to irradiation is that, at much lower total doses than are used to control malignant tumours, it is likely that the lens will develop a radiation cataract. This can be dealt with in a similar fashion to the common senile cataract but should not be allowed to occur unless it is totally unavoidable.

Larger volumes must be treated where one is endeavouring to eradicate a widely infiltrating glioma of the cerebral cortex. In such a case it may be necessary to treat virtually the whole of one cerebral hemisphere, sparing only the frontal or occipital poles. 5,000–5,500 rads is the usual dose range given in daily treatment over a six to seven week period.

A few brain tumours behave in an unusual fashion by the shedding of their cells within the cerebrospinal fluid allowing the development of metastatic deposits at distant parts of the central nervous system. Such a tumour is the medulloblastoma and improvement in the chances of survival can be offered if, in addition to 5,000 or 5,500 rads being given to the area of the cerebellum and fourth ventricle where the tumour

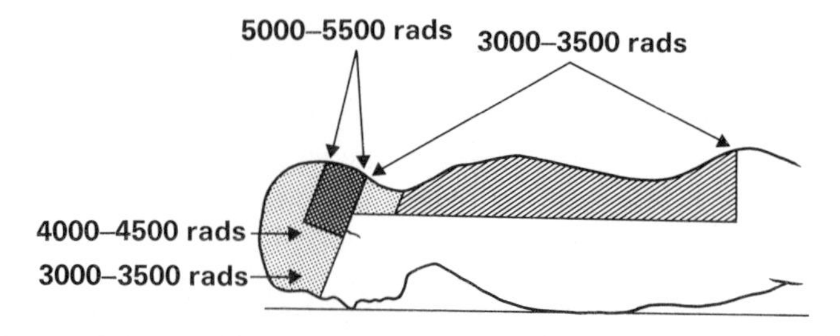

Figure 12.9 Whole central nervous system irradiation. In the technique illustrated, the whole cranium and upper cervical cord is first treated by radiation from each side. The high dose to the tumour bearing area is then continued using smaller fields. The remainder of the spine is treated by a direct posterior field.

originates, a smaller dose of irradiation (3,000–3,500 rads) is given to the whole central nervous system extending from the cranial vault to the end of the spinal theca at S_2 level.

Figure 12.9 shows one way in which such treatment can be administered. There are technical problems in avoiding irradiation to the lens of the eye and in protecting tissues of the mouth and nasopharynx without preventing irradiation reaching the brain stem area. Overlapping of the cranial and spinal fields could lead to overdosage of the cervical cord and so careful calculations of the gap between these fields as well as the provision of an immobilizing 'shell' for accuracy in each day's treatment must be made.

TONGUE

Lesions of the posterior third have already been mentioned and external radiotherapy by lateral fields which include the tumour site and its drainage lymph node areas is the usual plan of treatment.

The mobility of this organ presents particular problems when a carcinoma develops in its anterior two-thirds. If the lesion is accessible and confined to the tip or margin of the tongue, surgical excision may be appropriate. A more extensive lesion, especially if there is deep infiltration, is best treated by irradiation. External beam therapy allowing for movement of the tongue is difficult to perform satisfactorily without including the whole of the oral mucosa in the field. This is therefore a very suitable site for the insertion of radioactive sources into the tumour itself (Fig. 12.10).

Those most commonly used today are caesium needles and iridium wires. They are positioned in the operating theatre under general anaesthetic and sutured. After X-ray checks of their relationship, the physicist calculates how many days they have to be left in position to

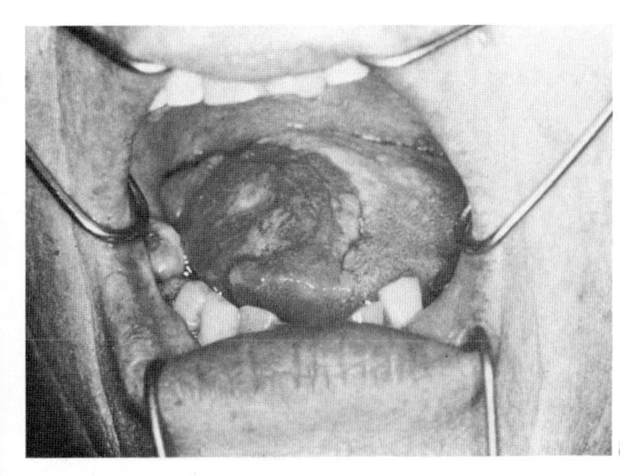

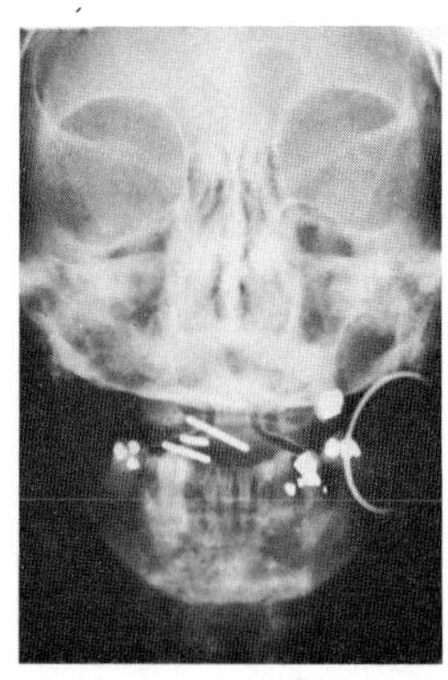

Figure 12.10 (a) Carcinoma of anterior two-thirds of right side of tongue which is inoperable. (b) X-ray of same patient as in (a) after insertion of caesium needles. The metal ring is a marker to aid dose calculations.

give adequate dosage. In the case of squamous cell carcinoma, one is usually aiming for a dose of 6,500 rads. The needles are removed after the appropriate interval and the patient's tongue will probably continue to be uncomfortable for a further seven to fourteen days during which time bland but nourishing food and good mouth hygiene will be important.

Depending on the site and extent of the primary tumour the lymph node areas of the neck may also require irradiation, by external beam therapy.

LARYNX

Where a carcinoma of this region commences on the vocal cord, it usually produces hoarseness at an early stage, and if this is investigated appropriately, treatment may begin before it has spread to involve other laryngeal tissues or regional lymph nodes.

Where this is the case, external beam irradiation is relatively straightforward. It is common to treat a field approximately 5 cm wide by 6 cm high on either side of the neck (Fig. 12.11(a)). A dose of 6,500 rads in six weeks using a cobalt unit is usually well tolerated and the oesophagus should not receive a high dose, nor should the spinal cord (Fig. 12.11(b)).

The majority of cases are cured at this dosage. If one treats to a higher dose, the chance of cure is even higher but the risk of complications such as radionecrosis of the laryngeal cartilages becomes unacceptably high.

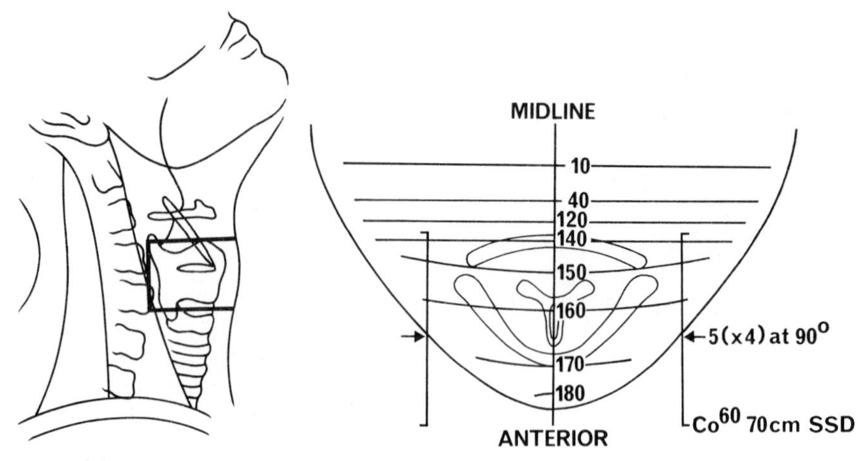

Figure 12.11 (a) Diagram to show the small size of field which may be used in radiation of a carcinoma of the larynx confined to the vocal cord. (b) Physicist's diagram of dose distribution when such a tumour is treated by two lateral fields. Note the rapid fall in dose received by adjacent tissues posteriorly.

Intrathoracic Tumours

CARCINOMA OF THE BRONCHUS

This is one of the most common cancers and is very frequently inoperable at the time of diagnosis. It therefore makes up a large proportion of a radiotherapy department's workload.

If the tumour is a squamous cell carcinoma, it tends to be moderately slow growing and late in spreading to distant sites. It is therefore common in a reasonably fit patient who shows no evidence of metastases to irradiate to a high dose such as 5,500 rads in six weeks. The first 3,000 rads may be given to a large area of the lung and adjacent mediastinum and then the last part of the treatment to a smaller volume, depending on the response as judged by serial chest X-rays. Where the treatment is regarded as palliative only, dosage may be limited to 4,000 rads in four weeks (or even more concentrated courses).

If the tumour is an 'oat cell' or poorly differentiated carcinoma, there is usually a good, though temporary, response to a dose of 3,500 rads in four weeks. Frequently, however, while a course of irradiation to the chest is continuing, enlarged cervical lymph nodes can become apparent, such is the rate of growth of these tumours. For this reason, it is customary to use a T-shaped field, to include the supraclavicular nodes on both sides of the neck as well as the primary tumour and adjacent mediastinum (Fig. 12.12).

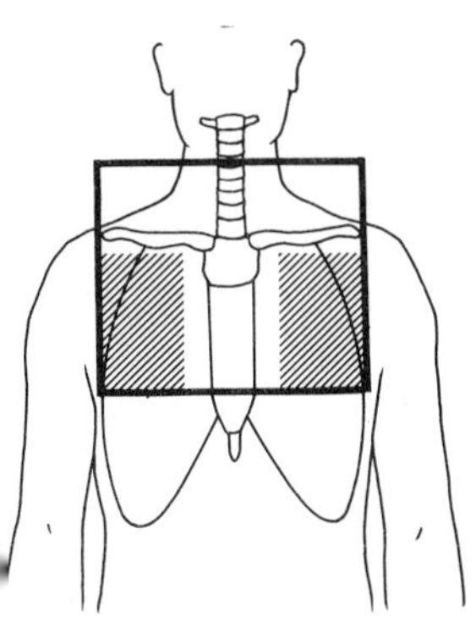

Figure 12.12 Diagram of T-shaped field used to treat a centrally placed, poorly differentiated carcinoma of lung.

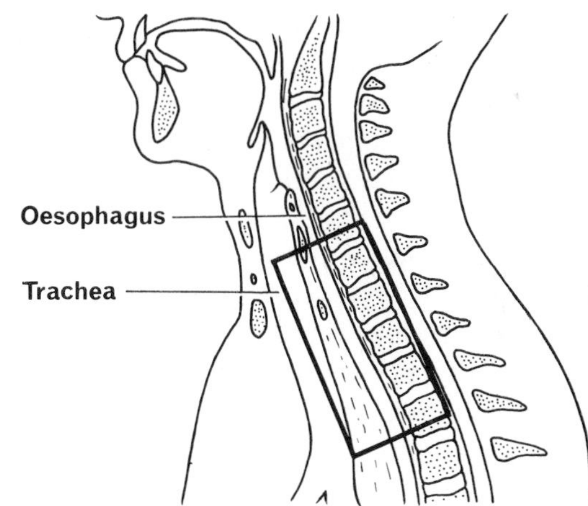

Figure 12.13 Diagram showing the position of the oesophagus and its varying depth in relation to the skin both anteriorly and posteriorly, making treatment planning for a tumour in its upper one-third (as marked by the rectangle) a complex exercise.

CARCINOMA OF THE OESOPHAGUS

In carcinoma of the upper third of the oesophagus, surgery is only possible if a very radical procedure is performed, and radiotherapy may be the preferred method of treatment. This is quite a challenge to the planning skills of the physicist and the radiotherapist, because of the high doses of irradiation which must be used for success (6,000 rads in six to seven weeks) and because of the irregular thickness of the patient and the proximity of the spinal cord to the very posteriorly situated oesophagus (Fig. 12.13). This is a good example of a tumour where several days of planning work may be necessary in making compensators which take these problems into account. The result may be treatment by four fields from different directions all at oblique angles to the patient. A considerable proportion of normal lung tissue will inevitably be irradiated in such a case and this can result in a degree of pulmonary fibrosis in the long term.

Tumours of the middle and lower third of the oesophagus tend to be advanced when referred for irradiation and palliative treatment by direct anterior and posterior fields to a dose of 4,000 rads in four weeks is not uncommon in an effort to relieve pain and swallowing difficulty.

Pelvic Irradiation

CARCINOMA OF THE BLADDER

Once a tumour of the bladder mucosa has begun to infiltrate the muscle wall, irradiation is likely to have a part in its treatment. If a superficially infiltrating tumour is solitary, small, but not at a suitable site for a partial cystectomy, it can be treated by the insertion of gold grains into its base at open operation after the surgeon has diathermied the surface bulk of the tumour. This is not a satisfactory form of treatment once the deep muscle of the bladder has been infiltrated. In such a case, one must use external beam therapy, including in the treatment volume the lymph node areas of the pelvis which have a high chance in such cases of being infiltrated also.

It is the practice in some departments, if the patient is fit for surgery, for 4,000 rads to be given by a field arrangement such as that shown in Fig. 12.14(a), prior to the surgeon operating to remove the bladder. If the patient is considered unfit for surgery a further 2,000 rads should be given. The volume is smaller for this second phase of treatment and the field arrangement may also be different in order to avoid undue irradiation to the femoral heads (Fig. 12.14(b)).

In pelvic irradiation one is always endeavouring to minimize dosage to the rectum because of the distressing symptoms high dosage can produce at the time, and the possibility of proctitis, rectal ulceration and stricture which can occur in the long term. Most patients will develop diarrhoea during such a course of treatment and urinary symptoms due to the tumour may be aggravated rather than diminished until treatment is over and recovery is occurring.

In cases where the tumour is cured without cystectomy, a small capacity bladder due to radiation fibrosis may lead to distressing urinary frequency months after treatment. (This fibrosis may be particularly noticeable where there has been a long history of cystodiathermy and other treatments for superficial bladder tumours.) Telangiectasia of the bladder wall due to irradiation damage of small blood vessels may result in haematuria months or years later.

CARCINOMA OF THE CERVIX

Where the tumour is confined to the cervix or immediately adjacent tissues without extension out to the pelvic side walls or downwards to the lower part of the vagina, it is customary to use local high dose irradiation by intracavitary sources followed by external beam irradiation to the whole pelvis.

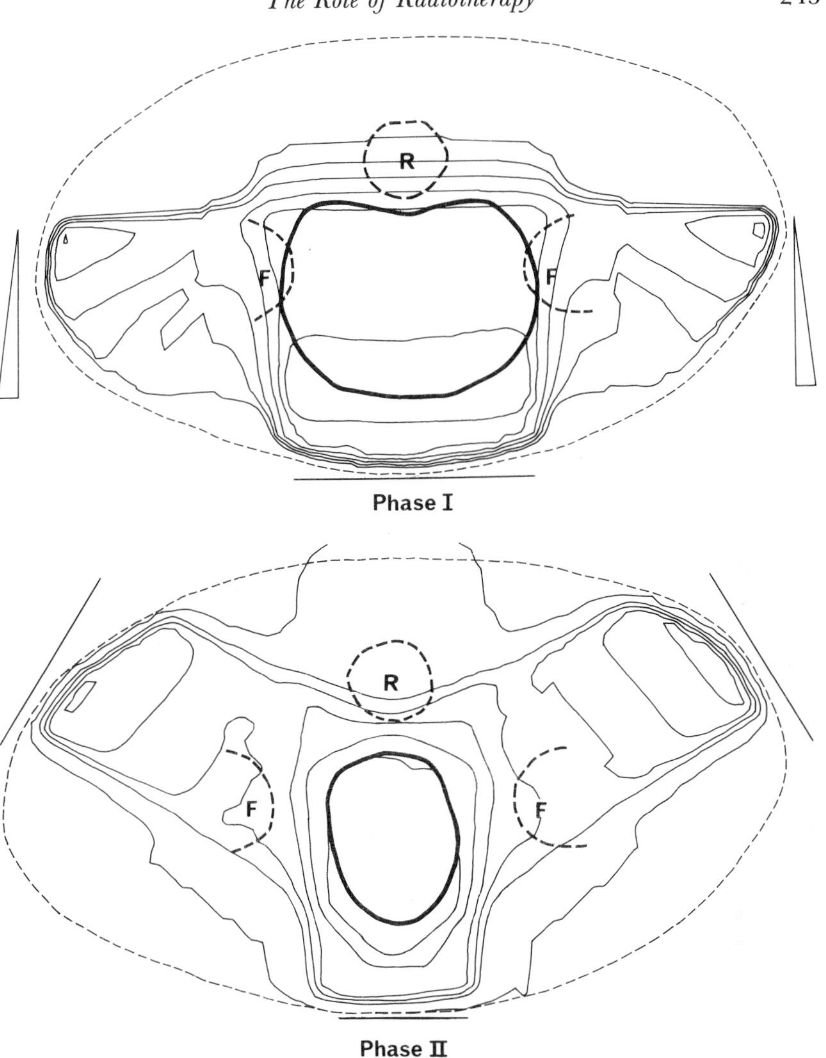

Figure 12.14 (a) Diagram of field arrangements to treat whole pelvis in carcinoma of bladder. (b) More limited volumes are treated in the second phase with a different field arrangement. (R = position of rectum, F = femoral heads).

There are many techniques of intracavitary irradiation but the aim is to include in the high dose area the whole uterine cavity as well as the cervix, paracervical tissues and upper vagina. This is achieved by the insertion of uterine sources of length appropriate to the size of the patient's uterus (usually between 4–8 cm). The sources are loaded in a fairly rigid plastic sheath and the string on the end of the sheath is attached with coloured tags indicating the number of sources and their strength. More sources are loaded in a separate plastic 'box' or 'tube' and positioned at the upper end of the vagina against the cervix or in the lateral fornices. Again, strings and tags are markers of the amount of irradiation in position.

The tubes and boxes are positioned (with the help of packing gauze in the vagina) in such a way that dosage to bladder and rectum are minimized. It is customary to divide the high dose given by this method into two, if not three, fractions each of twenty to thirty hours at weekly intervals depending on the dose to be given and the strength of the sources. The duration may be shortened if the position is such that the rectum is receiving an unacceptably high dose.

The nursing and other measures discussed in the section on radiation protection (Volume 2) must be applied when these sources are in position.

After this treatment is complete, the rest of the pelvis including lymph node areas where microscopic tumour deposits could be present is then irradiated, shielding the central pelvic structures including bladder, uterus and rectum. The pelvic tissues will have received doses of the order of 1,500 rads from the caesium insertions, in which case an additional dose of 3,500 rads should be given over about four weeks. The width of the shield must be such that none of the parametrial tissues gets less than 5,000 rads.

During this treatment most patients will develop diarrhoea, some slight, but others severe and debilitating. Mist Kaolin and Morph and Codeine Phosphate can usually control it without the need to interrupt treatment.

Bone

The commonest purpose in irradiating a bone is the relief of pain from its involvement with secondary malignancy. Where vertebral bodies are infiltrated with tumour, it is common practice to apply a direct posterior field to the patient, wide enough to include the full width of the vertebral body and its transverse processes and any associated soft tissue mass. The length of the field may include as many as two vertebrae above and two below the involved vertebrae. If the patient's condition is terminal, pain relief may be achieved quickly by a few large fractions. Where the patient's life expectancy is longer, one must consider the effects of the irradiation on the spinal cord. Depending on the length of the field a dose of 2,700 rads given over three weeks could be appropriate, treating three times per week.

Another common site of metastases is the bones of the hip joint. Here ıterior and posterior field are used to give a satisfactory midplane and because it is a weight-bearing joint the dose may be slightly ·r.

reful records, and check X-ray films, must be kept where patients multiple metastases which may require overlapping fields to be ed subsequently.

. here bones are the site of primary tumours, there is a wide range of dosage and technique used, depending on the type of tumour.

Whole Body Irradiation

Here there are problems of administration and dosage quite different in nature from the exposure of local volumes of tissue.

This method of treatment is sometimes used in disseminated lymphomas with the use of very small daily doses over several weeks. Because of the severe bone marrow depression and the gastrointestinal symptoms which may occur, this treatment has to be given with great care.

Radiation and Side Effects

Many of the side effects of irradiation at particular sites have already been mentioned, and it is not proposed to give a comprehensive list of these.

Many patients believe and are often told by their medical advisers, that they will vomit during radiotherapy. This is by no means universally so and depends on many factors, including the site being irradiated, the size of the volume, the dose given at each session, as well as on the general condition of the patient. It is common to be nauseated when the abdomen or lumbar spine is being irradiated, especially if a large volume is included.

Another commonly held fallacy has been derived from knowledge of the effect of atomic explosions, that irradiation causes hair to fall out. However, it only does so in areas which are in the direct path of the radiation beam and its occurrence is dose-dependent. The hair usually regrows over the months following, but may be delayed if the patient is continuing on cytotoxic drugs which cause epilation.

Depression and tiredness are often attributed to irradiation. It is hard to explain this and it is likely that radiation is one factor in it. But there are also many other factors involved, including the patient's general condition, the occurrence of recent surgery and anaesthetics, as well as the anxieties the patient has about his diagnosis.

We have not mentioned the damage which radiation is likely to cause to the kidney and liver at certain well-recognized dose limits. It is therefore usual practice to shield these organs as much as is consistent with effective treatment.

Where large areas of bone marrow (in adults mostly in the vertebral bodies, sternum and pelvic bones) are included in the treatment volume, there may be significant suppression of haemopoiesis, especially if the patient is also having cytotoxic drugs.

Radiation and Chemotherapy

With the increased use of combined treatment, more is being learned about the interactions of the two modalities and many of these have already been mentioned.

The use of Methotrexate seems to lower the skin dose of irradiation at which erythema occurs. Actinomycin-D sensitizes the liver and lung to irradiation and there are many other such interactions of which we must be aware.

Radiation and Children

Radiotherapy plays a part in the treatment of most malignancies of childhood but its use in children presents particular problems.

In general, the normal tissues of children are damaged by smaller doses of irradiation than one would expect with adults. This is true of the level of kidney irradiation at which changes of radiation nephritis may occur, as with the level at which radiation hepatitis can be seen when the liver is irradiated. Other tissues include the lens of the eye and the central nervous system, and these are particularly vulnerable and the younger the child the more likely is this susceptibility to become apparent. Doses are usually modified accordingly and it is fortunate that many of the tumours of childhood, being radioresponsive, do not require such high doses as most adult tumours.

Retardation or arrest of bone growth may occur if the growing ends of bones are irradiated in children, and this effect may be most marked if treatment is given at the time of the maximum growth spurts.

Most children are extremely resilient and tolerant of radiation treatment. In a very young child, sedation may be necessary for at least the first few treatments. In the toddler age group, and particularly if a precise treatment such as to the eye or brain is being given, a general anaesthetic is sometimes necessary on each occasion.

Chapter 13

Some Principles of Cancer Chemotherapy

BRIDGET T. HILL
Ph.D., F.R.I.C., C.Chem., M.I.Biol.
Senior Scientist
Laboratory of Cellular Chemotherapy
Imperial Cancer Research Fund Laboratories
London

and

L. A. PRICE
M.B., B.S., M.R.C.P.
Senior Lecturer in Medicine
Honorary Consultant Physician
Royal Marsden Hospital
London

The object of chemotherapy is to do the maximum amount of damage to the tumour and the minimum amount of damage to the patient. The application of certain concepts derived from fundamental studies of the growth characteristics and cell cycle kinetics of both normal and malignant cells has provided a logical basis for the design of selective cancer treatment protocols which attempt to achieve this objective.

Factors Influencing the Success of Chemotherapy

NUMBER OF MALIGNANT CELLS PRESENT

In experimental studies it has been shown that chemotherapy is most likely to be curative when the number of malignant cells present is smallest. Skipper and his colleagues developed a quantitative assay for determining the number of malignant cells in a mouse which could be killed by a given course of drug treatment. They were then able to demonstrate that the effect of an antitumour agent on malignant cells

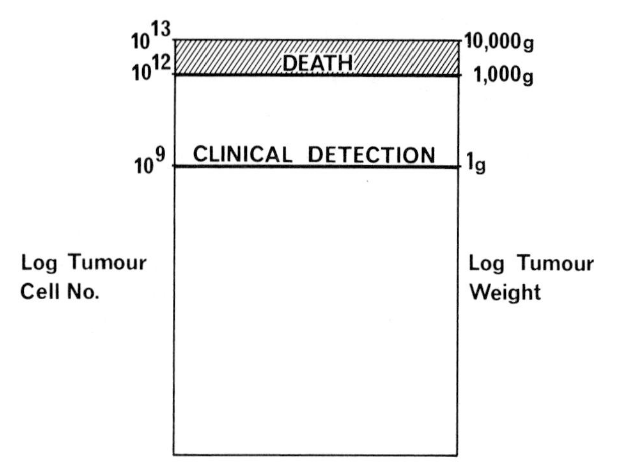

Figure 13.1 The relationship between tumour cell number, tumour weight, clinical detection and the death of the patient. Current methods of investigation allow detection of the tumour only when about 1 g of tumour is present and the tumour is already at least two-thirds of the way through its lifespan (from Hill and Price, 1977, courtesy of Heinemann (Medical Books)).

follows 'first order' kinetics. This means that for a given dose of a cytotoxic drug a fixed percentage of the total tumour cell population (not a fixed number) is killed. A simplified version of this concept is shown in Table 13.1 which gives the relationship between malignant cell number and eradication of the tumour. It is apparent that the same drug, achieving the same fraction of cells killed, given in the same manner, to animals bearing a similar type of tumour can either be completely useless when the number of malignant cells present is large

Table 13.1 *The relationship between cure rate and tumour cell number* (from Skipper *et al.*, 1965 and taken from Hill and Price, 1977, courtesy of Heinemann (Medical Books) London)

EFFECTS OF A DRUG WHICH ACHIEVES A 6 LOG CELL KILL (99·9999%)
'CURE' almost all animals with 10 thousand malignant cells
'CURE' 40% of animals with 1 million malignant cells
'CURE' NONE of animals with 1 billion malignant cells

or curative when the number of malignant cells present is small. These experimental data highlight the need to detect a tumour at an early stage in its development.

ABILITY TO DETECT A TUMOUR CLINICALLY

Unfortunately at the present time for most solid tumours the techniques available are unable to detect in man malignant cell numbers less than about 10^9 or 1 g of tumour (see Fig. 13.1). Since the patient will die when the total number of malignant cells increases to between 10^{12}–10^{13} (i.e. tumours weighing between 1 and 10 kg), it follows that at the time of detection the tumour has already passed through at least two-thirds of its lifespan. In biological terms, therefore, there is no such thing as an 'early' detectable lump. The same theoretical point applies to the detection of secondary deposits, i.e. it is likely that many patients with apparently 'local' tumours at presentation already have undetectable distant micrometastases. Therefore local treatment alone, such as surgery or radiotherapy, cannot hope to eradicate a disease whose true extent it is impossible to define accurately. To improve the 'cure' rate there is a need to integrate chemotherapy with the best methods of local treatment.

OPTIMAL THERAPY: A COMBINATION OF CHEMOTHERAPY AND LOCAL TREATMENT

Since antitumour drugs are most likely to be curative when the number of tumour cells in an animal is smallest, it follows that adjuvant chemotherapy should be given *immediately* after the bulk of the primary tumour has been removed or destroyed by surgery and/or radiotherapy. The application of this principle has markedly increased the cure rate in certain experimental tumours in animals, and is outlined diagrammatically in Fig. 13.2. This concept is now being tested in human disease (see Chapter 14).

In these types of studies the best results have generally been obtained by using full dose intensive chemotherapy following surgical procedures. The adoption of smaller doses of chemotherapy has been shown to be less effective. This principle is illustrated in Fig. 13.3 and is now starting to be applied in the treatment of human malignancies such as breast and lung cancers.

Kinetics of Tumour Growth

GROWTH RATE OF HUMAN TUMOURS

Several investigators have suggested that the growth rate of a tumour provides valuable prognostic information. Patients with 'rapidly growing' tumours are likely to survive for a shorter time than those

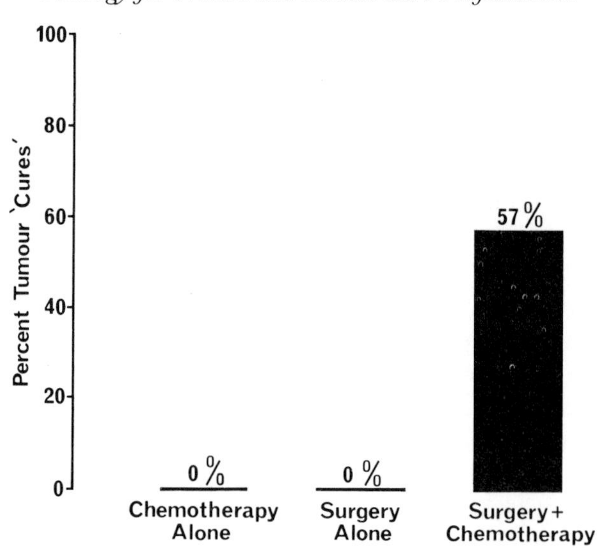

Figure 13.2 The advantages in terms of tumour 'cure' from combining local (surgery) and systemic (chemotherapy) forms of treatment in mice bearing the adenocarcinoma 755 (after Shapiro and Fugmann, 1957. *Cancer Research*, **17**, 1098, and taken from Hill and Price, 1977, courtesy of Heinemann (Medical Books)).

with 'slowly growing' tumours. Data are also frequently presented which suggest a correlation between high growth rate and favourable response to chemotherapy. It is suggested that these types of measurements may be useful as indicators for either commencing treatment and/or monitoring its effectiveness. However, it is essential that these claims are viewed in the light of all the limitations and criticisms of the techniques employed to measure these parameters which are discussed below. In particular, it should be remembered that these values are generally derived from heterogeneous lesions made up of different subpopulations with differing cell kinetic properties.

A characteristic feature of the growth of a tumour is the progressive increase in its cell number. In simple experimental systems such as tumour cells growing in suspension culture there is a constant relationship between increase in cell number and time, and these cells are said to grow exponentially. Under these circumstances if the tumour cell number has doubled in one day, it will have quadrupled in two days and by three days will have increased by a factor of eight. In most experimental animal tumours the growth of the tumour is also usually exponential, especially in the early part of its development. However, in most solid tumours, as the tumour mass increases in size and age there is a tendency for the rate of growth to slow (see Fig. 13.4).

Since in human solid tumours it is possible only to first detect a lump

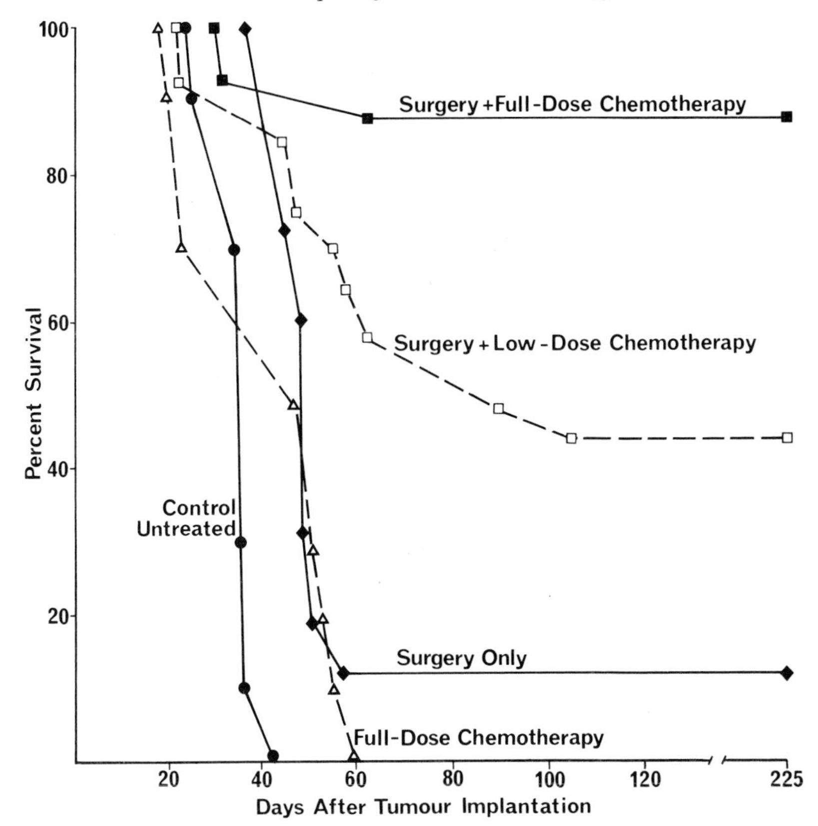

Figure 13.3 The advantages of using full dose intensive chemotherapy as adjuvant to surgical removal of primary C3H mammary adenocarcinomas, rather than compromising with low-dose chemotherapy (after Griswold *et al.*, 1969. *Cancer Chemotherapy Reports*, **53**, 345. Courtesy of Dr D. P. Griswold). Surgery on day 13; chemotherapy on day 17.

late on in its development, estimations of the rate of tumour growth are of necessity restricted to a short period near the end of the tumour's lifespan, where the rate of growth is not only likely to be atypical but is also liable to fluctuate. These limitations make it difficult to estimate the value or significance, if any, of attempts to determine the so-called 'growth parameters' of human tumours. For example, the 'growth rates' of tumours have been calculated from measurements of mean values of the diameter of the tumour as it increases with time. From these types of measurements, in breast cancer for example, the mean clinically observed 'doubling time' was 126 days (although the range was 23–209 days). However, when an autoradiographic technique was employed, the calculated 'doubling time' was only 43 days. Other published data have further emphasized the broad range of growth rates that have been observed: some solid tumours have a doubling time as short as a week, others in excess of a year, and the median value is approximately two months. These data at least serve to refute a common misconception: rapid growth is *not* a characteristic of primary tumours in man. Measurements of this type suffer from the following major limitations:

1. Observations on human tumours are of necessity limited with respect to site, time and number;
2. The majority of human tumours are inaccessible for measurement either directly or by X-ray or mammography;
3. Accurate measurements of irregularly shaped tumour masses are very difficult to achieve;
4. It is assumed that every tumour cell (i.e. 100 per cent) is engaged in mitotic activity which in human tumours is known not to be the case during the whole of their development; and
5. *No* account is taken of the considerable cellular heterogeneity of many tumours in clinically detectable stages of growth, which makes any average value obtained meaningless.

The clinical irrelevance of the above traditional cell kinetic measurements can be explained by some recent concepts of cell cycle kinetics.

THE CELL CYCLE

The introduction of the concept of the life cycle of a cell in 1953 has proved invaluable in extending our knowledge not only in fundamental cell biology concerned with understanding and manipulating growth in normal and malignant tissues, but has also shown how the treatment of human cancers can be improved.

Before the cell divides it must undergo certain stages in preparation. The sequence of changes or events which a cell undergoes between one division and the next is called the cell cycle. This consists of four phases (see Fig. 13.5). After cell division or mitosis (M) there is a period called the first gap or G_1 phase, during which the cell synthesizes both RNA and protein in preparation for DNA synthesis. DNA synthesis itself occurs only during the synthetic or S phase, and it is at this stage that the DNA content of the cell is doubled so as to allow the donation of the same amount of DNA as it has itself to each daughter cell after division. RNA and protein synthesis continue throughout S and on into the next phase of the cell cycle called G_2 or the second gap phase. During G_2 the cell prepares for mitosis. In M, when RNA synthesis ceases and protein synthesis is minimal, cell division occurs. This sequence of

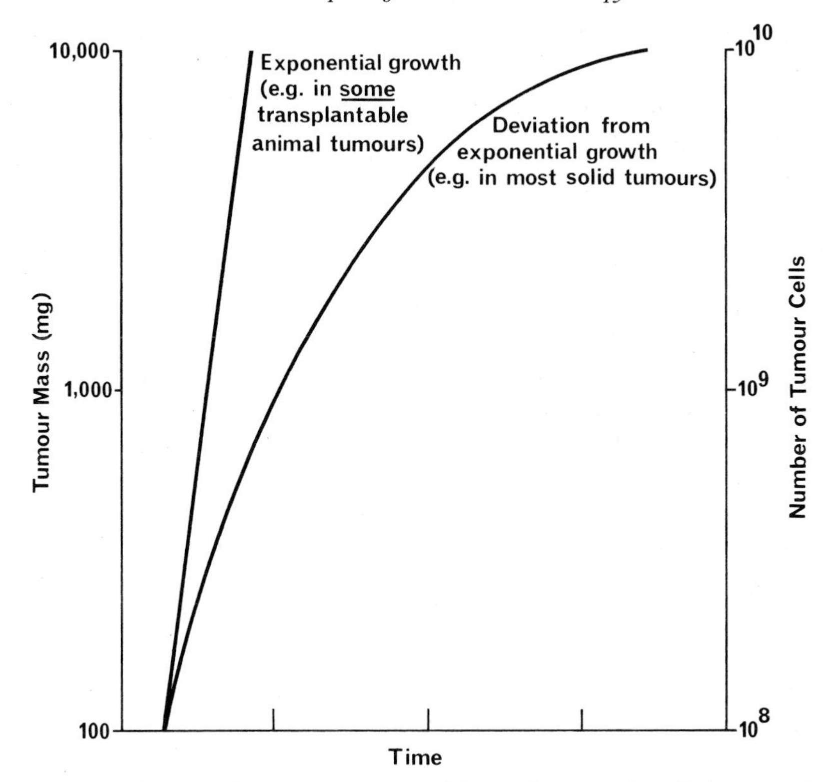

Figure 13.4 A comparison of true exponential growth, as seen in cells in suspension culture and in some transplantable animal tumours, with the type of growth curve most commonly observed in animal solid tumours. Notice that the deviation is greatest when more than 10^9 cells are present, which is at the level of clinical detection in man (see Fig. 13.1).

events leading up to and culminating in mitosis is very complex and all the processes involved are interrelated and interdependent. Therefore, any outside interference (e.g. from chemicals or irradiation), which either prevents cell division or interferes with or causes errors in synthesis or function of any macromolecule (e.g. DNA, RNA or protein), can lead to the death of the cell or its mutation or transformation.

The use of a radioactively labelled DNA precursor, usually tritiated thymidine, combined with autoradiography, enables one to label and recognize the cells in DNA synthesis. By following the passage of the radioactively labelled cohort of cells through successive mitoses (the technique of 'labelled mitoses') the *mean* duration of the cell cycle (or intermitotic time), its spread and the lengths of the different phases of the cell cycle can be estimated. However, the validity of this procedure for human tumours has been much discussed and criticized. In particular, there is once again the problem of obtaining a mean value representative of the majority of a cell population. This is made even more difficult since the interval between one mitosis and the next varies in different cells within a tissue and in both normal and malignant cells. The greatest variation is found in G_1 with estimated times varying from a few hours to several days. Therefore, depending on the length of the cell cycle, some cells are considered to be rapidly proliferating (with a short cell cycle time), while others have a slow turnover rate (with a longer cell cycle time). Neither state is specifically characteristic of normal or malignant tissues. Furthermore, care must be taken in talking of rapidly or slowly growing groups of cells or tissues since, in general, tissues, and tumours in particular, are composed of heterogeneous cell types with a wide spectrum of cell cycle times.

'RESTING' CELLS AND 'CYCLING' CELLS

Figure 13.5 also shows that at any one time not all cells are proceeding through the cycle since they may leave the cycle to rest entering a state called 'G_0'. This distribution of cells between 'resting' and 'cycling' states is important, since if cycling cells are destroyed by any means, for example by chemotherapy, more resting cells will be drawn back into cycle to restore the original population. In addition to 'cycling' and 'resting' cells there is another group of cells which are 'non-dividing' which have permanently left the cycle and are destined to die without dividing again.

FACTORS INFLUENCING THE GROWTH OF A CELL POPULATION

Therefore it follows that the growth of any cell population depends on at least three factors:

1. the length of the cell cycle(s);
2. the proportion of resting cells which can be brought back into cycle;
3. the extent of cell loss due to death, migration or exfoliation.

Attempts to measure these factors have met with very limited success. The term 'growth fraction' was introduced as a measure of the actual number of cells in a population which were 'cycling' (or proliferating). It has been suggested that tumours with a high growth fraction such as some transplantable ascites tumours and leukaemias, can be destroyed by cytotoxic drugs, but in most solid tumours the growth fraction is low

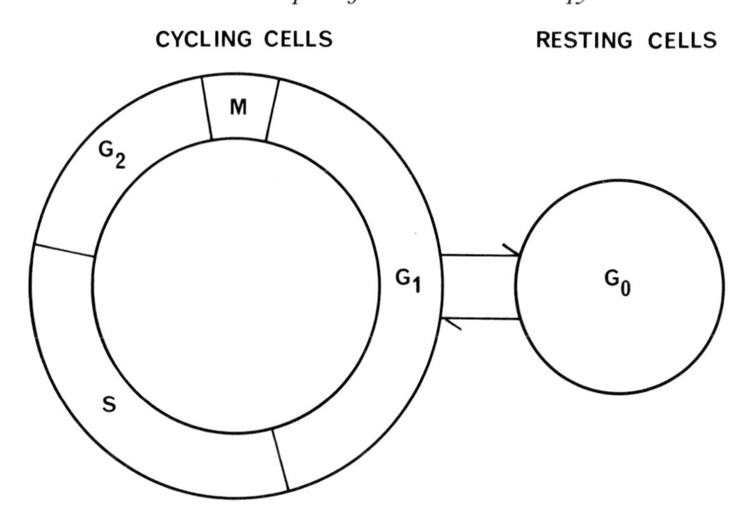

Figure 13.5 Diagrammatic representation of a cell system consisting of cycling (proliferating) cells and resting (non-proliferating) cells. The cycling cells traverse the four phases of the cycle moving after mitosis, through G_1, S and G_2 and so back to M. The G_0 cells have the capacity to re-enter the cycle in response to a suitable stimulus, for example, if many of the cycling cells are killed by chemotherapeutic agents.

and so only a small percentage of cells are susceptible to chemotherapy. Unfortunately, the use of this term in practice suffers from the major drawback that at present we do not have methods which enable us to distinguish accurately between 'resting' (or non-proliferating) cells and slowly or discontinuously cycling cells. Just as some resting cells can be triggered back into cycle, so cells proceeding slowly through the cycle may speed up their rate of transit in response to the appropriate stimulus. These events may occur in both normal and malignant cell populations.

Therefore the observations that the length of the cell cycle is not necessarily shorter in tumour cells than in normal cells, that a reduced growth fraction is not a consistent phenomenon in slower growing as opposed to more rapidly growing tumours and finally that increased cell loss is not a characteristic of malignant tissue, are not surprising. Measurements of these types have failed to provide any evidence of kinetic differences between normal and malignant cell populations which might be exploited clinically. They have also omitted to take into account the all important stem cell compartments which are responsible for maintaining the integrity and continued survival of any particular cell population.

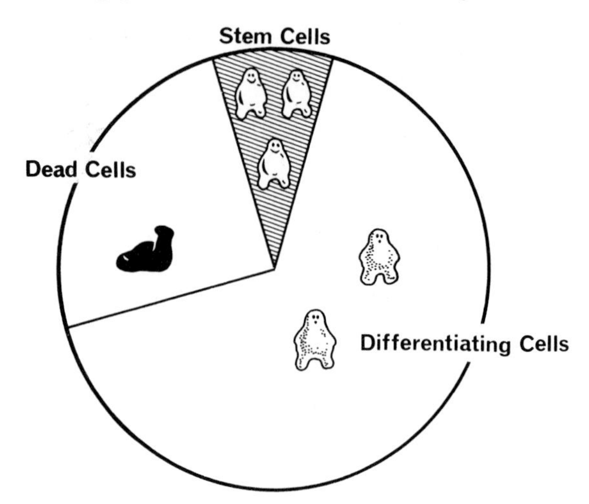

Figure 13.6 The three major components of a proliferating system.

STEM CELLS

Normal and malignant cell populations are characteristically heterogeneous systems consisting of many different cell types. In proliferating systems there are three major kinetic compartments: dead cells, cells that are differentiating and stem cells (see Fig. 13.6). The stem cell compartment is the smallest, and consists of cells which have the capacity to produce an indefinite number of like progeny; it is therefore the most important. A stem cell may divide into two other stem cells or may elect to differentiate so as to provide a feed-in system for the differentiating compartment.

Once the cell begins to differentiate it loses its capacity for indefinite proliferation and retains a capacity to divide only a certain limited number of times and will then die (see Fig. 13.7). In the differentiating compartment, e.g. in the bone marrow, there would be early, middle and late red and white blood cells. It is on this compartment that the histological assessment is made. If cells in the differentiating compartment are killed or damaged by any means, then more stem cells will differentiate so as to restore the original population. Both cells in the differentiating compartment and the stem cells can exist as either 'resting' or 'cycling' populations. The existence of stem cells in normal tissues is well established. However, evidence of malignant stem cells is more limited, being well documented only in experimental animal tumours. Definitive evidence of their presence in human solid tumours awaits the development of reliable assay methods. At present these cells can only be identified by a 'functional' assay procedure, that is by their capacity to produce a very large number of descendants in the form of

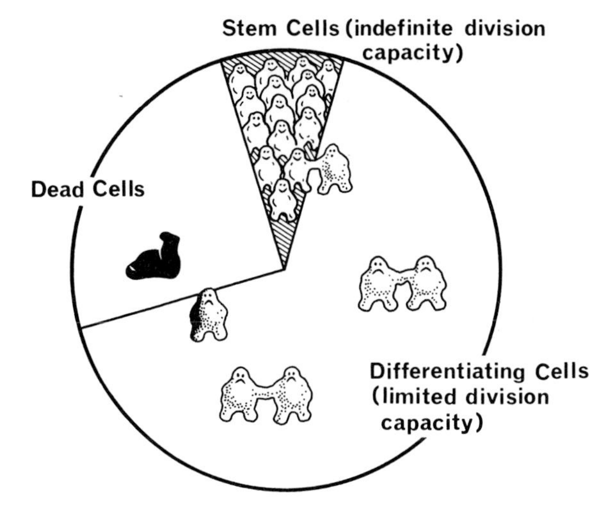

Figure 13.7 A diagrammatic representation of the *infinite* division capacity of stem cells and the *limited* division capacity of cells in the differentiating compartment.

'colonies' under defined conditions.

Once the importance of the stem cell population is appreciated it can be seen that the object of cancer chemotherapy becomes more precise, namely to kill the maximum number of malignant stem cells and the minimum number of vulnerable normal stem cells. Achieving this objective would allow the population of normal stem cells, such as the bone marrow, to recover before the malignant population, and perhaps eradicate the tumour without seriously damaging the host. In this way repeated courses of drug treatment could be given as soon as the normal marrow had recovered while the tumour stem cell population is gradually reduced and finally destroyed (see Fig. 13.8).

The Exploitable Kinetic Difference Between Normal and Malignant Stem Cell Systems

W. R. Bruce and his co-workers in 1966 were one of the first groups to highlight cell kinetic differences between normal and malignant stem cells. They developed a quantitative spleen-colony forming assay in the mouse for assessing the sensitivity of resting normal bone marrow stem cells and rapidly dividing clonogenic AKR lymphoma cells to a variety of cytotoxic agents. This enabled the design of successful regimens with a high degree of selective toxicity against the tumour, provided the agents were administered over short periods of time (namely twenty-four hours).

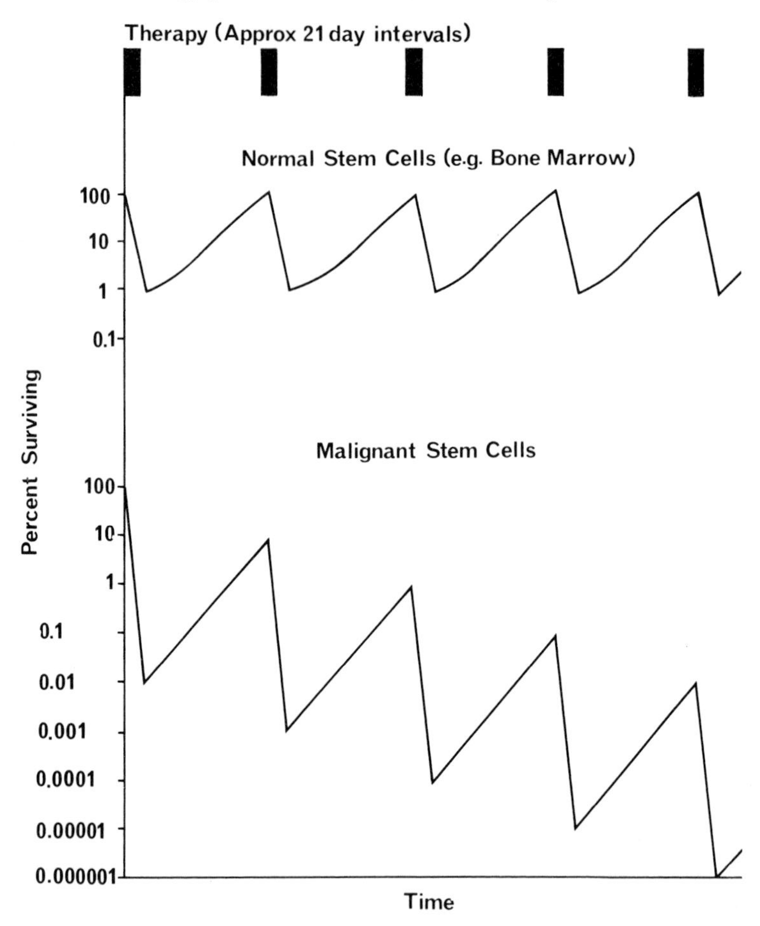

Figure 13.8 A theoretical representation of successful chemotherapy showing the effects of drug treatment on normal (e.g. haematopoietic) stem cells and malignant stem cells. Drug treatment on Day 1 reduces the number of normal stem cells to about 1 per cent, and approximately 21 days are required before these cells return to normal levels and permit a second course of therapy. However, the number of malignant stem cells are reduced by 99·99 per cent with each course, and regrow to only 10 per cent by the time the next course of treatment is given. Thus the tumour shrinks progressively.

Basically, these workers measured the effects of a twenty-four-hour exposure of various anticancer drugs on the normal bone marrow stem cells and lymphoma stem cells. They showed that the drugs fall into two main classes: those which do not increase bone marrow stem cell kill irrespective of dose (Class II or phase specific) and those where the bone marrow stem cell kill does increase with increasing dose (Class III or cycle specific). In both classes, there is maximal selective kill of malignant stem cells (see Fig. 13.9).

This selectivity of agents in both Class II and Class III appeared

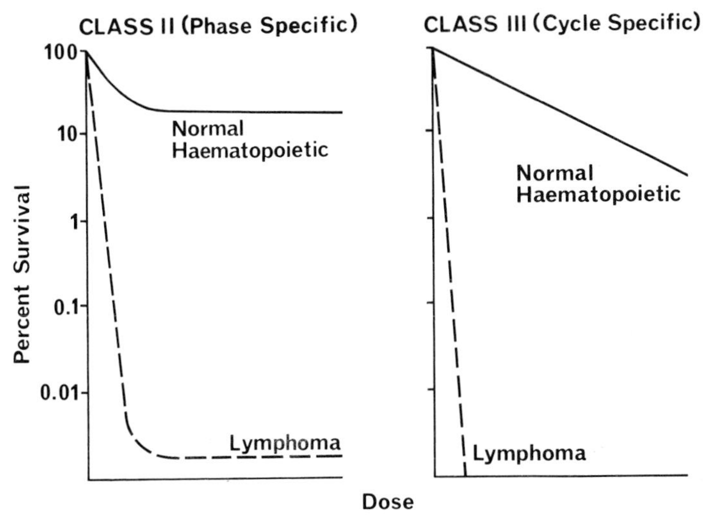

Figure 13.9 The basis of a Kinetic Classification of Antitumour Drugs. Dose–survival curves for both normal haematopoietic (——) and transplanted lymphoma (– – – –) colony forming units. Normal or tumour-bearing mice were given different doses of a given agent and their femoral marrows were assayed 24 hours later for their content of colony-forming units (after Bruce *et al.*, 1966, *J. National Cancer Institute*, **37**, 233).

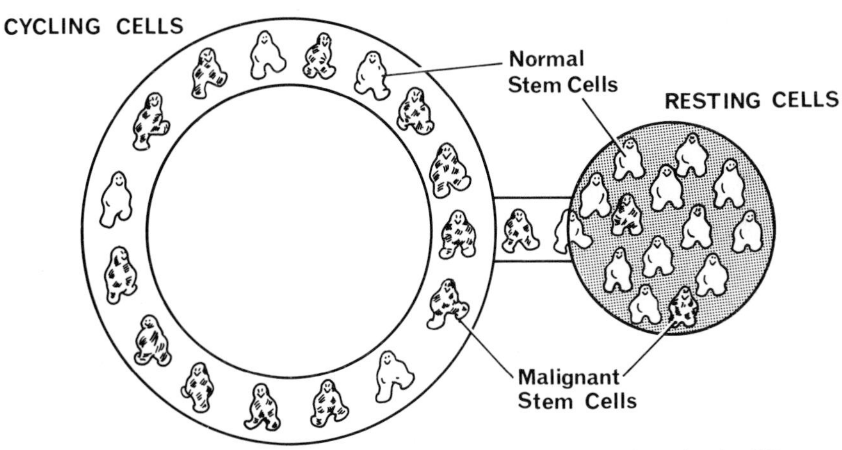

Figure 13.10 A diagrammatic representation of the exploitable kinetic difference between normal and malignant stem cells which exists over a 24-hour period – namely that during this time most normal stem cells are resting while most of the malignant stem cells are cycling.

to be associated with the fact that in untreated animals most of the normal stem cells were resting (G_0), while all of the detectable malignant stem cells appeared to be cycling (see Fig. 13.10). Therefore short courses (i.e. over twenty-four hours) of Class II and Class III agents, which preferentially kill cycling cells, would cause a much greater kill of malignant as opposed to normal stem cells. If the time of exposure is prolonged, however, this kinetic difference between normal and malignant stem cells is abolished and increasing damage to the bone marrow occurs. These initial studies have been extended to include other agents and form the basis for a kinetic classification of antitumour drugs. Examples of drugs in these two groups are given in Table 13.2.

Table 13.2 *Kinetic classification of some antitumour drugs*

Class II (phase specific)	*Class II (cycle specific)*
Cytosine arabinoside	Actinomycin-D
Hydroxyurea	Adryamycin
6-Mercaptopurine	BCNU
Methotrexàte	Chlorambucil
Vinblastine	*Cis*-platinum
Vincristine	Cyclophosphamide
	DTIC
	5-Fluorouracil
	Melphalan
	Myleran
	Nitrogen mustard

The application of this classification has enabled the effects of drugs on the bone marrow to be predicted, so toxicity can be reduced and *safer* chemotherapy can be achieved. From these original studies various predictions can be made, for example, addition of several Class III drugs to a combination will be additively toxic to the normal stem cells and so their doses should be reduced proportionately. However, the addition of Class II drugs to a combination will not increase the damage to the normal bone marrow provided they are given over no longer than one to two cell cycle times (i.e. approximately twenty-four to thirty-six hours in man) and full doses of these agents can be used.

These studies therefore demonstrated that the selectivity of cancer chemotherapy could be increased by giving drugs over twenty-four to thirty-six hours. Kinetic studies also showed that adequate time for recovery of the normal bone marrow following chemotherapy must be permitted before a further course of treatment was administered. Two patterns of recovery of marrow stem cells have been observed in the mouse and similar patterns have now been shown in humans. It is possible to divide chemotherapeutic agents into those that are associated with rapid recovery and others associated with delayed recovery, as shown in Fig. 13.11.

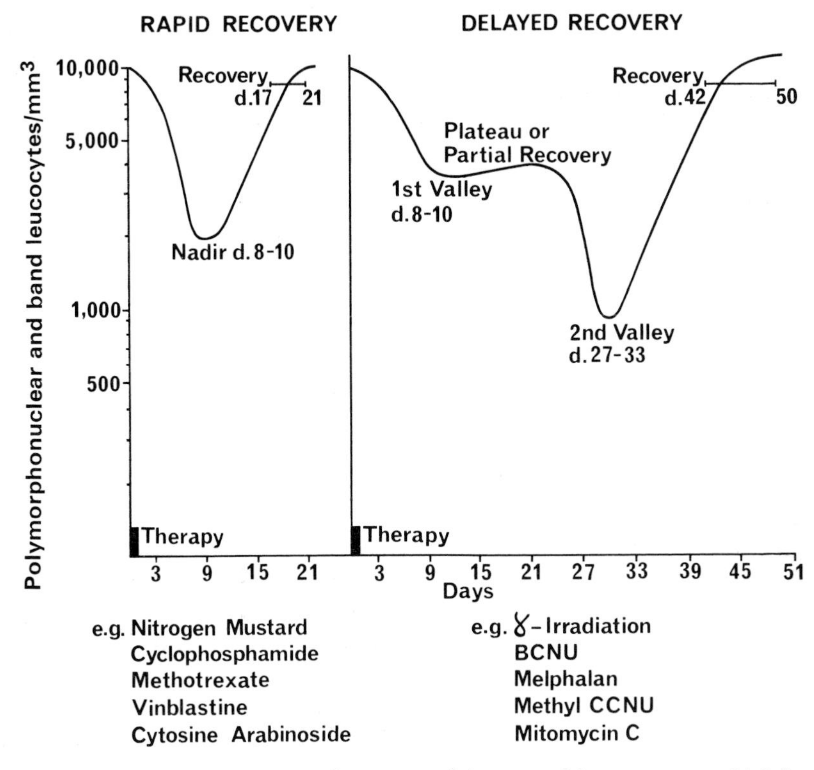

Figure 13.11 The two patterns of recovery of the normal bone marrow which have been observed in humans following chemotherapy. It is possible to divide drugs into those that are associated with rapid recovery, and others that are associated with delayed recovery (after Bergsagel, 1969).

Effects of Drugs on the Cell Cycle

The development of successful techniques for cell synchronization *in vitro* has enabled us to determine the phase or phases of the cell cycle where anticancer agents exert their effects on cells. In general, drugs exert two main types of effect: a delay or 'hold-up' in progression of cells through the cycle; and a lethal or cell killing effect. Examples of these effects are shown in Table 13.3 and Fig. 13.12. In general the use of lower drug concentrations for short periods of time results in the blocking effect, which is often reversible, while higher drug concentrations given over longer periods cause cell kill. The effectiveness of sequencing combinations may be influenced by using a drug which arrests cells at one stage of the cycle, to attempt partial tumour cell synchrony, followed by one which kills cells maximally at the point of the blockade itself or in the phase immediately succeeding it. For

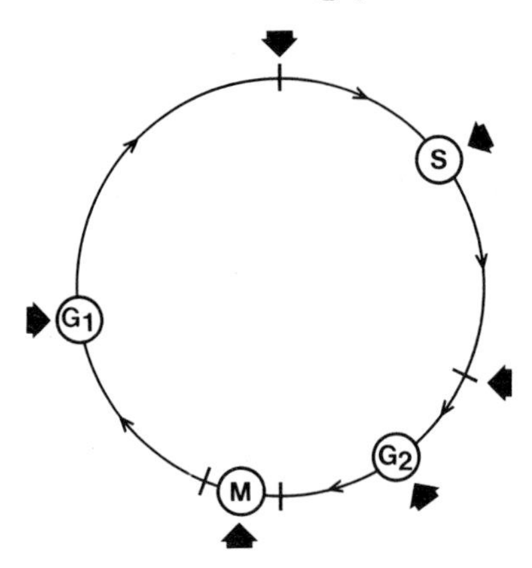

Figure 13.12 The phases of the cell cycle where antitumour agents exert their lethal effects (from Hill and Baserga, 1975 by courtesy of *Cancer Treatment Reviews*).

example, vincristine which holds cells up at M may be followed, six to twelve hours later, by a combination of bleomycin, which kills cells in mitosis, and methotrexate which kills cells in the succeeding G_1 and S phases of the cycle.

A major problem with these *in vitro* data is determining their relevance to man. There is a great need for further studies *in vivo* to confirm the phase specificity of drug action. The one important limitation in

Table 13.3 *Effects of some antitumour agents on the progression of cells through the cycle* (from Hill and Baserga, 1975, by courtesy of *Cancer Treatment Reviews*)

Phase of cycle where delay in progression or arrest occurs	*Antitumour drugs*
G_1	Actinomycin-D*; 6-Mercaptopurine
G_1/S 'boundary'	Actinomycin-D*; Cytosine arabinoside; 5-Fluorouracil; Hydroxyurea; Methotrexate
S	BCNU* (late); CCNU*; DTIC; Methyl CCNU*
S/G_2 'boundary'	Actinomycin-D*; Cytosine arabinoside*; Mitomycin C*; Bleomycin*
G_2	Actinomycin-D*; Adriamycin; BCNU*; Bleomycin*; CCNU* Cyclophosphamide; Methyl CCNU*; Mitomycin C*; Nitrogen Mustard
G_2/M 'boundary'	ICRF 159*; Puromycin
M	ICRF 159* (prophase); Vinblastine (metaphase); Vincristine (metaphase)

* Indicates more than one site of action of the agent.

attempting these *in vivo* studies is the shortage of available techniques for synchronizing cell populations *in vivo*. However, some advances have recently been made in this area using a combination of fasting and various drugs including cytosine arabinoside. Further studies are clearly needed to determine whether these kinetic findings can be generalized and extended to the use of other drugs in the treatment of a wide range of malignant diseases.

Experimental Predictions of Clinical Relevance

The experimental findings from these model systems have indicated that the following principles of cell cycle kinetics should be applied when attempting to design safer and more effective combination chemotherapy schedules:

1. Drug treatment should be administered when the smallest number of malignant cells are present. Therefore, where agents to which the tumour is sensitive are available, chemotherapy should be used either early in the disease, or *immediately* after primary local treatment, when surgery or radiotherapy has reduced the tumour mass.
2. Drugs should be given in short intensive courses using maximally tolerated doses on optimal schedules. A reduction in dosage is likely to compromise efficacy.
3. Chemotherapy should be given over periods of twenty-four to thirty-six hours in intermittent courses (at approximately three-weekly intervals), since this approach markedly reduces toxicity.
4. Treatment cycles should only be repeated when haematologic recovery has occurred. Therefore if agents are included which delay the recovery time of the normal bone marrow, treatment should only be repeated at approximately six-weekly intervals.
5. The toxicity of Class II (Phase specific) agents to normal stem cells (e.g. bone marrow) is not dose dependent. Class II agents may therefore be added to combinations without reducing their dose, provided the total treatment time does not exceed thirty-six hours.
6. Combinations of Class III (Cycle specific) agents will be additively toxic to normal bone marrow since toxicity is both time and dose dependent, therefore doses should be reduced proportionately.
7. The practice of giving small daily doses of drugs from either class should be avoided since under these conditions resting normal bone marrow stem cells will be drawn into cycle and killed and so the selective toxicity against malignant cells would be reduced.

8. When selecting drugs for combinations a knowledge of their cell killing effects and their ability to halt progression in different phases of the cell cycle may be helpful. Attempts to induce partial tumour cell synchrony by sequencing of agents within the twenty-four to thirty-six hour period could increase the selectivity against the tumour.

The successful clinical application of these experimental principles is outlined in Chapter 14.

References

Baserga, R. (ed.) (1971) *The Cell Cycle and Cancer.* New York: M. Dekker.

Bergsagel, D. E. (1969) Chemotherapy of cancer, *Modern Medicine in Canada*, **24**, 19–24.

Bruce, W. R. and Lin, H. (1969) An empirical cellular approach to the improvement of cancer therapy, *Cancer Research,* **29**, 2308–10.

Bruce, W. R. and Valeriote, F. A. (1968) Normal and malignant stem cells and chemotherapy, *The Proliferation and Spread of Neoplastic Cells*, pp. 409–20. (The University of Texas M. D. Anderson Hospital and Tumor Institute at Houston, Twenty-first Annual Symposium on Fundamental Cancer Research, 1967.) Baltimore, Maryland: The Williams and Wilkins Company.

Hill, Bridget T. (1976) Biochemistry of the cell cycle, *Scientific Foundations of Oncology*, pp. 63–72. T. Symington and R. Carter (eds.). London: W. Heinemann (Medical).

Hill, Bridget T. and Baserga, R. (1975) The cell cycle and its significance for cancer treatment, *Cancer Treatment Reviews*, **2**, 159–75.

Hill, Bridget T. and Price, L. A. (1977) Concepts and prospects in adjuvant chemotherapy, *Secondary Spread in Breast Cancer*: Vol. 3. *New Aspects of Breast Cancer*, pp. 193–212. B. A. Stoll (ed.). London: W. Heinemann (Medical).

Lamerton, L. F. (1972) Cell proliferation and the differential response of normal and malignant tissues, *British Journal of Radiology*, **45**, 161–70.

Schabel, F. M., Jr. (1969) Cellular kinetics and its implication in cancer chemotherapy, *Neoplasia in Childhood*, pp. 61–78. (The University of Texas M. D. Anderson Hospital and Tumor Institute.) Chicago: Yearbook Medical Publishers.

Skipper, H. E. (1968) Kinetic considerations associated with therapy of solid tumors, *The Proliferation and Spread of Neoplastic Cells*, pp. 213–33. (The University of Texas M. D. Anderson Hospital and Tumor Institute at Houston, Twenty-first Annual Symposium on Fundamental Cancer Research, 1967.) Baltimore, Maryland: The Williams and Wilkins Company.

Steel, G. G. (1975) Cell kinetics and cell survival, *Medical Oncology*, pp. 49–66. K. D. Bagshawe (ed.). Oxford: Blackwells.

Chapter 14

The Role of Chemotherapy

L. A. PRICE
M.B., B.S., M.R.C.P.
Senior Lecturer in Medicine
Honorary Consultant Physician
Royal Marsden Hospital
London

and

BRIDGET T. HILL
Ph.D., F.R.I.C., C.Chem., M.I. Biol.
Senior Scientist
Laboratory of Cellular Chemotherapy
Imperial Cancer Research Fund Laboratories
London

The exact role of chemotherapy is not known for most malignant diseases at the present time. This is because most of the available anticancer drugs have never been adequately evaluated in most common cancers. Table 14.1 shows the thirty anticancer drugs commonly available and Table 14.2 the number of drugs which have been properly tested for effectiveness against the common so-called 'solid' tumours.

It is obvious that a large number of drugs which have been available for many years, have not yet been properly tested against many types of cancer. Even so, from the trials conducted so far, the role of chemotherapy has become sufficiently clear to use it routinely in some tumours. Table 14.3 shows the current status of chemotherapy.

In some malignant disease, certain drugs have become part of the routine management of the disease. Drugs are usually regarded as effective if they produce a response rate of 20 per cent or more when given alone. Such agents can then be used as 'building blocks' for combination chemotherapy. At present it is customary to give several drugs together since the response rates can often be improved by this approach. Currently, at different centres around the world, there is a

Table 14.1 *Commonly available anticancer drugs*

Drug	*Abbreviation*		
Cyclophosphamide	CYC	Adriamycin	ADR
Mechlorothamine	HN2	Bleomycin	BLM
Chlorambucil	CHL	Mitomycin C	MTC
Melphalan	MPL	BCNU	BCNU
Busulfan	BUS	CCNU	CCNU
5-Fluorourocil	5-FU	Methyl-CCNU	MCCNU
Methotrexate	MTX	Streptozotocin	STZ
6-Mercaptopurine	6-MP	DTIC	DTIC
6-Thioguanine	6-TG	Hexamethylmelamine	HXM
Cytosine arabinoside	Ara-C	Dibromodulcitol	DBD
Vincristine	VCR	Hydroxyurea	HYD
Vinblastine	VBL	Procarbazine	PCB
Actinomycin D	ACT	L-Asparaginase	L-ASP
Mithramycin	MTH	Dibromomannitol	DBM
Daunorubicin	DNR	5-Azacytidine	5-AZC

Table 14.2 *Drug evaluation in common 'solid' tumours*

Tumour	*No. of drugs (of 30) adequately evaluated*	*No. of drugs with evidence of antitumour effect*	*No. of drugs ineffective*	*No. of drugs (of 30) never adequately evaluated*
Bladder	3	3	None	27
Brain	8	7	1	22
Breast	24	13	11	6
Cervix	10	10	None	20
Colon	25	7	18	5
Oesophagus	1	1	None	29
Head and neck	16	12	4	14
Kidney	8	2	6	22
Lung	22	14	8	8
Melanomas	23	6	17	7
Pancreas	3	2	1	27
Prostate	5	3	2	25
Ovary	11	9	2	19
Sarcomas	11	8	3	19
Stomach	8	6	2	22
Testicle	6	6	None	24
Uterus	1	1	None	29

Table 14.3 *The role of chemotherapy in different malignant diseases*

1. *Disease-free survival possible for long periods*	2. *Significant chance of objective regression with increased survival*	3. *Transient regressions in some patients but increased survival not established*
Blood and associated diseases	*Blood and associated diseases*	*Blood and associated diseases*
Acute lymphocytic leukaemia	Non-Hodgkin's malignant lymphoma	Blast crisis of chronic granulocytic leukaemia
Stage III and IV of Hodgkin's disease	Multiple myeloma	
Burkitt's lymphoma	Acute myeloid leukaemia	
	Chronic lymphocytic leukaemia	
Adult solid tumours	*Adult solid tumours*	*Adult solid tumours*
Trophoblastic carcinoma (choriocarcinoma)	Carcinoma of the breast	Carcinoma of the lung
Testicular tumours	Carcinoma of the ovary	Adenocarcinoma of the gastrointestinal tract
	Squamous cell carcinoma of the head and neck	Carcinoma of the prostate
*Paediatric solid tumours**		Carcinoma of the bladder
Wilms's tumour	*Paediatric solid tumours**	Carcinoma of the thyroid
Ewing's sarcoma	Neuroblastoma	Soft tissue sarcoma
Embryonal rhabdomyosarcoma	Osteogenic sarcoma	Malignant melanoma
Retinoblastoma		

* The best use of chemotherapy in these diseases is in combination with radiotherapy and/or surgery.

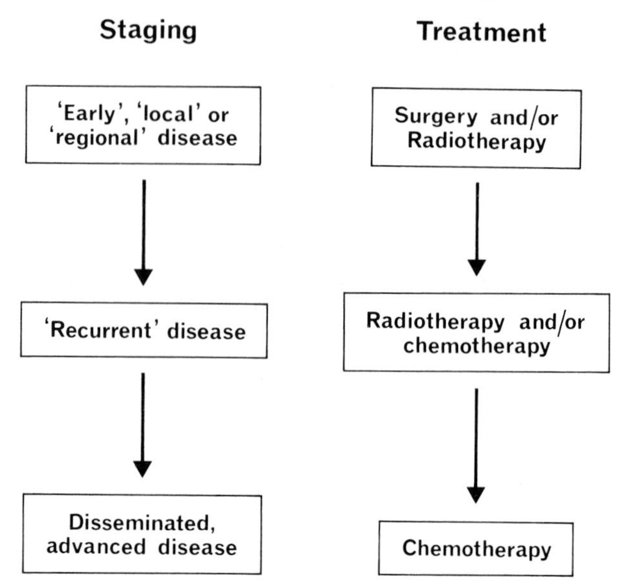

Figure 14.1 Traditional approach to solid tumour therapy.

bewildering variety of combination schedules for many tumours, using different drugs, scheduling and doses. It would be futile to attempt to summarize these, since they are changing so rapidly. However, some drugs are now widely accepted as having a part to play in the management of various cancers and these are summarized in Table 14.4.

Some Recent Concepts in Cancer Chemotherapy

Over the past few years it has become obvious from certain well-established experimental principles and some preliminary clinical studies that the traditional role of chemotherapy in the overall management of cancer should be critically re-evaluated. In the past it was usual to reserve antitumour drugs until all other kinds of treatment had failed, i.e. they were used only as a last resort when surgery or radiotherapy had failed to cure the primary tumour. This concept is illustrated in Fig. 14.1.

The reasons why one cannot be complacent about the traditional approach fall into two groups, practical and theoretical. Practical reasons are that surgeons and radiotherapists have the privilege of curing most of those cancer patients who are cured, although it is an unfortunate fact that using these modalities alone there has been no improvement for several decades in the overall survival rates for common lethal tumours such as breast, lung, stomach and squamous cell

Table 14.4 *Common drugs in the management of various cancers*

Cancer type	*Useful drugs*	*Other drugs with some effect*
	(i) *Blood and associated diseases*	
Acute lymphocytic leukaemia	Vincristine, Prednisone, Methotrexate, 6-Mercaptopurine, Cylcophosphamide	Asparaginase, Cytosine arabinoside, Thioguanine, Adriamycin, BCNU
Acute myeloid leukaemia	Cytosine arabinoside, Cyclophosphamide, Thioguanine, Adriamycin, Methotrexate, 6-Mercaptopurine	5-Azacytidine, Prednisone, Asparaginase
Chronic lymphocytic leukaemia	Chlorambucil, Cyclophosphamide, Prednisone	Cytosine arabinoside
Chronic myeloid leukaemia	Busulphan, Hydroxyurea	Adriamycin, 6-Mercaptopurine, Melphalan, Dibromomannitol
Multiple myeloma	Melphalan, Cyclophosphamide, Prednisone	Chlorambucil, BCNU
Hodgkin's Disease	Nitrogen mustard, Vincristine, Prednisone, Procarbazine, Vinblastine, Adriamycin, Bleomycin, Chlorambucil, Cyclophosphamide	BCNU, DTIC, Methotrexate
Non-Hodgkin's lymphoma	Cyclophosphamide, Vincristine, Prednisone, Adriamycin, Bleomycin, Procarbazine, Chlorambucil, Vinblastine	Methotrexate, Nitrogen mustard
Burkitt's lymphoma	Cyclophosphamide	
Mycosis fungoides	Methotrexate	

Table 14.4—*contd.*

Cancer type	*Useful drugs*	*Other drugs with some effect*
	(ii) *Adult solid tumours*	
Breast cancer	Adriamycin, 5-Fluorourocil, Vincristine, Methotrexate, Cyclophosphamide	Melphalan, BCNU, Vinblastine, Dibromodulcitol, Hexamethylmelamine, Bleomycin
Ovarian cancer	Chlorambucil, Melphalan, 5-FU Methotrexate, Adriamycin, Hexamethylmelamine	Platinum compounds
Lung cancer	Cyclophosphamide, Nitrogen mustard, 5-FU, Procarbazine, Methotrexate	Adriamycin
Adenocarcinoma of the GI tract (colon, stomach, pancreas)	5-FU, Methyl CCNU, Mitomycin-C	Cyclophosphamide
Prostate	5-FU, Adriamycin	Cyclophosphamide, Nitrogen mustard
Bladder	5-FU, Methotrexate, Mitomycin-C, Adriamycin	
Squamous cell head and neck	Cyclophosphamide, Hydroxyurea, 5-FU, Bleomycin, Methotrexate, Vinblastine	6-Mercaptopurine, Adriamycin
Squamous cell cervix	Cyclophosphamide, 5-FU, Adriamycin, Bleomycin	Methotrexate, Chlorambucil
Testicular seminoma	Cyclophosphamide, Melphalan	
Testicular tumours, teratoma	Vinblastine, Actinomycin-D, Methotrexate, Bleomycin, Platinum compounds	
Trophoblastic neoplasms	Methotrexate, Actinomycin-D, Vinblastine	
Renal cell carcinoma	Vinblastine	Hydroxyurea, Methyl-CCNU, DDMP*

Misc. sarcomas	Cyclophosphamide, Actinomycin-D, Vincristine, Adriamycin	Chlorambucil
Primary brain neoplasms	BCNU, CCNU, Methyl-CCNU, Vincristine, Methotrexate	Procarbazine
Oesophagus	Bleomycin	
Melanoma	DTIC	Actinomycin-D, CCNU, Dibromodulcitol
	(iii) *Paediatric solid tumours*	
Wilm's tumour	Actinomycin-D, Adriamycin, Vincristine	
Ewing's sarcoma	Cyclophosphamide, Actinomycin-D, Adriamycin, Vincristine	
Embryonal rhabdomyosarcoma	Cyclophosphamide, Adriamycin, Actinomycin-D, Vincristine	Methotrexate
Neuroblastoma	Cyclophosphamide, Adriamycin, Vincristine	Vinblastine, Prednisone
Retinoblastoma	Triethylmelamine, Cyclophosphamide, Dibromodulcitol, Vincristine	

* DDMP is not listed in the table of standard agents since it is still under investigation.

carcinoma of the head and neck, etc. For example, a woman who contracts breast cancer has an 80 per cent chance of dying eventually from that disease and this is the same risk as fifty years ago. Since many of these tumours recur, even though they have apparently been totally removed or cured by local radiation, it is obvious that local treatment is very often leaving behind a certain number of malignant cells, since by definition if all malignant cells were killed or removed by local treatment all the patients would be cured. The reason why these cells are left behind is that, as pointed out in the previous chapter, current techniques are unable to detect small cell numbers. Thus one of the reasons for the failure of purely local treatment to improve survival times lies in the fact that the true extent of the disease at presentation cannot be detected by present means. Many cancers therefore, such as those of the breast and the lung, should be regarded as being widely disseminated at presentation and it seems unlikely that survival times will be increased in these diseases unless a systemic component (i.e. anticancer drugs) is added to the initial treatment. The theoretical objections to the traditional role of cancer chemotherapy have been outlined in the previous chapter. It is common experience that chemotherapy does not cure advanced tumours with a few very rare exceptions. This is because anticancer drugs are much more effective when the total number of malignant cells present is small. Thus an optimum dose of a given drug which would kill 99.9 per cent of cancer cells would, if given to a metastasis consisting of 10^{10} cells, still leave 10 million viable cancer cells present. However, if it were given to a micrometastasis of a hundred cells it would suffice to destroy all the cells and cure the patient. Clinically, it is obvious that the number of tumour cells present is smallest immediately after the surgeon has removed the primary tumour or the radiotherapist has killed most of the cells present. These facts, together with the supporting experimental arguments from the previous chapter, overwhelmingly indicate that cancer chemotherapy should be regarded as part of the initial attack on tumours provided two conditions can be met: the proposed drug treatment must be known to have some effect in advanced disease; and treatment must be safe. This concept is outlined in Fig. 14.2.

Adjuvant Chemotherapy

The reasoning outlined above has inevitably led to the concept of adjuvant chemotherapy, i.e. the administration of anticancer drugs simultaneously with, or immediately after surgery or radiotherapy.

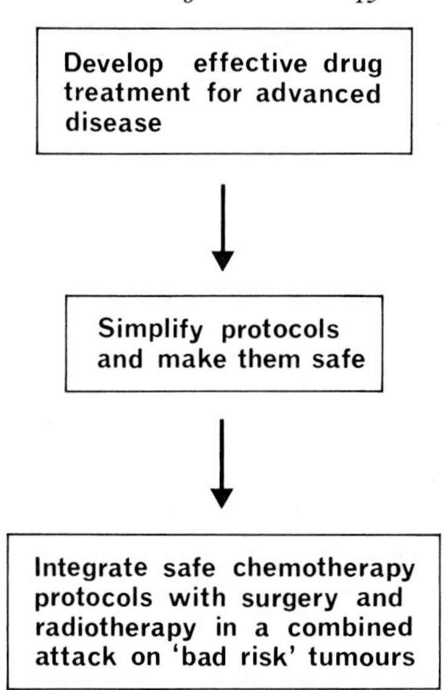

Figure 14.2 Logical approach to solid tumour therapy.

The object of adjuvant chemotherapy is nothing less than to increase the percentage of cures in patients at high risk for recurrence. Thus adjuvant chemotherapy should be given optimally, i.e. in maximum doses designed to kill the maximum number of malignant cells. In experimental systems compromising the dose by reducing it, say by 30 per cent, often makes the difference between curing the animal and not curing it at all. Thus we should not be surprised if some current clinical studies of adjuvant chemotherapy which are using suboptimal doses are not very effective when they are finally analysed.

Certain objections have been raised to the use of adjuvant chemotherapy and have to be considered. The principle among these is that anticancer drugs will almost inevitably produce very severe side effects. This belief is a complete delusion. Although certain side effects are inevitable, they can be very greatly reduced by the use of the kinetic principles referred to in the previous chapter. The clinical application of this approach is widely misunderstood; however, a scientific and logical basis now exists for the design of anticancer drug schedules which will make them safer than chemotherapy has usually been in the past. This approach has been applied successfully using combinations of cyclophosphamide, vincristine, 5-FU and methotrexate to miscellaneous solid tumours and breast cancer and with other drugs to testicular teratomas and head and neck cancer. In all cases the administration of drugs over a period of twenty-four hours or so proved to be far less toxic than when these agents are given over five or eight days as is the usual practice. Confirmation of the clinical success of this approach has now come from Germany and from other centres in the United Kingdom. The practice of administering antitumour drugs over periods of several days, usually five, should be reconsidered or at least some logical explanation should be advanced as to why this is done. The advantages of the twenty-four-hour approach to the patient are enormous. He spends only one or two nights every month in hospital; there is no severe bone marrow depression so that the requirement for intensive supportive therapy using platelets and antisepticaemia regimens is drastically reduced; and intensive treatment can be offered without ruining the quality of the patient's life.

This approach should be tested much more widely in view of its enormous potential advantage for large numbers of patients and specifically for its application to adjuvant chemotherapy. There is now much more confidence about the use of intensive adjuvant chemotherapy in patients who are at high risk for relapse but in whom no detectable disease is present, since these combinations can now be given safely. There is, in any event, in oncological circles something of a double standard about side effects. While some unpleasant side effects from drug treatment inevitably occur, it cannot be argued that radical mastectomy followed by removal of the ovaries and adrenals is always perfectly safe. Even radiation therapy is not totally free from adverse effects. Even so, adjuvant chemotherapy does involve giving drugs to patients who might actually be cured, though they are only a small percentage, and it is essential to emphasize that it is not yet known for certain whether the addition of drugs to primary treatment in solid tumours actually does improve the survival time. There is therefore no case whatever at present for the mass use of adjuvant chemotherapy in solid tumours. However, there is a major requirement for carefully conducted clinical trials carried out at specialized centres with proper controls which will definitively answer once and for all the question 'Does the addition of drugs to standard local treatment improve the survival time in these patients?' Several trials of this nature are currently underway and in our opinion it is the function of specialized centres to carry out such studies. For the practising clinician, however, the standard treatment should not be altered until the proposed new treatment has been definitely shown to be clinically superior in terms of survival.

Other objections to adjuvant chemotherapy, such as the possible development of second tumours, the long term effects of the immunosuppression which the drugs may produce, etc. may be valid but until the studies are actually carried out with long term follow-up it is impossible to balance these theoretical risks against any proven practical gain. It is often overlooked, however, that where adjuvant chemotherapy has been tested it has quite markedly improved the survival time in certain paediatric tumours, such as Wilms's tumour. The cure rate in this disease with surgery with or without radiotherapy, used to be between 17–23 per cent. When actinomycin-D was added to the protocol, given almost simultaneously, an 80 per cent cure rate was obtained in this previously highly incurable disease. In Ewing's tumour, which is highly sensitive to radiation therapy, the primary can be completely eradicated but 80–90 per cent of the patients will go on to die from metastases elsewhere even though they appeared to be completely free from disease other than the primary tumour at the time radiation was given. However, when the therapeutic dose of radiation therapy was given to the primary, and this was followed immediately by adjuvant chemotherapy with a combination of cyclophosphamide, vincristine and sometimes actinomycin-D and adriamycin, excellent results were achieved ranging between 55–70 per cent long term disease-free survival, many of which are presumed to be cures. Preliminary results in embryonal rhabdomyosarcoma and osteogenic sarcoma suggest that adjuvant chemotherapy significantly prolongs disease-free survival. Considering that the adjuvant chemotherapy in many of these studies is not given in the very best way and yet still achieves results there is all the more reason to suppose that optimally given adjuvant chemotherapy would be still more effective.

Prospects for the Future

Although several promising new agents, e.g. platinum compounds, are being developed, it is much more likely that improvements in the treatment of cancer will come from a more intelligent use of the drugs already available rather than by the sudden discovery of some spectacular new compound. Much therapeutically relevant knowledge which has been available for some time has unfortunately been neglected by many physicians.

It seems likely that an increasing number of patients with cancer will be receiving drug therapy in the next ten years and it is fortunate that a logical scientific basis exists now for the design of safe combination schedules. Combination drug treatment which is superior to single agent therapy now exists for cancers of the breast, stomach, testicular teratomas, colon, head and neck, 'oat cell' carcinoma of the lung and various bone cancers. The approach outlined in Fig. 14.2 may well lead to an improved cure rate in these tumours in the next ten years. Provided that surgeons, radiotherapists and chemotherapists co-operate in a combined initial attack on bad risk diseases using adjuvant chemotherapy given optimally, then it is quite possible that in the next decade we will see for the first time for over fifty years significant increases in the survival times and even the cure rates of certain common cancers.

References

Carter, S. K. and Soper, William T. (1974) The integration of chemotherapy into combined modality treatment of solid tumours, *Cancer Treatment Reviews* **1**, i.

Burchenal, Joseph H. (1976) Adjuvant therapy – theory, practice and potential, *Cancer*, **1**, 37, p. 46.

Price, L. A. (1973) The application of a kinetic model to clinical cancer chemotherapy, *Proceedings of the Third Eli Lilly Symposium*, W. H. Shedden (ed.).

Price, L. A. and Goldie, J. H. (1971) Multiple drug treatment of disseminated solid tumours, *Brit. Med. J.*, **4**, 336.

Price, L. A., Hill, Bridget T. and Calvert, A. H. *et al.* (1975) Kinetically based multiple drug treatment for advanced head and neck cancer, *Brit. Med. J.*, **3**, 156.

Chapter 15

Endocrine Therapy

T. J. POWLES
B.Sc., Ph.D., M.R.C.P.
Senior Lecturer in Medicine
Honorary Consultant Physician
Royal Marsden Hospital
Surrey

Introduction

The development of many types of malignant tumours, particularly those which arise in tissues normally under endocrine control, may be influenced by manipulation of the hormone status of the host. This has been used as a basis for treatment of patients with carcinoma of the breast, prostate, thyroid and uterus. Remissions in patients with renal carcinoma and malignant melanoma have also occurred with endocrine treatment. The treatment of each tumour will be discussed under separate headings. Treatment of lymphoma and leukaemia with corticosteroids is effective, although this is probably a cytoxic effect and not a hormone effect on abnormal haemopoietic cells and will be dealt with elsewhere.

Normal Endocrine Physiology

Hormones are substances, produced by various glands in the body, which circulate in the blood and affect other tissues. They are used to control various functions of the body. The hormones which are of most importance in cancer therapy are those produced in the hypothalamus, anterior pituitary, adrenals and gonads (Fig. 15.1). The hypothalamus produces small polypeptide (protein) hormones such as corticotrophin releasing factor (CRF), thyrotropin releasing factor (TRF), luteinizing hormone releasing hormone (LHRH) and others which pass through special blood vessels to the anterior pituitary to cause production and release of more complex protein hormones such as adrenalcortico-

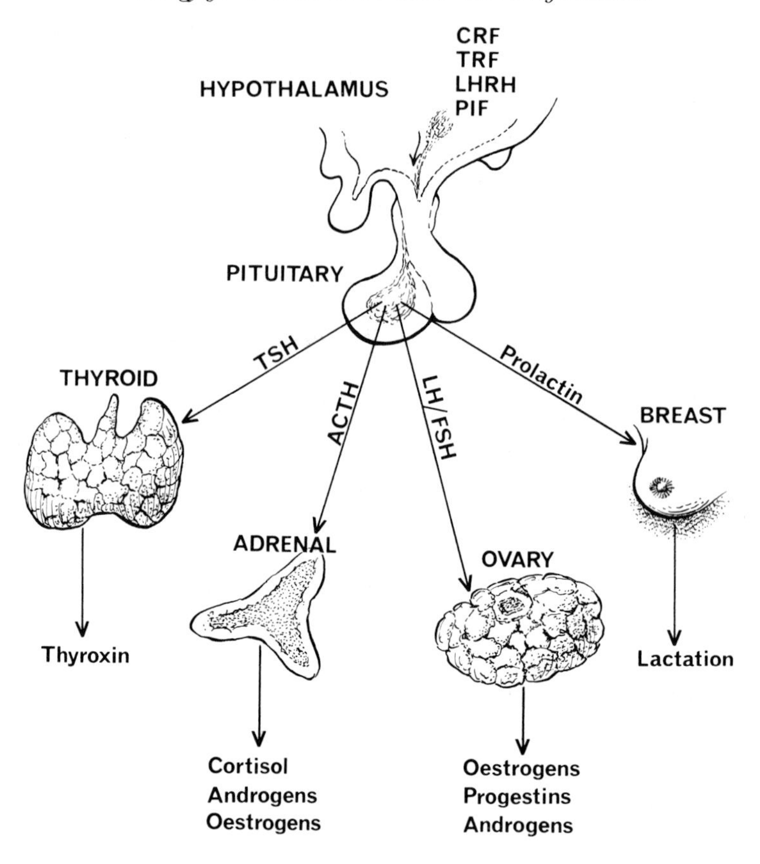

CRF	**Corticotrophin Releasing Factor**
TRF	**Thyrotropin Releasing Factor**
LHRF	**Luteinising Hormone Releasing Factor**
PIF	**Prolactin Inhibitory Factor**
TSH	**Thyroid Stimulating Hormone**
ACTH	**Adrenal Cortical Stimulating Hormone**
LH/FSH	**Luteinising Hormone/ Follicle Stimulating Hormone**

Figure 15.1 Hormones released by the hypothalamus and pituitary.

trophin hormone (ACTH), thyroid stimulating hormone (TSH) and luteinizing and follicle stimulating hormones (LH/FSH). These respectively stimulate the adrenal glands to produce and release corticosteroids, and the ovary and adrenal glands to release oestrogens, androgens and other sex hormones. These hormones not only stimulate development and function of various tissues such as the prostate and uterus, but also have more general effects on growth, development and metabolism of the whole body. Control of these processes depends on the ability of the steroid hormones to 'feedback' and 'switch off' production of hypothalamic and pituitary stimulating hormones when sufficient effect has occurred.

Hormone Receptors

Hormones generally act inside the nucleus of cells. Protein hormones, which are unable to cross the cell membranes, attach to specific membrane receptors on the outside of the cell to stimulate the required process within the cell. Each hormone has its own special receptor and therefore only cells with this receptor can be affected by the hormone. This allows a hormone to have a selective effect on certain tissues (those which possess the special receptor). For example, ACTH produced by the pituitary will only stimulate the adrenal gland because only these cells have the ACTH receptor.

Steroid hormones are able to pass through the cell membrane, but need to combine with specific receptors within the cytoplasm of the cells in order to pass into the nucleus and become effective. This allows for the selective effect of these hormones on various tissues of the body.

Steroid Hormones

All steroid hormones are structurally related to cholesterol (Fig. 15.2). The most important hormone produced by the adrenal gland is hydrocortisone (cortisol), which has an effect on the general metabolism of all tissues of the body and is essential to life. Cortisone is an inactive synthetic drug which is converted to the active hydrocortisone by the liver. Prednisolone, dexamethasone and betamethasone are similar drugs which act like hydrocortisone.

The adrenal cortex also produces small amounts of androgens and oestrogens which, in normal health, are not nearly as important as those produced by the gonads. The most important hormones produced by the testes are androgens. These hormones not only stimulate development and function of the male genitalia, and the development of the body hair (androgenic effect), but they also stimulate development of muscle and skeletal tissues (anabolic effect). Some androgen-like drugs such as naladrone (Durabolin) have anabolic but few androgenic effects. The testes also produce small amounts of oestrogens.

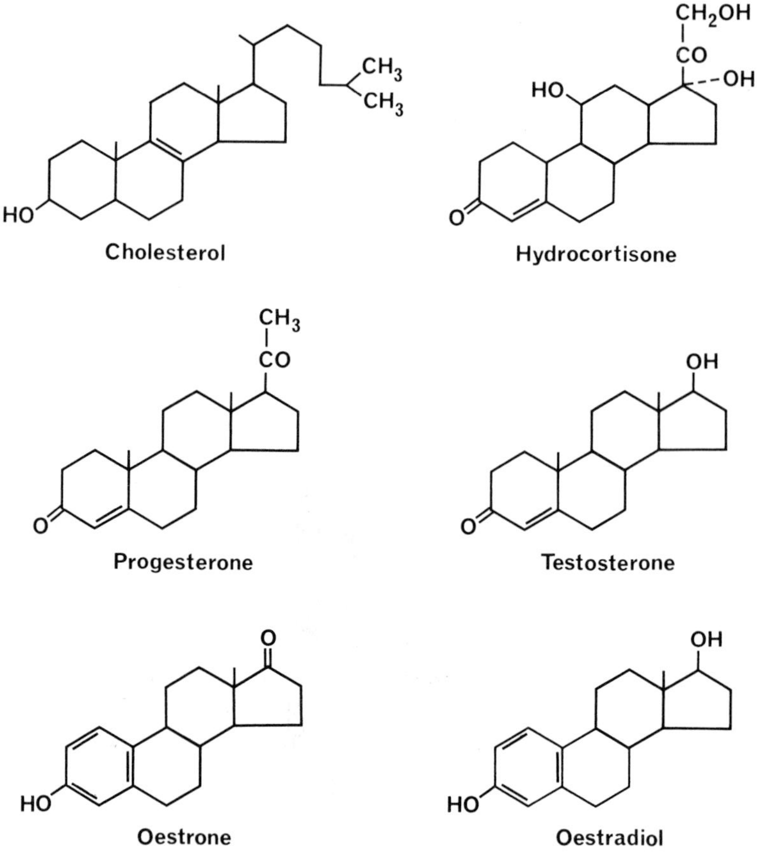

Figure 15.2 Chemical structure of various steroid hormones in relation to cholesterol.

The most important hormones produced by the ovaries are oestrogens and progesterone which are concerned with development of secondary sexual characteristics including breast development, menstruation, lactation and pregnancy. Drugs like stilboestrol, ethinyloestradiol and hexoestriol are oestrogenic, whereas norethisterone and medroxyprogesterone (Provera) are similar to progesterone.

Breast Cancer

Development of the female breast and lactation may be stimulated or influenced by many hormones, particularly oestrogens from the ovary and prolactin from the pituitary. Corticosteroids from the adrenal, progestins and androgens from the ovary, oestrogens and androgens from the adrenal glands, growth hormone from the pituitary, various hypothalamic polypeptide hormones and the thyroid hormones may also be involved. It is therefore not surprising that the development of some breast cancers may be influenced by administration of various hormones, or by ablation of various endocrine glands.

Patients with breast cancer may be divided into those whose disease is considered 'local' and who should have local treatment such as mastectomy, and those who have or subsequently develop metastases. Local treatment for these patients, although perhaps important for control of symptoms from the breast tumour, will not influence the metastases which will eventually kill them. For this it is necessary to use general treatment such as chemotherapy or hormonal therapy. Patients with metastatic disease are seldom, if ever, 'cured' by these treatments but the progress of the metastatic disease can be dramatically influenced in many cases, not only to prolong survival, but also to improve the quality of life.

About 30 per cent of the patients with metastatic breast cancer will respond to primary endocrine therapy. Patients who have slowly growing tumours (for example, those who have a long interval between development of a primary tumour and metastases) are more likely to respond than those with rapidly growing tumours (for example, those who present with metastatic disease).

Response also varies according to the site of metastases. For example, bone metastases are more likely to respond to endocrine ablation therapy than liver metastases. The age of the patient is another factor which will influence response. Young and old patients respond better than those in middle age, particularly at the time of the menopause.

Possible response to hormone therapy may be indicated by detection of oestrogen receptors in the tumour cells. This is done by a special test in the laboratory on samples of tumour from biopsy specimens. 90 per cent of patients whose tumours contain this receptor will respond to endocrine therapy compared to less than 10 per cent of those with no receptor.

Response to endocrine therapy is usually clinically obvious by four to six weeks, although response sometimes occurs very rapidly, particularly relief of pain from bone metastases after successful endocrine ablation. The mean duration of response to endocrine therapy is about twenty months which is considerably longer than for chemotherapy (approximately eight months), and the quality of life, particularly after successful ablation therapy, is usually excellent and much more satisfactory than after current chemotherapy.

Endocrine therapy therefore plays an important part in the management of patients with established metastatic disease. However, a major risk which occurs frequently with endocrine therapy, especially with hormone administration, is activation of tumour growth. If this occurs it indicates hormone sensitivity by the tumour cells and alternative endocrine therapy should be considered.

PRIMARY ENDOCRINE THERAPY

Ovarian Ablation

The level of circulating oestrogens seems to be the most important factor and this varies according to the menopausal status of the patient. In premenopausal patients the ovaries are actively producing large quantities of these hormones and therefore bilateral ovariectomy (oophorectomy) is the usual primary hormone treatment for patients with metastatic breast cancer. Alternatively, ovarian function, particularly hormone production, may be prevented by radiotherapy, the so called 'radiation menopause'. This is advantageous because it does not involve a surgical operation, but has the disadvantage of taking time to be effective, and denies the surgeon the opportunity of examining the abdomen for metastases.

Oestrogen Therapy

Postmenopausal patients, on the other hand, generally have low levels of circulating oestrogens and therefore administration of these hormones is considered the best treatment for patients with metastatic disease, except those with involvement of bones. Whether these hormones act directly on the tumour cells, or indirectly on the brain to influence production of hypothalamic or pituitary hormones, is not known except that ovariectomy or oestrogen therapy is seldom, if ever, effective in posthypophysectomy patients.

Ethinyloestradiol 0·3 mg/day or stilboestrol 15 mg/day are the most commonly used agents, but Premarin 7·5 mg/day, a mixture of 'conjugated' oestrogens extracted from pregnant mare's urine, is as effective, with fewer side effects. The most important side effects from oestrogen therapy are:

1. Nausea and vomiting.
2. Fluid retention. This may precipitate cardiac failure which may give rise to severe pulmonary oedema causing shortness of breath and even death.
3. Vaginal bleeding.

4. Hypercalcaemia. This serious complication frequently occurs in patients with bone metastases, particularly those treated with oestrogens. Curiously, although bone metastases are likely to respond to ovariectomy (40 per cent), adrenalectomy (40 per cent), pituitary ablation (50 per cent) or androgens (20 per cent), the response to oestrogen therapy is poor (less than 10 per cent) and therefore this risk of hypercalcaemia (approximately 20 per cent) mitigates against use of this treatment as primary therapy for patients with bone metastases. Hypercalcaemia is caused by an excessive release of calcium from the bones into the circulation, which gives rise to constipation, increased thirst and urine output and general malaise which may progress rapidly to coma and death. This metabolic complication should always be remembered in patients with breast cancer, particularly those on oestrogen therapy.

SECONDARY ENDOCRINE THERAPY

Patients who relapse after a response to primary hormone therapy are more likely to respond to subsequent endocrine manoeuvres. For example, a patient who has previously responded to bilateral ovariectomy is four times more likely to respond to bilateral adrenalectomy than someone who has not.

There is often a 'withdrawal' response after cessation of hormone treatment, particularly after a response and then relapse on oestrogen therapy. This is usually not as good or as long as the initial response, but it is unwise to start alternative hormone treatment until at least six weeks after stopping previous hormones unless there is obvious clinical deterioration.

Adrenalectomy

Removal of the adrenal glands may induce remission of metastases particularly in bone. It is most effective for premenopausal patients who have previously responded to ovariectomy (approximately 50 per cent) and postmenopausal patients (approximately 40 per cent). Perimenopausal patients respond poorly (< 10 per cent) as do patients who have been on corticosteroid therapy for more than three months. About 60 per cent of patients have significant and rapid relief of pain from bone metastases and although many will not subsequently have an objective remission of tumour, this palliative subjective effect will usually justify the procedure.

The adrenal glands may be removed through an anterior abdominal incision or from behind through two loin incisions.

Production of corticosteroids and aldosterone by the adrenal glands is essential to life. All patients therefore require replacement therapy usually with cortisone acetate 50–75 mg per day or prednisolone 7·5–10 mg per day, and fludrocortisone 0·1 mg on alternate days *for life*. In times of physical stress (infections, operations, etc.), higher doses of cortisone are required.

Instead of surgical removal of the adrenals, attempts have been made to interfere with adrenal steroid production by drug therapy ('medical' adenalectomy) using cortisone which inhibits ACTH release from the pituitary, or with aminoglutethimide, an agent which blocks synthesis of steroids by the adrenals. Response to cortisone is low (approximately 10 per cent) and even this may in part be a direct cytotoxic effect of the steroid on the tumour cells. Aminoglutethimide is more promising as an 'antiadrenal' agent with the added advantage over surgical adrenalectomy that its effect is reversible.

Pituitary Ablation

Ablation of the pituitary gland is an *alternative* procedure to adrenalectomy, usually reserved for premenopausal patients who have previously responded to ovariectomy, or postmenopausal patients who have previously responded to oestrogen or androgen therapy. It may be used for patients with visceral or lymph node metastases, but is particularly useful for those patients with bone metastases or local recurrent disease.

Choice of adrenalectomy or hypophysectomy depends on several factors. Adrenalectomy is contraindicated in patients who have had prolonged corticosteroid therapy or gross liver or peritoneal involvement. Hypophysectomy is contraindicated in patients with bone metastases in the base of the skull. Adrenalectomy is undertaken by most 'general' surgeons but hypophysectomy is only available in specialized units.

The hypophysis may be removed by a neurosurgeon through a frontal craniotomy or by an ENT surgeon through the sphenoidal sinus. Alternatively the gland may be destroyed by implanting radioactive yttrium (^{90}Y) into the gland or by freezing the gland with a 'cryoscope'. All of these procedures have been used with variable success.

After successful pituitary ablation, the patient must have 'replacement' therapy with cortisone acetate 50–75 mg per day or prednisolone 7·5–10 mg per day. Thyroxine 0·2–0·3 mg per day is also required because pituitary control of thyroid function has ceased. Fludrocortisone is not required because although the adrenal glands fail to produce hydrocortisone after pituitary ablation, aldosterone, which is not under pituitary control, is still produced. In many respects 'replacement' therapy is easier in posthypophysectomy rather than postadrenalectomy patients.

Subsequent hormone therapy with oestrogens (and perhaps with androgens) is unlikely to be successful in postadrenalectomy or post-hypophysectomy patients.

Androgen Therapy

This is principally reserved for postmenopausal patients, often as primary therapy for bone metastases. In premenopausal patients it is usually used after relapse of successful ovariectomy induced remission of bone metastases.

Therapy usually consists of an intramuscular injection of 100 mg of nandrolone phenyl propionate (Durabolin) once per week. Masculinization especially facial hirsutism, plethora, acne and voice change are problems in approximately 40 per cent of patients, but hypercalcaemia is relatively uncommon. Testosterone propionate and methyl testosterone have also been extensively used but masculinization and possibly hypercalcaemia occur more frequently with no increase in response. Fluoxymesterone 20–30 mg daily by mouth is an alternative androgen with relatively little virilizing properties.

Androgen therapy is also useful for treatment of bone marrow metastases associated with thrombocytopenia and leucopenia. The response may depend not only on an antitumour effect, but also the anabolic stimulus to marrow function. For this reason, it has frequently been used in combination with marrow-depressing chemotherapy.

Progestin Therapy

Norethisterone acetate 40–60 mg per day and medroxyprogesterone acetate 300–400 mg per day are both progesterone-like agents used in treatment of metastatic breast cancer. Generally the response to these hormones is poor except for local recurrent disease in the chest wall and soft tissue nodules where responses of up to 30 per cent have been reported.

'Anti'-oestrogens

Tamoxiphen (Nolvadex) 20–40 gm per day is an oestrogen-like agent which has very little oestrogenic activity but can bind to the 'oestrogen receptor' in tumour cells and prevent more active oestrogens from binding. It is not clear if this prevention of oestrogen binding is the mechanism of action – it seems more likely that this agent is acting, like other oestrogens, as a cytotoxic agent, certainly in the post-menopausal patient. It is therefore used for the most part in older patients, particularly those with soft tissue and visceral disease. It causes less fluid retention, nausea and hypercalcaemia than ethinyloestradiol, though possibly no less than Premarin. Photosensitivity of the skin can be a problem.

Corticosteriod Therapy

These agents can cause objective regression of tumour in about 15 per cent of patients with metastases. It is not known if this is a direct cytotoxic effect on the tumour cells or an indirect endocrine effect perhaps by inhibition of pituitary or hypothalamic hormone secretion.

Symptom of pain in bone metastases, shortness of breath from lung metastases, itching from skin metastases and raised intracranial pressure from cerebral metastases, may be rapidly relieved with corticosteroids in approximately 80 per cent of patients with these problems. It is supposed that this results from the anti-inflammatory properties of these agents, and although usually of short duration, it is of great therapeutic benefit in 'buying time' before the effect of alternative therapy can occur (with chemotherapy for example).

These agents are also of particular use in the management of terminal disease where a combination of euphoria with relief of unpleasant symptoms is welcome to patient and physician alike.

Cortisone acetate 40–200 mg per day by mouth, hydrocortisone 50–200 mg per day by mouth or injection, and prednisolone 5–20 mg per day by mouth may be used. The higher doses will cause symptoms of Cushing's syndrome, particularly truncal and facial obesity, plethora, hypertension and possible hirsutism and acne. Dexamethasone 2–4 mg per day, the most powerful anti-inflammatory corticosteroid available, is used for CNS metastases causing raised intracranial pressure or cord compression, particularly to cover the period of radiotherapy.

Hypercalcaemia is caused by metastatic destruction of bone and release of calcium into the circulation. This may be relieved in most patients by corticosteroid therapy and adequate rehydration.

MANAGEMENT OF PERIMENOPAUSAL PATIENTS

Patients within five years of the menopause respond poorly and with less certainty to endocrine therapy than older or younger patients. This is in part related to their uncertain endocrine state, but even when levels of oestrogens and gonadotrophins are measured the responses are still poor. Ovariectomy, sometimes with adrenalectomy, is the usual primary endocrine treatment, especially for patients within one year of the menopause.

INTEGRATION OF CHEMOTHERAPY AND HORMONE THERAPY IN THE OVERALL MANAGEMENT

As discussed above, the duration of remission for chemotherapy is generally shorter than for hormone therapy, and the quality of life even for complete remission is usually better with endocrine therapy, especially ablative treatment, than with chemotherapy. For this reason most physicians trained in endocrine therapy generally prefer it as primary treatment. On the other hand, chemotherapists trained as haematological oncologists tend to confine their management to the use of cytotoxic agents. A balanced approach is probably of more benefit to the patient (Fig. 15.3).

The primary treatment for young and old patients with bone metastases and relatively slowly growing tumours should be endocrine therapy, whereas perimenopausal patients with rapidly developing visceral or soft tissue disease should probably be treated initially with chemotherapy. Management of patients between these two extremes must be based on a balance of the various factors outlined above.

At present it is unwise to use chemotherapy and hormone therapy at the same time because the possible interactions of these two types of treatment is not understood.

Male Breast Cancer

Endocrine therapy is also effective in men with metastatic breast cancer. Approximately 70 per cent of patients will respond to orchidectomy for an average duration of approximately 30 months. Patients with bone metastases and those with a long interval between primary treatment and development of metastases respond best.

Oestrogen and progesterone therapy is relatively ineffective and androgens frequently exacerbate pain from bone metastases. Corticosteroid therapy on the other hand will often relieve the pain of bone metastases.

Adrenalectomy but not hypophysectomy is often used as second line treatment in patients who have previously responded to orchidectomy. The efficiency of aminoglutethimide has not yet been established.

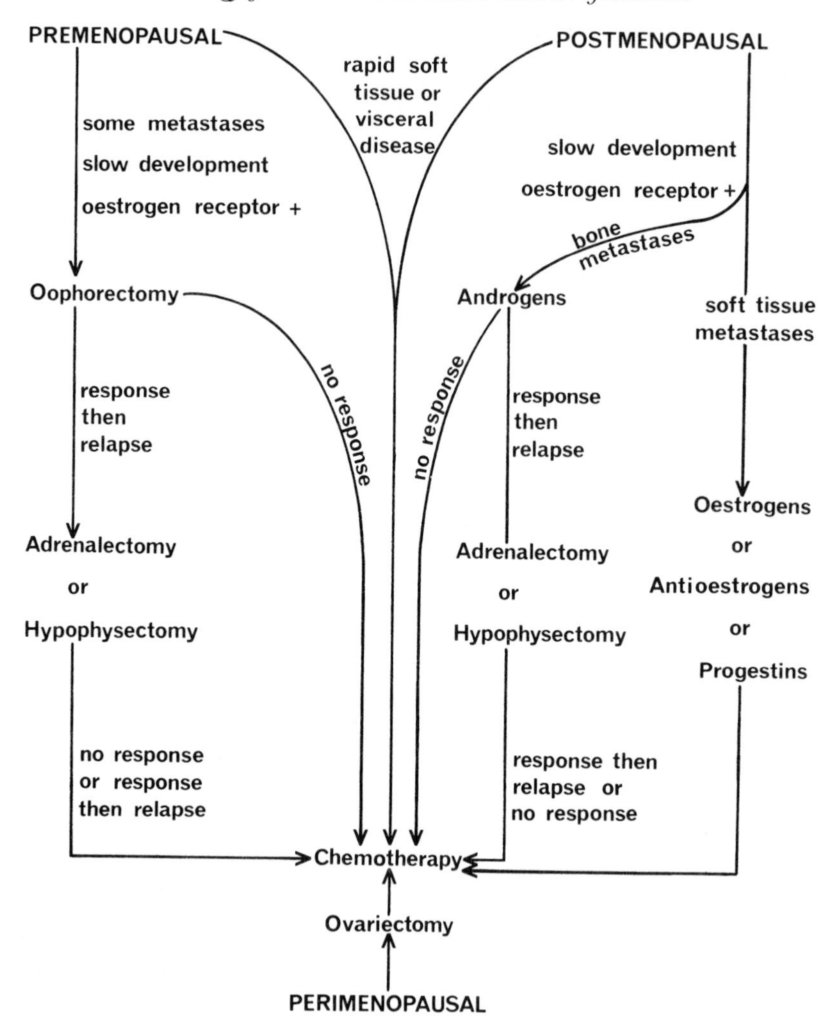

Figure 15.3 A plan for primary and subsequent therapy for patients with breast cancer.

Prostatic Cancer

The prostate gland fails to develop in the absence of testosterone or the presence of oestrogens. It is therefore not surprising that development of most prostate tumours may be influenced by changes in circulating levels of these hormones.

Endocrine treatment is usually reserved for patients with metastatic or locally recurrent disease and is most useful for control of urinary symptoms and pain from bone metastases. No patients are 'cured' by endocrine therapy but remissions may be maintained for many years.

Generally, evaluation of response rates is difficult, because the disease tends to be slowly progressive and occurs in older patients. Therefore most patients die of other causes even if untreated for prostatic cancer.

PRIMARY ENDOCRINE THERAPY

Orchidectomy

Response to removal of the testes occurs in approximately 80 per cent of patients. Relief of pain or urinary symptoms may occur very rapidly and the duration of response may last for many years. It is most useful for management of younger patients, because their relatively more aggressive disease often responds well with good and prolonged symptomatic relief. Unfortunately these are the patients who are the most hesitant to accept emasculation. Technically the operation is easy and long-term side effects apart from impotence are few.

Oestrogen Therapy

These hormones have a similar effect to orchidectomy. They may act by inhibiting gonadotrophin release from the pituitary and thereby reducing androgen secretion from the testes. Alternatively, they may antagonize the effects of androgens on the tumour cells or they may be directly cytotoxic.

Response rates are high (approximately 80 per cent), especially in older patients. Side effects from oestrogen therapy can be troublesome and unpleasant. Nausea and vomiting occur in a large number of patients who are given stilboestrol and therefore ethinyloestradiol 0·3 mg/day or Premarin 5–15 mg/day are preferable.

Impotence usually occurs and gynaecomastia may become troublesome and require mastectomy. Feminization may cause considerable psychological problems and embarrassment.

Hepatotoxicity occurs occasionally but is not usually a problem with oral administration of ethinyl oestradiol or Premarin. Oedema and congestive cardiac failure can be a problem especially in the old and frail. The most serious side effect of oestrogen therapy is the stimulation of blood clotting and increased risk of cerebral and myocardial infarction. It has been claimed that the increased risk of death from cardiovascular causes may more than outweigh any benefit from the treatment.

SECONDARY ENDOCRINE THERAPY

These measures are used only after relapse of successful remission from primary endocrine therapy.

Androgens and Progestins

Generally speaking, use of these agents is dangerous in this disease. They have, however, been used in a limited manner in conjunction with high doses of radioactive phosphorus in an attempt to stimulate uptake of the isotope in bone metastases. They have also been used before oestrogen therapy in patients who have become resistant to this treatment. Occasional responses to progestins have also been reported.

Adrenalectomy

The results are poor by comparison with breast cancer and the mortality and morbidity are higher because of the age of the relapsing patients. Pain relief, although infrequent, can sometimes be dramatic, not necessarily associated with objective regression of disease. Post-adrenalectomy patients must have replacement therapy with cortisone and fludrocortisone for life.

Pituitary Ablation

Hypophysectomy or pituitary destruction by implantation of radioactive yttrium (^{90}Y) into the gland is associated with good responses. In patients who have previously responded to oestrogen therapy and then relapsed, approximately 60 per cent will have relief of bone pain from bone metastases for up to three years, although this is not usually associated with objective regression of metastases. Patients must have cortisone and thyroxine replacement therapy for life.

Corticosteroid Therapy

Remissions, particularly relief of urinary symptoms and bone pain, occur in about 30 per cent of patients not usually associated with tumour regression. Although this is not as good as other endocrine manoeuvres it is well tolerated in the old and sick and frequently associated with euphoria. Prednisolone 20–30 mg/day is usually used and when relapse after symptomatic response occurs, then reduction of the steroid dosage associated with increase of other analgesics and euphorients, is usually associated with a quick and painless demise.

CONCLUSIONS

Endocrine therapy has a considerable place in the management of patients with metastatic prostatic cancer. Symptomatic relief occurs in a large proportion of patients which is of particular use because other therapy such as cytotoxic therapy is of little use in these patients.

Endometrial Cancer

Clinical, histological and biological evidence indicates that endometrial hyperplasia and cancer arise as a result of long continued oestrogen stimulation in the absence of progesterone. It was, therefore, not surprising that administration of progestins could inhibit metastatic endometrial carcinoma. Approximately 30 per cent of patients respond to this treatment, especially those with lung or bone metastases but not pelvic deposits. Those with slowly growing or histologically well-differentiated tumours respond best. Maximum response may not be achieved for several months and may last for many years. 17α-hydroxyprogesterone derivatives, particularly medroxyprogesterone acetate have been used (400–1,000 mg/month) but it seems that a 'loading' dose of approximately 5 g in the first three weeks is necessary to induce remission.

There are some indications that progestin therapy may be useful as an adjuvant to local therapy for the prevention of metastases in patients with primary disease.

Renal Cancer

Approximately 15 per cent of patients with metastatic renal cancer respond to treatment with medroxyprogesterone. Although responses have generally not been good or prolonged it is worth trying because of the very poor response to cytotoxic therapy. Men respond two or three times more frequently than women. There is inadequate evidence of response to other hormone manoeuvres.

Thyroid Cancer

Papillary carcinoma of the thyroid is usually under the control of TSH released from the pituitary. This TSH secretion can be inhibited by administration of the thyroid hormone thyroxine (or dessicated thyroid) and it is therefore not surprising that this hormone will cause remissions in more than 50 per cent of patients with this tumour. Female patients between puberty and forty years of age respond best, especially those with irradiation-induced tumours.

Generally, if the primary tumour cannot be removed easily by surgery, or if metastases are present, it is better to start treatment with thyroxine (0·3 mg/day) rather than with radioactive iodine which may change the tumour into a non-responding anaplastic carcinoma. Response may take several months to achieve and arrest of growth rather than regression of tumour may occur. Remission lasts indefinitely once achieved as long as thyroxine treatment is continued.

Other Tumours

Although malignant melanoma may regress during pregnancy and changes in growth rate have been noted at puberty, the menopause and periodically with menstruation, response to hormone manipulation is very rare. Regressions have been reported with oestrogen, progestin and major ablation therapy, but are so unusual that they play no part in the management of this disease.

Leukaemias and lymphomas may respond to corticosteroid therapy, but this is almost certainly a direct cytotoxic effect and not a hormone effect.

Conclusions

Manipulation of hormone status by hormone administration or endocrine gland ablation can give rise to useful remissions in patients with metastases from breast, prostatic, thyroid and endometrial cancer. The remissions are usually longer, better and the morbidity less than for alternative therapy and therefore play an important part in the management of patients with these diseases.

Chapter 16

Immunotherapy

R. L. POWLES
M.D., B.Sc., M.R.C.P.
Senior Lecturer in Medicine
Honorary Consultant Physician
Royal Marsden Hospital
Surrey

The enthusiasm for giving 'immunotherapy' to patients with cancer is not so much proportional to claims of therapeutic success in this field, but more a result of pessimism for other methods of treatment. This 'demand' for different (and thus possibly successful) methods of treatment for cancer is not new and attempts at a variety of procedures including immunotherapy have been tried for almost a century. The somewhat disappointing results currently being obtained with cytotoxic chemotherapy of solid tumours have once again led to increased interest in the use of the immune system for attacking cancer in man. However, it is a pity that the motivation for testing such new methods is charged with unfair expectations because true evaluation becomes impossible.

The purpose of this chapter is to illustrate the small but definite progress that has been made in understanding the host response against cancer and how this has been harnessed for preliminary studies of applied methods of treatment for these patients. Two independent approaches to this problem have been adopted, animal work and human studies, and although these two disciplines are largely interrelated it is convenient for the purpose of this chapter to discuss them sequentially.

Animal Work

During the first four decades of this century there were several hundred reports of experiments which showed that animals could be made to resist developing cancer following the injection of live cancer cells (see Hauschka, 1952; Southam, 1960). One of the earliest of these studies was by Clowes and Baeslack, who, in 1905, observed that mice could be implanted with cancer (from other mice) and occasionally the tumour would stop growing and then be spontaneously rejected. If these mice were then reinoculated with the same cancer it failed to grow and so it could be assumed that these animals had become resistant to that particular form of cancer. Despite the many experiments during this early period of tumour immunology it was not until 1935 that any clear principles could be determined about the mechanism by which these animals resisted cancer. Besredka and Gross (1935) discovered that it was not necessary for an animal to spontaneously reject a tumour before it became immune; an animal could be immunized with a finely ground preparation from the tumour and then, when injected with live cancer cells, tumours did not develop, i.e. the animal was immune to cancer. Unfortunately, these early studies all had one very serious experimental defect which invalidated them, namely that if tissue (not cancer) is taken from one animal and implanted into another animal, then rejection of that tissue occurs just like an unrelated kidney graft in man. All these early experiments were in situations where the cancer cells had been taken from an unrelated animal and injected into the experimental animal and so rejection, if it occurred, was simply due to transplantation antigens and this applied equally to both normal and neoplastic tissue. These experiments, therefore, had little or no relevance to human disease, where transplantation antigens on the surface of cancer cells are not recognized by the patient because the cancer cells are of his own tissue.

Interest in the field was revived when this transplantation problem was overcome in the early 1940s by Leonell Strong who developed inbred mice colonies at Yale University, USA. A strain of mice was created which had been bred by continuous brother to sister mating for more than twenty years with deliberate selection of only those with similar characteristics, and thus all these mice acquired a remarkable genetic uniformity that may for practical purposes be considered like identical twins. This meant that normal tissues could be transplanted from mouse to mouse without rejection.

Thereafter followed a series of experiments showing that animals immunized before being given their tumour could be protected against subsequent growth (and death), and then in 1943 the more important experiments were designed to show that animals with established tumours could be protected against spread by immunization, i.e. treatment rather than prophylaxis, a situation much more relevant to man. The principal investigator of immunotherapy as treatment of cancer in mice was Ludwig Gross who used an inbred mouse strain to study transplantation into these animals of a chemically induced sarcoma originally produced in an animal of the same line. This tumour (and subsequent animal tumours) could be preserved in the laboratory simply by transplanting from one animal just before it died into a new animal and theoretically the tumour could be kept alive for ever – immortal death; and experiments involving this tumour became easy and repeatable. These mice always died of disseminated cancer after being implanted with this tumour.

If subsequent rejection occurred after suitable immunization, then the possibility that the immunity to the tumour was caused by 'transplantation antigen' differences between the tumour cells and those of the host were eliminated because all tissues came originally from the same strain of mouse. Gross found that by inoculating tumour-bearing animals with a suspension of this sarcoma, 20 per cent of the animals showed tumour regression. It could thus be inferred that these mice had been vaccinated in such a way that they had developed immunity against their own tumour (as we would like to achieve in man) and subsequently rejected the cancer.

Why an animal should recognize its own cancer as foreign became apparent by the late 1950s when carefully conducted animal experiments showed that tumour cells which had been induced by chemical carcinogens, by viruses or by physical carcinogens had on their surface substances which were not present on normal cells. Like a bacterial infection, the host recognizes these substances as foreign and reacts against them by producing an immune reaction to reject them, i.e. antibodies and cell-mediated immunity. (These are the two independent but often complementary systems whereby the immunity of the body attacks foreign invaders, including cancer cells, both of which need to be instructed what to do by either prior experience with the antigen or by immunization. Antibodies are proteins in the blood and the cell-mediated immunity consists of clones of cells, lymphocytes and macrophages, which can migrate to and kill the invader.) Subsequent attempts in carefully controlled animal systems to treat by immunological methods tumours known to have these foreign substances on their surface were disappointing and in an authoritative review in 1964 Old and Boyce wrote 'Despite the evident antigenicity of a variety of experimental tumours, it is a fact that no immunological manoeuvre is known that will cause the rejection of an established malignant tumour, primary or transplanted, regardless of its size.' However, in the same year, Haddow and Alexander (at the Chester Beatty Cancer Institute) were able to show that primary sarcomas in rats which had been induced by implanting a pellet of the carcinogic chemical 3,4-benzpyrene could be controlled by two types of immunological treatment after the bulk of the tumour had been removed either by surgery or by radiotherapy (which in itself was insufficient to cure these animals). The residual tumour cells could be held in check either by active immunization with irradiated tumour cells derived from the tumour to be treated or by injection of lymphocytes obtained from other animals that had been immunized previously with a piece of the same tumour. It was quickly shown that these immunotherapy procedures were also effective against leukaemias in mice.

At first it is difficult to see why this immunization works when the tumour itself does not cause its own rejection. The explanation is that by the time the growing tumour has made the host immune it is such a size that control and rejection is impossible. A similar situation occurs with tuberculosis, an organism which man recognizes as foreign and to which he can raise a strong immunity yet most untreated patients ultimately succumb to the disease. Immunization, even after contact, can boost the immune system much more quickly than the infection itself and the disease is eradicated. However, the immunization material must have on its surface the same 'foreign' molecules as the disease and the injections must be in sites, such as the skin, so that the lymph nodes and immune system are stimulated.

The unresolved question was whether such immunological manoeuvres had a role in the treatment of human malignant disease. This concept was not a new idea, anecdotal attempts to influence the course of cancer in man by a variety of immunological methods have been reported for more than eighty years (see Currie, 1972), and the first recorded attempt to treat acute leukaemia was by Tyzzer as long ago as 1916.

Methods of Immunotherapy in Man

There are several distinct ways in which the immune system may be used to modify the response of man against malignant disease. These methods have been grouped together as follows: Active immunotherapy occurs if the host's own immune system is stimulated to attack the tumour; adoptive immunotherapy signifies the transplantation into the tumour-bearing host of immunocompetent (normal) cells directed against the tumour, and passive immunotherapy is the injection of antisera or other serum factors. These methods are specific rather than non-specific if tumour antigen has been involved in obtaining the effect.

NON-SPECIFIC PASSIVE IMMUNOTHERAPY

This least important method of immunotherapy consists of giving non-specific normal serum factors to patients who are suspected of having low levels. In cancer patients limited trials (see Southam, 1961) have shown no striking or sustained effect on blood levels or tumour growth.

SPECIFIC PASSIVE IMMUNOTHERAPY

This method of immunotherapy, more commonly known as serotherapy, has a very long history. In general, animals are immunized with human tumour material and the antiserum so produced is then used for treatment. An early example of such an experiment was in 1895 by Hericourt and Richet, who treated fifty patients, many of whom had both objective and subjective improvement. These workers further went on to state that normal animal serum did not have any beneficial effect and thus concluded that they were using a specific form of immunotherapy. Many similar attempts followed all with poor or uninterpretable results (see Currie, 1972) and it was not until 1960 that alternative methods of serotherapy were tried. The first of these by Sumner and Foraker (1960) involved transfusing blood from patients with malignant melanoma, whose tumours had regressed, into patients wide widespread melanoma. One of the two patients studied had a long-lasting regression.

More recently antisera to normal transplantation antigens (i.e. HLA antisera) have been used to treat patients with leukaemia. The antisera were produced by immunizing normal volunteers with normal lymphocytes and the resulting HLA antibodies were injected into three patients with chronic lymphatic leukaemia and it was noted there was resulting lymphopenia and a reduction in the lymph node size. Sera from unimmunized donors did not cause the same effect.

NON-SPECIFIC ADOPTIVE IMMUNOTHERAPY

This form of 'treatment' is based upon the administration of lymphocytes from unrelated donors into patients with cancer. The idea is that the lymphocytes grow as a foreign graft and attack and reject all the host tissues (including the cancer) in the so-called graft versus host reaction. It would be an understatement to say that such methods of treatment will not be without side effects. Woodruff and Nolan attempted this procedure in man in 1963, and they noticed both subjective and objective improvement in eight patients with advanced malignant disease. However, the evidence that either a graft versus host reaction existed or that regression was directly the result of the transferred lymphocytes is far from convincing, as all these patients were also receiving other forms of treatment. Similarly, in 1966 Schwarzenberg and his colleagues treating patients with leukaemia with white cell transfusions from patients with chronic granulocytic leukaemia (which contain normal lymphocytes) noticed that the patients with acute leukaemia who had modified graft versus host disease also attained some form of remission from their disease. This observation was not supported by the leukaemia patients treated by the Seattle group who developed graft versus host reactions following bone marrow transplantation.

SPECIFIC ADOPTIVE IMMUNOTHERAPY

In this form of treatment the principle is to transfer lymphocytes from donors who have been immunized against a tumour into the person bearing the tumour. Although the injection of cancer cells into normal people is not possible, Nadler and Moore in 1969 designed a study that was ethically feasible, by cross-immunizing a pair of patients with tumour and subsequent transfusion of their stimulated peripheral blood lymphocytes into each other. Most of the patients had malignant melanomas and only occasional regressions were recorded. Andrews in 1967 used thoracic duct lymphocytes and in spite of being able to use enormous numbers of cells no therapeutic effect was detected. Recently, Bagshawe (1974) has suggested a novel approach of using patients with chorionepitheliomata as a model system for detecting an effect of adoptive immunotherapy. This disease circumvents the ethical problem of immunizing normal volunteers with tumour cells because chorionepithelioma cells are of foetal origin and carry normal transplantation antigens (from the 'father' of the tumour) on their surface and these antigens are thus represented on the normal tissues of the 'father'. By using a cross-over arrangement with the 'husbands' of two patients, each immunized with the other's normal tissues, it is possible to design a very elegant method of adoptive immunotherapy that is ethically justifiable. Hyperimmune lymphocytes are produced in each husband which can then be injected directly into the appropriate (opposite) tumour-bearing wife. The very sensitive urinary gonadotrophin marker of tumour activity in these patients showed transient but definite tumour regression using these methods.

NON-SPECIFIC ACTIVE IMMUNOTHERAPY

The principle of this method is to immunize patients with material which boosts the immune system generally and provides a non-specific increase in immunity. The rationale for this was based on the findings in animals first made by Halpern (1959) and then widely confirmed that inoculation with BCG (as used for preventing tubercle) increases the capacity of these animals to resist all infections. He noticed these animals also resisted inoculation with cancer cells. The effect was weaker and occurred less frequently when the BCG was given to animals already bearing tumours, i.e. therapy as opposed to prophylaxis, and was interpreted as meaning that the BCG could only overcome a few malignant cells. Many tumours did not respond at all to such treatments. When BCG is introduced directly into an established tumour, either by injection or by lymphatic drainage, it causes an intense inflammatory reaction, during the course of which some tumours regress. It is not clear whether this regression of local tumours is in the strict sense immunotherapy, since the reaction is probably not directed against the tumour-specific antigens.

ACTIVE SPECIFIC IMMUNOTHERAPY

In man (as in experimental animals) it has been shown that the injection of killed tumour cells subcutaneously at multiple sites into patients with cancer heightens their reaction to the tumour antigens and the consequent attack on the tumour is termed active specific immunotherapy. This increased antitumour reaction of the host occurs because the injected cells stimulate distant lymph nodes and bring them into play to produce antibodies and cell-mediated responses. Alexander *et al.* (1969) have shown that the nodes draining the tumour even when they are not involved are partially paralysed and the magnitude of the host response without immunization is, therefore, very limited. This adds to the other reason stated before as to why the patients do not overcome unaided the growth of the tumour.

Yet another reason for tumour growth in spite of the presence of tumour antigens is that the immune reaction is 'blocked' by material circulating in the blood which has been released by the tumour itself – soluble tumour antigen – and this neutralizes the circulating antibody directed against the tumour. One of the most effective ways of removing soluble tumour antigen from the circulation is by combining it with antibody whereupon it is removed in the form of antibody–antigen complexes. In our laboratory it has been shown in a number of systems, both in man and in experimental animals, that immunization with killed tumour cells leads to disappearance of antigen from the circulation due to an increased antibody production which results from the stimulation of distant lymphoid tissues.

In man the use of active specific immunotherapy for malignant disease has a long history. For instance in 1902 von Leyden and Blumenthal described tumour cell immunotherapy given to patients with advanced metastatic disease, and reported disappointing results. Various attempts at immunotherapy since 1902 (see Currie, 1972) have produced only anecdotal results and it is now obvious that to show immunotherapy procedures are clinically useful requires carefully conducted clinical trials.

Methods for Clinical Trials

At this point a word must be said about how a physician can be sure that a treatment programme given to a patient has been responsible for a clinical effect seen. At first sight it seems obvious that if a patient is given something and he gets better then the treatment must have been responsible, but unfortunately (for the investigating physician, not for the individual patient) cancer behaves in odd ways and sometimes patients temporarily rally and get better without any treatment being given and all patients behave in an individual and variable way. This means that to truly assess the effectiveness of a new treatment programme the test material (say immunotherapy) must be given not to one, but many patients and their overall results compared with a group of patients who are studied at the same time, but given no treatment. So as not to bias the results by deliberately putting the best patients into the test group, all the patients in the study must be allotted to either the treatment or no-treatment groups in a random fashion, i.e. by tossing a coin. Such studies are called controlled trials. Alas, even now, very few workers conduct controlled clinical trials in cancer.

Acute Lymphoblastic Leukaemia (ALL)

The modern era of immunotherapy for treating cancer started in Paris in the mid-1960s when Mathé decided to attempt to control the disease process of patients with acute leukaemia using such procedures. He chose leukaemia as a suitable disease to study because the animal results showed clearly that immunotherapy, if it had any effect at all, was only of a very weak nature, and the amount of active disease it could overcome was minimal. Thus leukaemia was an obvious choice to study because cancer drugs could be given to these patients so that they had no detectable leukaemia remaining (so-called remission) although we know a few hidden leukaemic cells were still present because left without further treatment the florid disease inevitably returned. Mathé chose acute lymphoblastic leukaemia (ALL) as the disease to study because many children were available in his practice, but, as will be explained below, this form of leukaemia may not be the optimum one to produce therapeutic results.

In his first study (Mathé, 1969) he selected a group of thirty children with ALL, all of whom had been in remission for at least two years (Fig. 16.1). For some all treatment stopped and the rest were given weekly Pasteur BCG, killed leukaemia cells, or both BCG and cells. All ten of the untreated patients relapsed within 130 days, whereas half of the twenty immunotherapy patients remained in remission for greater than 295 days, some of them for many years. The numbers were too small to decide which of the immunological regimes was best.

Several attempts have been made to confirm the value of BCG alone in ALL during remission. In Britain the Medical Research Council arranged a trial (MRC, 1971) which compared the use of twice weekly methotrexate with BCG and no treatment. Figure 16.2 summarizes the results of this study in which it was found that the duration of remission for eighteen patients who received no further treatment after an initial five and a half months of chemotherapy was not significantly different from a similar group of fifty patients given weekly Glaxo BCG. Patients who received further chemotherapy (methotrexate) during the period following the initial five and a half months had longer remissions. Further follow-up of these patients five years later confirms these initial findings and only one patient in each of the BCG and no treatment arms remains in first remission. Of interest there is no difference in the overall survival curves of these three groups of patients. A similar study in the USA by Leukaemia Study Group A (Heyn *et al.*, 1975) was based upon similar lines to the British study comparing BCG with no treatment (and with maintenance methotrexate). No difference in remission duration could be detected between those patients receiving Chicago BCG and those untreated, although those patients given methotrexate during remission tended to stay longer in remission. In this study the initial randomization was after three and a half months of chemotherapy but the patients receiving maintenance chemotherapy were further randomized after another eight months into BCG, no treatment or methotrexate maintenance. This further

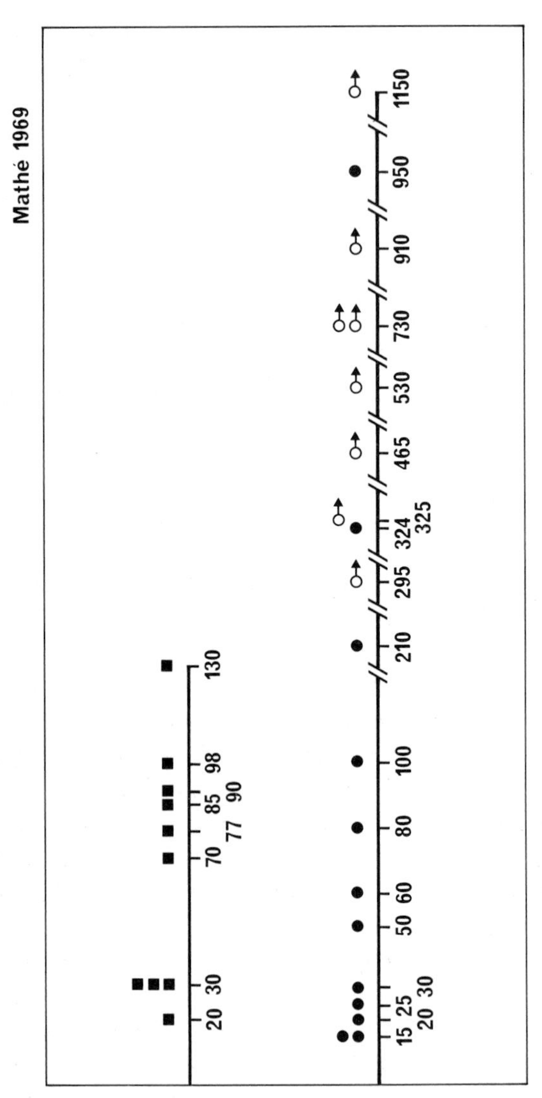

Figure 16.1 Moving left to right the black squares (upper group) represent the time (in days) at which ten patients relapsed following unmaintained remission. The lower group of patients show that eight of twenty who received BCG remained in first remission for between 295 and 1,150 days. Pasteur BCG was given using scarification. (Courtesy of the *British Medical Journal* and Professor Mathé.)

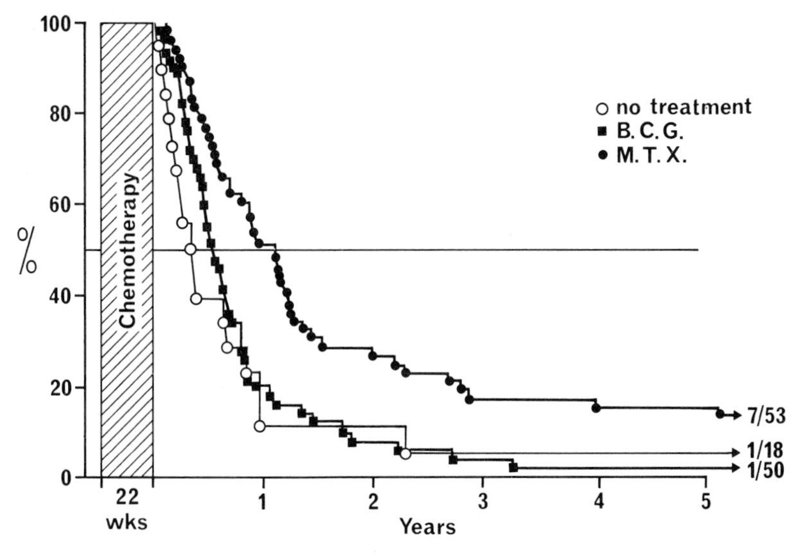

Figure 16.2 Remission duration of all randomized patients still in remission at the end of twenty-two weeks chemotherapy. (Courtesy of Raven Press.)

randomization showed no therapeutic advantage of BCG over no treatment for maintaining remission.

These three studies raise many questions. Table 16.1 summarizes the details and differences of Mathé's study from the two subsequent attempts designed to test his claim. It can be seen that Mathé's study only included patients that had already been on chemotherapy and in remission for two years and this may be a factor in selecting patients with less residual leukaemia than in the other two studies. Animal studies show that immunotherapy is only effective if the tumour mass is very small and recent chemotherapy programmes (Simone, 1974) confirm that chemotherapy of less than two years is associated with very early relapse presumably due to a large number of remaining leukaemia cells. However, this is not the whole answer, because although the control arms in the British and American studies relapsed very quickly (Table 16.1) so did those in Mathé's control arm (median remission duration of the ten patients two months after two years of chemotherapy). Other factors that may be important for the variance between Mathé and the other groups is that the BCG was different for the three studies, and Mathé used cells in addition to BCG for some (and ultimately all) of his patients. Another important factor in making interpretation of these early studies difficult is failure to treat the central nervous system of these children. We now know that nests of leukaemia

Table 16.1 *Immunotherapy for acute lymphoblastic leukaemia of childhood*

				Number of patients in each treatment group (bracket – median remission lengths)			
Study	*Duration induction chemo-therapy*	*CNS prophyl-axis*	*BCG used*	*BCG*	*BCG + cells*	*No treat-ment*	*Metho-trexate*
Mathé	24/12	No	Pasteur		20	10	
					(7)	(2)	
MRC	$5\frac{1}{2}/12$	No	Glaxo	50		18	53
				(6)		(4)	(14)
Heyn	$3\frac{1}{2}/12$	No	Chicago	34		31	285*
				(4)		(4)	(8)
Heyn	*$11\frac{1}{2}/12$	No	Chicago	44		52	57
				(5)		(6)	(14)
Poplack		Yes	Pasteur		21		35

* Patient in this arm still in remission after 8 months further randomized into study below.

cells remain hidden in the brain of children even when following chemotherapy they are in remission and this is because many cancer drugs (and immunotherapy) cannot pass across the blood–brain barrier. Even if these patients remain on chemotherapy (or immunotherapy) to 'maintain' their remission these nests of leukaemia cells can proliferate and ultimately overcome and disseminate into the body whereupon subsequent successful treatment is very difficult. Modern practice therefore uses irradiation just after remission to sterilize the brain (and spinal canal) of remaining nests of leukaemia cells. Clearly, failure to irradiate prophylactically the CNS is something that should not be allowed to influence possible future studies although careful inspection of Heyn's and MRC's results does not suggest this factor unfavourably biased the results against a possible therapeutic effect of BCG. Many of these objections could have been clarified by a study from Washington (Poplack *et al.*, 1977) in which Pasteur BCG and (live) leukaemia cells were used for immunotherapy for twenty-one children with chemotherapy-induced remission (including CNS prophylaxis – see Table 16.1). The immunotherapy was given for two-month periods interspersed with four months of chemotherapy and the whole cycle was repeated. Alas the thirty-five patients in the control arm were given methotrexate instead of no treatment during the corresponding two-month period when the treatment group was being immunized. Both arms were indistinguishable for length of first remission and thus a definitive conclusion about the usefulness of immunotherapy in this study is impossible; either immunotherapy is as effective as methotrexate for maintaining remission, or both treatments have no benefit at all.

As mentioned above the correct method to determine if a new treatment programme is useful is to randomly allocate the patients being studied into two groups, those receiving treatment and those not, and to compare the subsequent results. Unfortunately, because it is sometimes difficult to make such studies possible, some physicians resort to a trick whereby they give all the patients they see over a set period the test treatment and compare this with previous results (i.e. historical controls) obtained using other methods either in their own or other institutes. Alas, this method of analysis is fraught with hazard mainly because other general aspects of the management of cancer patients (i.e. antibiotics, etc.) are improving with time which may inadvertently account for a possible beneficial result. Also, there is an inherent mathematical weakness in analysing the results of studies only just completed because it makes these patients appear to be responding much better than expected as many of them will not yet have had a chance to die unlike those to whom they are being compared in the historical more distant control group.

Thus in a non-randomized (historical controls) study the Houston Group has used Pasteur BCG for the maintenance of remission of all forms of adult leukaemia, and although it reports benefit with acute myelogenous leukaemia (see below), there is no evidence that Pasteur BCG prolonged remission in ALL. However, the number of patients studied was small and was a sequential series of patients using historical controls and is thus open to the above criticism.

In the related disease Burkitt's lymphoma, Ziegler used Pasteur BCG given to the patients by scarification for ten weeks after cyclophosphamide-induced remission. He reports that eleven of the twenty-one BCG treated patients have relapsed which is no different from eleven of the nineteen control patients. However, it is always difficult to evaluate negative studies, particularly involving small numbers of patients having a disease with many staging parameters. For example, six of the eleven patients that relapsed in the BCG group did so in the CNS, compared with only one of the eleven patients in the control group; although this was attributed to an imbalance of the distribution of stage B patients in the original randomization, it nevertheless detracts from the significance of the data and it is probably futile to attempt to draw any conclusions from this study concerning BCG, one way or the other.

At present the place of immunotherapy alone for the maintenance of remission in ALL must remain speculative since only Mathé has reported a therapeutic effect and no other study has done exactly as he did in giving Pasteur BCG and cells after two years of chemotherapy. It seems unlikely that it is at present necessary to use immunotherapy alone as the primary method of treatment for ALL in the face of the outstanding results produced by intensive combination chemotherapy with prophylactic treatment of the CNS as developed by Pinkel and his colleagues (Simone, 1974), but the possibility of chemoimmunotherapy as used in adult myelogenous leukaemia deserves careful consideration in properly controlled studies and this has yet to be done.

Acute Myeloblastic Leukaemia (AML)

Following the confused results obtained in the empirical clinical studies in ALL, it soon became apparent that a rationale must be developed for decisive studies in the future and this would depend upon the ability to measure in the test-tube the reaction that was occurring in individual patients – the equivalent of measuring the blood sugar to determine the best way to manage patients with diabetes. The key to such scientific studies was to measure in the laboratory the host response to leukaemia cells following immunization. From such studies (Powles *et al.*, 1971) we learned:

1. man recognizes his own leukaemia cells as foreign;
2. that to alter the test-tube response of the patient to leukaemia cells required an injection of at least one gram of irradiated leukaemia cells; and
3. the effect was transient so repeated injections were required to obtain a sustained effect (i.e. up to one pint of cells might be required for a course of treatment).

It thus became apparent that the limiting factor to a therapeutic programme of active immunotherapy would be the availability of a large bank of immunizing cells. It was this consideration that led us to concentrate our efforts in clinical immunotherapy on AML. To obtain the bank of leukaemia cells depended upon collecting the leukaemia cells from the blood of new patients and, because AML primarily affected adults, as much as two pints of packed leukaemia cells could be removed from a single patient presenting with a high blood count. However, collecting these cells depended upon a special machine, the

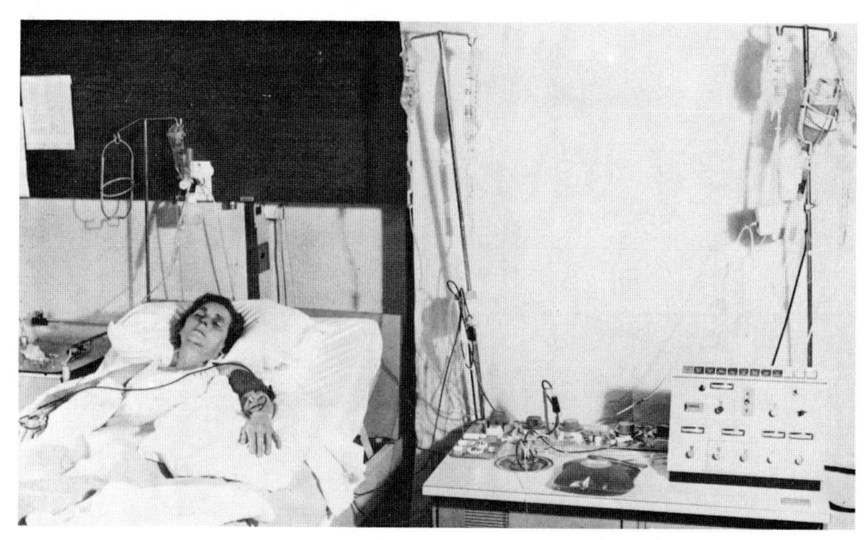

Figure 16.3 Leukaemia cells being removed from the blood by centrifugation using the IBM blood cell separator.

NCI/IBM blood cell separator (Powles *et al.*, 1974) which is a centrifuge (see Fig. 16.3) which concentrates the leukaemia cells from the blood. Using this machine for children is technically very difficult so it is not logistically feasible to treat ALL. Cells removed from the patients at presentation were stored in a viable form by freezing in liquid nitrogen (Powles, 1973; Chapuis *et al.*, 1977) until required for immunotherapy, and luckily we found that the immunizing cells did not necessarily need to be the patient's own so this avoided the difficulty of individual patients running out of cells. Other reasons for studying patients with AML were:

1. that chemotherapeutic agents, notably cytosine arabinoside and daunorubicin, had become available which meant approximately 50 per cent of all patients could be brought into a true haematological remission, but these remissions were very short. Nevertheless, these short remissions represented a state of 'minimal residual disease' in which, from the animal data, immunotherapy might be expected to work;
2. intradermal and subcutaneous injections of large numbers of cells are very painful and this to some extent precludes childhood ALL as a disease for multiple protracted immunization;
3. immunological studies of remission patients suggested AML patients might be more immunocompetent than ALL patients and thus be able to respond better to immunotherapy (Powles, 1976).

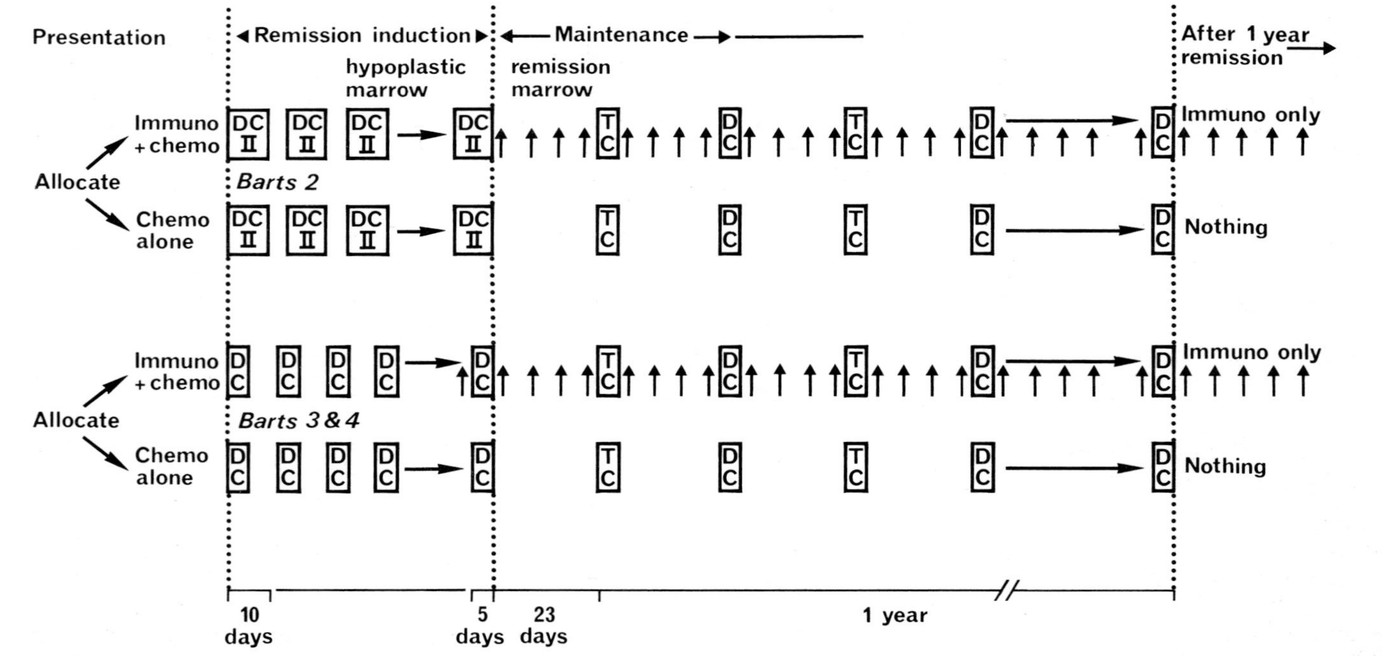

Figure 16.4 Squares containing DCII: cytosine arabinoside i.v. injection eight-hourly ×6. Total dose in 48 hours 4 mg/kg. No treatment then for 72 hours. Then cytosine arabinoside 2 mg/kg i.v. injection daily for three days and daunorubicin 1·5 mg/kg i.v. fast infusion on the first of these 3 days. Squares containing DC: cytosine arabinoside 2 mg/kg i.v. daily for five days with daunorubicin 1·5 mg/kg i.v. on the first of these days. Squares containing TC: cytosine arabinoside 2 mg/kg i.v. daily and 6-thioguanine 2 mg/kg orally daily, both for five days concurrently. Vertical arrows: Immunotherapy consisting of weekly (a) Glaxo BCG 1×10^6 live organisms percutaneously given using a multipuncture Heaf gun (40 punctures) and (b) irradiated allogeneic myelogenous leukaemia cells, 1×10^6 intradermally and subcutaneously at three sites.
Bart's 4 trial differs from Bart's 3 trial in excluding all patients over 60 years of age. (Courtesy of the *British Journal of Cancer*.)

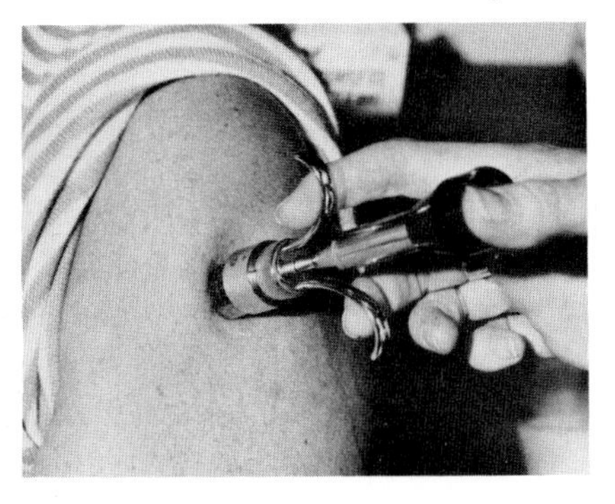

Figure 16.5 A Heaf gun used to administer BCG.

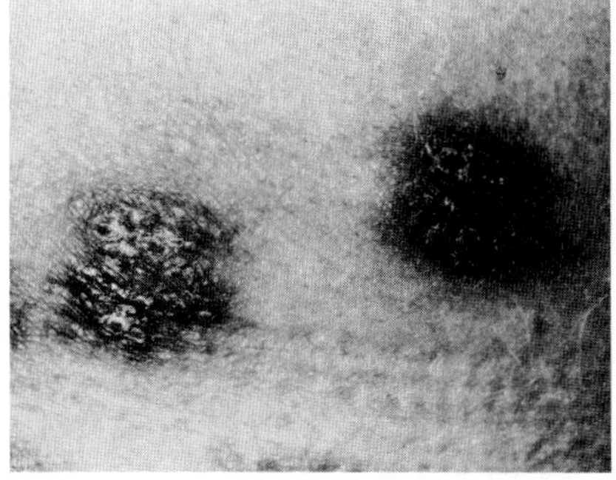

Figure 16.6 A typical BCG reaction.

The Barts/Marsden Study

Thus in 1970 a joint immunotherapy study was devised between the Royal Marsden Hospital in Sutton, Surrey and St Bartholomew's Hospital in London, the protocol of which is shown in Fig. 16.4. All patients received the same initial treatment consisting of cytosine arabinoside and daunorubicin, and approximately half attained clinical remission. In remission these patients were randomized to receive either chemotherapy alone or chemotherapy plus immunotherapy for the maintenance of their remissions.

The maintenance chemotherapy consisted of courses of five days of treatment with cytosine arabinoside together with either daunorubicin or 6-thioguanine. There was a gap of twenty-three days between courses. Immunotherapy consisted of weekly BCG and irradiated myeloblastic leukaemia cells. The BCG was from Glaxo and administered using a Heaf gun (Fig. 16.5) which gave a dose of 10^6 live organisms. All four limbs received BCG in turn once weekly and 1×10^9 stored leukaemia cells were injected into the three limbs not receiving BCG that week. A typical BCG lesion is shown in Fig. 16.6. Usually a vesicular lesion would appear at about three days and this would become erythematous and sometimes break down finally healing after about four weeks. No scarring should remain.

When patients relapsed, the initial induction treatment with daunorubicin and cytosine arabinoside was repeated whenever possible. If no regression of leukaemia was seen the treatment was usually changed to a combination of cyclophosphamide and 6-thioguanine. If remission occurred, then maintenance treatment was modified to a single injection of daunorubicin and three days of cytosine arabinoside followed eleven days later by three days of oral cyclophosphamide and

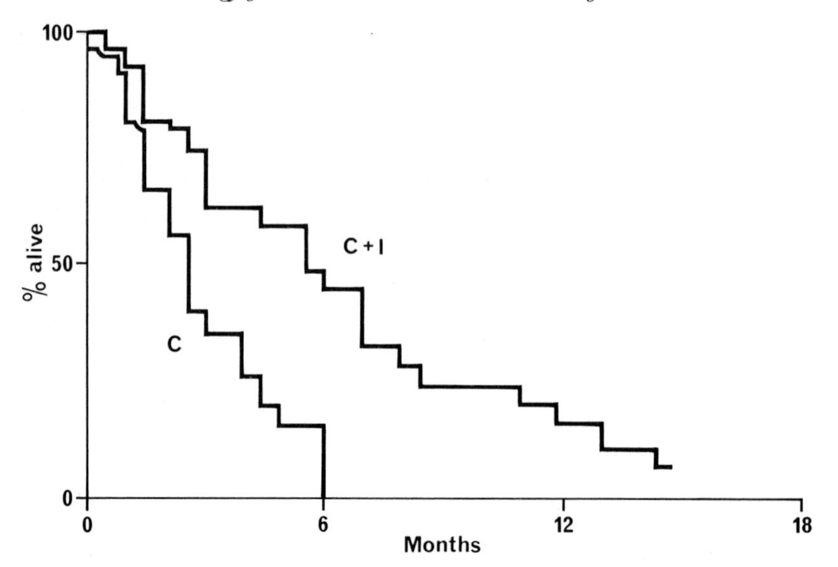

Figure 16.7 Twenty patients who previously received only chemotherapy and relapsed all died and their median survival (after relapse) was only twelve weeks, compared to twenty-three weeks for the twenty-eight patients (twenty-three dead) who received immunotherapy. (Courtesy of the *British Journal of Cancer*.)

6-thioguanine. After another eleven-day gap, the whole cycle was repeated with maintenance chemotherapy for three days every fortnight. Those patients who previously received immunotherapy were given further treatment with BCG and irradiated AML cells.

This study which was started in October 1970 was completed at the end of 1973. A preliminary analysis of the data was published in 1973 (Powles, *et al.*, 1973). The data as at August 1975 can be summarized as follows: of the fifty-three patients who achieved full remission, twenty-two were in the arm of the trial which received chemotherapy alone; twenty-eight in the arm which received chemotherapy plus immunotherapy; and three were excluded (for further details see Powles *et al.*, 1977). Of the twenty-two patients who received chemotherapy alone, twenty have died with a median survival of 270 days, twenty-three of the twenty-eight patients who received chemotherapy plus immunotherapy have died, with an estimated median survival of 510 days. Statistical analysis calculates that there are less than three chances in 100 that this difference occurred by chance alone. Twenty-seven of the twenty-eight patients in the chemotherapy plus immunotherapy group have relapsed compared with twenty of the twenty-two chemotherapy alone patients. The median duration of remission was 191 days for the chemotherapy alone patients compared with 305 days for the chemotherapy plus immunotherapy patients, but this difference was not statistically secure. The reason the overall survival was significantly different between the two groups was because survival consists of two summative components, remission duration and survival of patients after they relapse, and in this study by far the most significant effect of the immunotherapy was upon this latter component. Figure 16.7 shows that the twenty patients who previously received only chemotherapy and relapsed all died and their median survival (after relapse) was only twelve weeks, compared to twenty-three weeks for the twenty-eight patients (twenty-three dead) who received immunotherapy. The statistical chance for this difference not being true is 5 chances in 10,000.

Two studies have attempted to exactly repeat this Barts/Marsden study described below (Table 16.2). In a three-centred trial conducted by the Medical Research Council of Britain, during 1973 and 1974, seventy-one remission patients were entered into two treatment groups identical with the Barts/Marsden study; twenty-four patients receiving maintenance chemotherapy alone and forty-seven patients chemotherapy plus immunotherapy. At a follow-up time to September 1976, fifty-seven of these patients had relapsed and although preliminary, the results appear to confirm the findings of the earlier study – that is, like the Barts/Marsden study, survival after relapse appears to be most significantly effected by immunotherapy.

The other study to attempt to exactly repeat the Barts/Marsden study is by the Swedish group (Reizenstein *et al.*, 1977) who only varied this study by giving live rather than irradiated cells because of logistic difficulties in irradiating them. They found overall survival was significantly prolonged for patients who received immunotherapy, and once again the main reason for this effect was due to prolonged survival of the immunotherapy patients after relapse.

The mechanism of action in these three studies is obscure because for technical reasons it has not been possible to measure the immune reaction of the host directed against the leukaemia cells. Two possible mechanisms deserve consideration; the first is an increased immune reaction against the leukaemia cells produced by administration of cells which would account for the prolongation of first remission, but it is difficult to see how such a mechanism could be involved in the prolongation of survival after relapse. A second mechanism which could produce this latter effect is a non-specific stimulation of the bone marrow which permitted immunotherapy patients who had relapsed to tolerate the high doses of cytotoxic chemotherapy which were then required. Such an effect would be effective because patients who have relapsed usually die due to bone marrow failure.

Table 16.2 *Three separate studies showing remission patients, some receiving maintenance chemotherapy alone and some receiving chemotherapy plus immunotherapy*

	Duration initial induction chemo.	*Maint. chemo.*	*BCG used*	*AML cells used*	*Number of patients Chemo. alone*	*Chemo. plus immuno.*	*Duration (weeks) Remission C*	*C + I*	*Survival C*	*C + I*	*Survival after relapse C*	*C + I*
Powles	up to 3/12	Yes	Glaxo	Irradiated allogeneic	22	28	27	43	39	73	12	23
M.R.C.	up to 3/12	Yes	Glaxo	Irradiated allogeneic	24	47	21–40	32	44	70	14	23
Reizenstein	up to 3/12	Yes	Glaxo	Viable allogeneic	14	16	23	36	40	80		

An obvious question concerns the relative importance of the BCG and cells and to answer this would require three arms to a trial, i.e. chemotherapy alone, chemotherapy plus BCG, and chemotherapy plus BCG plus cells. This was not possible in the initial study because of the limited number of patients available.

BCG Alone for Immunotherapy of Acute Myeloid Leukaemia

The use of BCG alone without the use of cells for treating patients with AML has been tried by four groups (Table 16.3). The first study was reported initially in 1974 by Vogler and his colleagues when it was seen that patients who had their maintenance chemotherapy stopped (about five months after being in remission) and were given Tice BCG twice weekly for four weeks and then were put back on chemotherapy, maintained longer remissions than those patients who were given methotrexate instead. However, there are some points difficult to understand in this study; only 58 of the 351 patients ever reached the maintenance part of the study; the controlled section of the study compared immunotherapy *with* chemotherapy which is not an interpretable comparison; and lastly, the remission curves for the two arms cross over at ten months making statistical interpretation impossible. The data concerning survival of patients after relapse are not yet available.

Following this study the Houston Group (Gutterman *et al.*, 1974) suggested there was a distinct benefit from the use of immunotherapy in maintaining adult patients with acute leukaemia. This study consisted of twenty consecutive patients who received intermittent chemotherapy (cytarabine, vincristine and prednisolone, OPA) and liquid Pasteur BCG administered weekly by scarification. The duration of remission of these patients was compared with that of a previous group of thirty-three consecutive patients maintained on OAP alone. Eleven of the twenty OAP plus BCG treated patients remained in remission with an estimated median duration of ninety-one weeks, whereas only fourteen of the thirty-three patients maintained on OAP remained in remission with a median duration of fifty weeks. Alas, although these results were said to show a significant advantage for the use of BCG upon remission length subsequent analysis shows this difference to be no longer significant (Hersh, 1977) and highlights the pitfalls of using historical controls. When sufficient time has elapsed to rectify the bias due to historical controls in this study it will be of interest to see if this immunotherapy prolonged survival after relapse of these patients.

A more recent study in the same area as the Houston Group (South-

Table 16.3 *Results of BCG alone without the use of cells for treating patients with acute myeloid leukaemia*

	Duration initial induction chemo.	*BCG used*	*Maintenance chemo.*	*Number control pts*	*Number immuno pts*	*Duration (weeks)*					
						Remission		*Survival*		*Survival after relapse*	
						C	*C + I*	*C*	*C + I*	*C*	*C + I*
Vogler	at least 5/12	Tice (Twice weekly for 4 weeks)	Not during BCG*	33	25	33·5 (13·3)	40·9 (24·9)	78·1	93·2		
Hewlett	3/12	Pasteur scarified	OAP	25	20	55	59	74	55+		
Whittaker	3/12	Glaxo monthly I.V.	Monthly DNR + ARA-C	19	18	27	34	50	69		
Gutterman†	3/12	Pasteur scarified	OAP	33	20	50‡	91†	—	—		

* Those patients not receiving BCG received Methotrexate. † Sequential study with historical controls. ‡ Results 1974.

West Co-operative Group – Hewlett, 1977) attempted to repeat exactly the Gutterman study using OAP and Pasteur BCG, but conducted its study as a randomized trial rather than using historical controls. Its results shown in Table 16.3 and published recently (Hewlett, 1977) showed no advantage for remission length, survival (and presumably survival after relapse) for patients who received BCG in addition to OAP, rather than those who received OAP alone.

The fourth of the BCG alone studies for AML (Whittaker *et al.*, 1977) has been giving intravenous BCG to remission patients in conjunction with maintenance chemotherapy (Table 16.3). Although remission length appears to be longer for the eighteen patients who received BCG and chemotherapy than for the nineteen patients who received only chemotherapy, the greatest and most significant effect is upon survival and we must conclude that this study has produced an effect very similar to that seen in the original Barts/Marsden study.

Summarizing the seven studies in AML so far described, in all three studies where patients received BCG and cells, there was a therapeutic effect seen whereby survival was prolonged, and the major contributory factor to this was prolongation of survival after relapse. In the four studies using BCG alone, only one shows convincingly a therapeutic effect (Whittaker, 1977), and again this was similar to the BCG and cell studies. It must be concluded that the observation that immunotherapy prolongs survival after relapse in patients with AML is a real effect, and it seems probable that cells and BCG are better for gaining this effect than BCG alone.

Variations of Immunotherapy for AML

Variations of methods for immunotherapy are now becoming numerous throughout the world and there are under way several excellent studies testing some of the more ambitious approaches. For example, there is evidence to suggest that after sialic acid has been removed from tumour cells using neuraminidase, they become more immunogenic (Currie and Bagshawe, 1963). A controlled trial is now under way (Holland, 1977) in which cells so treated are used for immunotherapy and although some of these patients also received Methanol Extract Residue of BCG (MER), it would appear that the therapeutic effect seen is predominantly upon survival and due largely to the cells. A separate study by Leukaemia Study Group B (Cuttner, 1977) involving some of the same workers as in the neuraminidase study, describes over a hundred patients in remission, all of whom received maintenance chemotherapy, but fifty-seven of whom also received immunotherapy with MER. Preliminary results suggest that those patients receiving the MER are having longer remissions than the controls.

Another attempt to increase the specific antigenicity of the immunizing cells comes from the Swiss Group recently reported by Sauter *et al.* (1977). Augmentation of the immunogenicity of tumour associated antigens by infection with viruses has been claimed by several laboratories (Boone and Blackman, 1972; Lindenman, 1974) and an avian influenza A virus (FPV) has been found to be a suitable virus for use with AML cells (Gerber *et al.*, 1973). In their study forty-four patients were randomized to two maintenance arms, twenty-two for monthly chemotherapy and twenty-two for monthly chemotherapy plus virus treated cells. They found no difference between the two groups for remission duration and survival, and this study has an average follow-up of thirteen and a half months.

The St Bartholomew's-Royal Marsden Group has recently completed a controlled study attempting to increase the antigenicity of the immunizing AML cells by using BCG as a 'classical' adjuvant and mixing it with the cells before injection. This study finished nearly one year ago and compared one group of fifteen patients who received immunotherapy alone for maintenance of remission (given as in the Bart's/Marsden Study), with a second group of patients given identical immunotherapy, but also given on four occasions early in their remission the BCG and cells mixed together. Any difference between these two groups would only be attributed to the mixed cells and BCG, and at present four patients remain in remission (on a plateau) in the mixed arm and all have relapsed in the non-mixed arm. Within a year this study can be fully analysed. Two other studies have recently been reported where AML patients have been given non-specific immunostimulation other than BCG. The first of these is from the Sloan Kettering Institute (Gee *et al.*, 1977) and followed the fascinating observation upon a group of untreated AML patients given a vaccine to protect them against *Pseudomonas* infections prior to induction chemotherapy. This study was conducted eight years ago and of fifteen of these patients who subsequently passed into remission, retrospective analysis showed that seven of them became long term survivors seemingly on a plateau of survival. This group now has a controlled prospective study underway with twenty-five remission patients already included and it is hoped it will not be long before this mode of treatment can be properly assessed.

Immunotherapy for AML Before Remission

The possibility of treating AML patients while they still have detectable disease has also been explored. In a preliminary study Fairley (1975) collected all patients with acute myelogenous leukaemia who had been admitted to St Bartholomew's Hospital in London in recent years and who were alive three months after starting chemotherapy (even if they were not in remission).

The survival data of these patients show that patients given immunotherapy as part of their maintenance survive significantly longer than those receiving only chemotherapy; indeed it made little difference to survival whether the patient was in so-called 'complete remission' or only in partial remission more than three months from the onset of treatment. Patients not in complete remission, who had immunotherapy, fared better than those in complete remission who only had chemotherapy. Eleven patients who were not in complete remission more than three months after the onset of treatment were given immunotherapy (BCG mixed with allogeneic non-irradiated leukaemic cells) without further chemotherapy. These patients were fit and had only a small number (between 6–10 per cent) of blast cells in the marrow. Five patients achieved complete remission from two to six months after the cessation of chemotherapy and the beginning of the immunotherapy. The duration of these remissions ranged from six weeks to four and a half months. This is the first definite clinical indication of a direct effect of immunotherapy on the malignant cell population.

Future Prospects for AML

It would be an understatement to say that future prospects are somewhat uncertain at present, but we can be optimistic that clinical trials will be more effective if they are based upon a scientific rationale and so efforts in basic research must continue. It now seems that two important aspects must be examined; the non-specific bone marrow stimulation effect which involves rescreening all the previously tried immunotherapy agents with suitable monitoring of effects, and the further investigation of the specific antitumour effect directed against the tumour, the key to which is the isolation and characterization of the tumour antigens on the leukaemia cells.

There are three entirely new approaches which might soon deserve consideration in clinical studies. Specific antisera (raised in animals) are now available for acute leukaemia cells and although this has immediate application for monitoring the disease process, the possibility of using such material for passive serotherapy should be considered as their specificity would overcome many of the problems previously encountered with such methods. Another exciting recent development has been the isolation of molecules in human leukaemia cells which appear to have a common identity with a monkey virus. Once the relevance of these claims to pathogenesis has been established, the possibility of an immunological (and chemotherapeutic) approach to their presence could be considered.

Third, in a rat leukaemia model, thymosin – a hormone extracted from the thymus – has been found to be effective in bringing about total remission and when this material becomes available in larger quantities the possibility of clinical evaluation may not then be too distant.

Immunotherapeutic Effect of Bone Marrow Grafting for AML

It is now possible to consider bone marrow transplantation for patients with acute leukaemia (Thomas *et al.*, 1976), a procedure known to be effective for treating aplastic anaemia.

The technique of transplantation is simple and belies the immunological problems that follow. Red marrow is aspirated at multiple sites from a suitable anaesthetized donor using a syringe and biopsy needle until 400–500 ml have been collected. This suspension is then infused intravenously into the recipient where it passes first to the lungs and then ultimately settles into the marrow space.

If the graft is not rejected, polymorphs appear in the blood of the recipient in about ten to fourteen days, and platelets will be found by the end of one month. A cytogenetic sex marker, if present, will show these blood cells to be of donor origin and if the graft is not followed by any complications then donor cells will constitute the entire blood population thereafter.

To stop graft rejection the donor has to be matched (in practice a sib who is HLA identical), and the recipient must be immunosuppressed, usually by giving massive doses of cyclophosphamide or total body irradiation just prior to grafting. This chemotherapy and/or irradiation would normally kill the recipient by destroying the remaining normal bone marrow cells leading to infection and haemorrhage, but the new bone marrow graft acts as a rescue procedure by providing functioning new marrow within two weeks.

Grafting was introduced into the management of acute leukaemia because without it the limiting factor for giving antileukaemic chemotherapy is bone marrow failure. Thus the possibility of rescue using bone marrow transplantation after deliberate excessive treatment has obvious and sensible appeal. Luckily this deliberate excessive treatment is the same as is required to immunosuppress the recipient prior to transplantation. The Thomas Group has suggested the best conditioning combination is cyclophosphamide (65 mg/kg) given for two days, followed by total body irradiation to 1,000 rads and then the marrow. Its results up to October 1975 (followed up to 1 February 1977) showed that only 15 per cent of 110 patients (10 received only radiotherapy) with matched sib grafts have survived on a 'plateau', but even this would not have occurred if they had been treated by drugs alone as they were all relapse patients. There were, in February 1977, eight acute lymphoblastic leukaemia and six acute myeloblastic leukaemia patients living longer than 600 days. However, it must not be forgotten that the treatment is heroic and 50 per cent of the patients are dead within 180 days of grafting and the problems of graft versus host syndrome, infection and recurrent leukaemia are horrendous. Following these very difficult problems the 15 per cent of long term survivors in this group may seem small, but they are important because they raise the possibility that the graft has an antitumour action. Mathé suggested that patients with graft versus host (GVH) tended to do better in terms of their leukaemia provided they survived the GVH, but this is not the experience in Seattle, USA. Because of the distinct nature of tumour antigens it is not necessary to postulate that a graft versus tumour action has to be indistinguishable from the GVH syndrome, and it is possible that there can be an antitumour action from the graft in the absence of GVH.

As far as the future is concerned for transplantation of leukaemia patients, a few specific topics seem important. First, the plateau of survival must be shown to be real because survival curves are difficult to analyse with confidence until much time has elapsed. If it is shown that a subgroup of long term survivors does exist this would be dissimilar from anything seen previously using conventional chemotherapy and two possible mechanisms deserve consideration – either the intensive anticancer preparation that is required to immunosuppress the patient prior to grafting has eradicated the leukaemia, or there has been a direct action of the graft against the leukaemia. The former is unlikely, because 1,000 rads (even though as a single dose it is equivalent to perhaps 2,000 rads in fractionated treatment) would not be expected to eradicate all leukaemia. If, however, these long term survivors are the result of an antitumour action of the graft, then it is vital a definitive test of this mechanism is established. It is now possible to collect and store leukaemia cells in liquid nitrogen such that they can be recovered and grown in proliferative cultures. It therefore seems a relatively simple procedure to use the circulating 'graft' cells and/or serum of the grafted patient to see if there is an antitumour action. Such tests have been used for some time in non-grafted patients and no antitumour action has been clearly established, but until these experiments have been repeated for these long term graft survivors, we can say little about the possibility of an antitumour action of the graft. Whichever of the possible mechanisms is involved in producing these survivors, it is vital that we see if it can be exploited in ungrafted patients. If high dose cytotoxic chemotherapy with or without total body irradiation is responsible for these survivors then we might have more courage to pursue such treatment in ungrafted patients, and obviously massive support would be required. If, however, it is due to an antitumour effect of the graft, then we might feel more encouraged to explore similar forms of 'immunotherapy' in ungrafted patients. It would be misleading to discuss the possible antileukaemic action of the graft without a note of caution concerning the two cases reported by Seattle of leukaemia occurring in the grafted cells of transplanted patients with acute lymphoblastic leukaemia. This raises the very important question of the aetiology of acute leukaemia being a host environmental defect rather than a potentially eradicatable, spontaneous mutation of a single cell. However, this concept does not counter the possibility that bone marrow transplantation may reconstitute the host in a way in which the original person was lacking so removing the underlying aetiological defect. The small but encouraging success rate for long survival of grafted patients with acute leukaemia confirms our belief that specialized units should continue with this method of treatment. But, it must not be forgotten that at present this treatment is highly experimental and if we are to ethically justify the appalling manmade consequences that ensue for the majority of grafted patients, then we must include a scientific programme of research to advance the subject so that ultimately the majority will benefit. This will only be possible by understanding the biological nature of the methods we are using.

Lung Cancer

In the opening part of this chapter various methods of immunotherapy were discussed which were applicable to man following observations in animals of systemic approaches to treatment. The concept of a local immunotherapeutic effect did not seem to be worth pursuing because the problem with cancer is metastasis, not the control of the primary tumour. A recent study in lung cancer, however, has led to some reservation concerning the futility of 'local' immunotherapy. This study by McKneally and his colleagues (McKneally *et al.*, 1976, 1977) followed the observation first made a decade ago (Krant *et al.*, 1968) that patients who develop empyema after surgical resection for lung cancer seem to survive longer than patients without this complication. To mimic this effect McKneally *et al.* decided to deliberately introduce living bacilli (Tice BCG) into the pleural cavity of patients following surgery for lung cancer in an attempt at producing a local inflammatory response. Since April 1973 they have treated with surgery ninety-five patients with anaplastic, adeno-, and squamous cell lung carcinomas, but not 'oat cell' tumours. Following surgery they were staged 'blind' and randomized (after statification) into two treatment arms, one group to receive the BCG the other to receive no further treatment. Analysis for significant prognostic factors such as age, extent of surgery, etc., shows the randomization was fair and a statistical comparison was possible. The Tice BCG was given through the thoracic surgical drainage tube used for the lung resection as a single intrapleural injection of 1×10^7 live organisms just prior to the tube being removed, i.e. four to six days after surgery. Fourteen days later isoniazid was given to all patients (including controls) and this was continued for twelve weeks. Ninety-five patients have so far been included in the study (sixty-two followed up for more than one year), and fifty-eight of these patients are Stage I with a median follow up of twenty months. Of these fifty-eight patients, twenty-six have received BCG and two have recurrences (at ten and sixteen months) and one has died, whereas nine of the thirty-two control patients have relapsed (and all but one died). The difference between these two groups is highly significant. Although the number of patients is small, it seems that Stages II and III patients accrue no benefit from the BCG. A similar study from Japan (Yamamura, 1977) involving the use of an oil-attached cell wall skeleton of BCG given in many different ways including into the pleural fluid of Stages III and IV lung cancer patients claims that benefit occurs. Thirteen patients so treated were compared with sixteen controls and the median survivals of the two groups were 11·0 months and 5·6 months respectively. Although sufficient time has elapsed because only two patients remain alive, more details of the exact staging criteria and statifications are required, and clearly in a disease as protean as lung cancer the number of patients is at present far too few to draw any worthwhile conclusions.

The possible mechanism of action of intrapleural BCG deserves some consideration. In McKneally's study the BCG was shown to have been recognized systemically in that thirty of the thirty-two patients given the bacillus converted to a positive skin reaction to tuberculin. Although direct absorption of BCG through the pleural cavity into the blood-stream is possible, it seems most likely that the main reason for this conversion (and thus the antitumour effect) is due to entry of the BCG (with or without macrophages) into the regional mediastinal lymph nodes. Here a direct killing of residual malignant cells would be possible. Time will need to elapse before it will be possible to assess the effect of this form of immunotherapy upon distant metastasis but such therapeutic effect if it occurred could either be due to the destruction of malignant cells in the nodes before they spread systemically, or due to specific cytotoxic antibody and/or mononuclear cells being released from the mediastinal nodes because the presence of tumour cells and BCG within the node have invoked a specific immune response directed against the tumour. Clearly this therapeutic study of McKneally's, if it is substantiated, has introduced a fascinating new insight into host responses to tumours.

Two studies investigating active specific immunotherapy for lung cancer have been reported (Stewart *et al.*, 1977; Takita *et al.*, 1977). The Stewart study involved thirteen Stage I and II patients who, following surgery, were given a soluble extract of lung cancer cells and intermittent high dose methotrexate and they were compared with ten randomized controls. There were also sixteen non-randomized patients who did not receive chemotherapy or immunotherapy, and sixteen patients (randomized with the chemotherapy patients) who received only immunotherapy. Grouping all immunotherapy versus non-immunotherapy patients together in this study, the immunotherapy patients survived significantly longer than the non-immunotherapy patients, but obviously such an analysis is open to some criticism as very few patients are so far dead and the number of patients in the truly controlled chemotherapy versus chemoimmunotherapy section of the study is so few that time must elapse before fruitful interpretation of this study is possible.

A similar criticism can be directed at the controlled Takita (1977) study from Roswell Park, whereby Stage III patients have been treated with a tumour cell vaccine (tumour cells treated with concanavalin A and neuraminidase and injected with Freurd's adjuvant). Although seven of the fifteen immunized patients remain alive with an estimated median survival of 34·8 months and only three of the fifteen controls with a median of 12·1 months and this is reported as significant at the 5 per cent level, many more of the control patients had pneumonectomies rather than lobectomies and no valid information can usefully be drawn from this study at present.

In summary, local intrapleural immunotherapy for lung cancer opens up a new and unexpected 'biological' approach to the management of this disease and clearly such studies are worth pursuing particularly if a scientific rationale for better methods of treatment can be developed and exploited. But on the evidence so far available the future for active specific immunotherapy for lung cancer must remain, at the very least, highly speculative.

Immunotherapy for Other Malignancies

Claims of active immunotherapy for treating melanoma have followed the observation that tumour nodules in the skin shrink and disappear after being injected with BCG – more importantly, occasionally nodules at distant sites also regress. Unfortunately, the obvious explanation for the inoculated nodule shrinking is simply due to a direct toxic effect of the BCG (such as would occur if nitric acid were injected) and the claimed distant effect simply represents the known natural history of this disease whereby nodules may spontaneously (transiently) regress in the face of other nodules progressing.

As yet there are no convincing reports of active specific immunotherapy having any place in the management of other cancers although numerous 'adequate' studies appear to have been conducted. In many respects this is disappointing, but as has been stressed by Currie (1976), unless attempts are made to measure (and monitor) the host reaction to his tumour then it is unlikely that a useful method of treatment will be developed. Pure empirical studies cannot be expected to reveal this obviously weak (but perhaps useful) host response to tumour cells.

Conclusions

The overall results so far obtained in man for controlling cancer using immunotherapy are clearly disappointing, but it must be remembered that only ten years have elapsed since Mathé first attempted to treat patients with leukaemia and this is only the very beginning of an understanding of this discipline. There seems no doubt that the observation made in prolonging survival of patients with acute myelogenous leukaemia following their relapse is a real one, because it has been repeated by many centres. It must be remembered that never before has any form of treatment been given to patients with acute myelogenous leukaemia in remission that has in any way altered the natural history of the disease, and the fact that the immunotherapy given has produced a therapeutic result may give a clue to the very nature of the disease process involved. It is becoming increasingly clear that AML is quite different from ALL, and it may not be unreasonable to regard it in many respects as a unique disease which affects not a single malignant clone of cells, but more the very soil of the marrow itself and that recurrent mutations and malignant clones of cells are an inevitable consequence. Thus, it is possible that AML is chemotherapeutically incurable using the sort of agents we have available at the moment, and this in many respects is supported by the extremely dismal long term results obtained using these drugs. Perhaps an attack on the host biological control mechanisms (even outside that of the immune system, i.e. CSF) may be the long term chemotherapy approach that pays dividends, and obviously anything that has altered the biology of the disease will help elucidate this possible mode of attack. Obviously future immunotherapy programmes will help in this aim, and the isolation and characterization of the leukaemia antigen therefore remains a vital goal in developing a rationale for these trials.

Concerning other cancers, the only other convincing data to suggest immunotherapy has had any effect is the local response to BCG in patients with resected lung cancer. Although it seems obvious at first sight this is due to local inflammatory responses, it does not exclude the possibility that active specific immunotherapy may also be involved, particularly if the BCG has activated nodes containing microscopic deposits of cancer cells, this specific immune reaction then being disseminated systemically. Again, it is hoped that the positive results seen so far will be confirmed and that in conjunction with careful laboratory investigations they will help reveal the exact underlying biological nature of this response.

There now seems little doubt that tumour antigens exist in many solid tumours and if progress is to be made these antigens must be defined and characterized. Attempts must be made to exploit their presence for active systemic immunotherapy, but if no benefit occurs then they may still be exploited for possible immunodiagnosis and immunoprophylaxis in high risk groups of patients.

Acknowledgement

I am indebted to the Leukaemia Research Fund for support for all my projects.

References

Currie, G. A. (1972) Eighty years of immunotherapy; a view of immunological methods used for the treatment of human cancer, *Brit. J. Cancer*, **26**, 427.

Hauschka, T. S. (1952) Immunological aspects of cancer: a review, *Cancer Research*, **12**, 9, 615.

Old, L. J. and Boyce, E. A. (1966) Scientific antigens of tumours and leukaemias of experimental animals, *Med. Clin. N. Amer.*, **50**, 901.

Proceedings of the Washington Congress November 1976, *Immunotherapy of Cancer*. W. Terry (ed.). Raven Press (in press).

Powles, R. *et al.* (1977) Immunotherapy for acute myelogenous leukaemia: a controlled clinical study two and a half years after entry of the last patient, *Brit. J. Cancer*, **35**, 265.

Southam, C. M. (1960) Relationship of immunology to cancer: a review, *Cancer Research*, **20**, 3, 271.

Southam, C. M. (1961) Applications of immunology to clinical cancer: past attempts and future possibilities, *Cancer Research*, **21**, 1302.

Table of Contents of the second volume of this two-volume work

Oncology for Nurses and Health Care Professionals

Editor ROBERT TIFFANY
Director of Nursing, The Royal Marsden Hospital, London

Volume 2 *Care and Support*

Chapter 6 Rehabilitation
Patricia A. Downie, F.C.S.P.
A Winston Churchill Fellow 1976

Chapter 7 Teaching Patients and Relatives
Patricia MacMillan, S.R.N., R.M.N., R.C.I.(Edin.)
Senior Lecturer in Applied Social Studies,
Hammersmith and West London College

Chapter 8 Pain and its Management
A. T. Mennie, M.B., M.Ch.
Law Hospital, Carluke, Scotland

Chapter 9 Care of the Dying
D. H. Summers, S.R.N., R.N.T.
Co-ordinator of Studies,
St Christopher's Hospice, London

Chapter 10 Domiciliary Care
Charlotte R. Kratz, S.R.N., S.C.M., H.V.Cert., D.N.Tutor,
B.Sc.(Soc), Ph.D., Queen's Nurse

Chapter 11 Services Available for the Cancer Patient
J. E. C. Baldwin, B.Com., A.I.M.S.W.
Principal Hospital Social Worker,
Royal Marsden Hospital, London and Surrey

Chapter 12 Cancer Education
R. L. Davison, M.Ed., Dip. Adult Ed., M.I.H.E.
Executive Director,
Manchester Regional Committee for Cancer Education

Index

Note Where the letter p is shown after a page number, it indicates a relevant illustration.